ELECTROCARDIOGRAPHY
FOR HEALTHCARE PROFESSIONALS

Third Edition

Kathryn A. Booth, MS, RN, RMA (AMT), RPT, CPhT

Facilitator/ Instructor, Military to Medicine
INOVA Health System
Falls Church, Virginia

Thomas E. O'Brien AS, CCT, CST, CRAT

Central Florida Institute
Palm Harbor, Florida

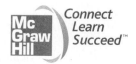
Connect
Learn
Succeed™

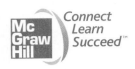

The McGraw-Hill Companies

Connect
Learn
Succeed™

ELECTROCARDIOGRAPHY FOR HEALTHCARE PROFESSIONALS
Published by McGraw-Hill, a business unit of The McGraw-Hill Companies, Inc., 1221 Avenue of the Americas, New York, NY, 10020.
Copyright © 2012 by The McGraw-Hill Companies, Inc. All rights reserved. Previous editions © 2001 and 2008. No part of this publication may be reproduced or distributed in any form or by any means, or stored in a database or retrieval system, without the prior written consent of The McGraw-Hill Companies, Inc., including, but not limited to, in any network or other electronic storage or transmission, or broadcast for distance learning.

Some ancillaries, including electronic and print components, may not be available to customers outside the United States.

This book is printed on acid-free paper.

Printed in the United States of America.

5 6 7 8 9 0 DOW/DOW 1 0 9 8 7 6 5 4

ISBN 978-0-07-337435-2
MHID 0-07-337435-0

Vice president/Editor in chief: *Elizabeth Haefele*
Vice president/Director of marketing: *John E. Biernat*
Publisher: *Kenneth S. Kasee Jr.*
Senior sponsoring editor: *Debbie Fitzgerald*
Director of development: *Sarah Wood*
Managing developmental editor: *Kimberly D. Hooker*
Developmental editor: *Katherine Pidde*
Editorial coordinator: *Jenna Skwarek*
Marketing manager: *Mary B. Haran*
Lead digital product manager: *Damian Moshak*
Director, Editing/Design/Production: *Jess Ann Kosic*
Lead project manager: *Rick Hecker*
Senior buyer: *Michael R. McCormick*
Senior designer: *Srdjan Savanovic*
Senior photo research coordinator: *Lori Hancock*
Media project manager: *Brent dela Cruz*
Cover design: *Alexa Viscius*
Typeface: *10.5/13 Melior*
Compositor: *Laserwords Private Limited*
Printer: *RR Donnelley*
Credits: The credits section for this book begins on page PC-1 and is considered an extension of the copyright page.

Library of Congress Cataloging-in-Publication Data
Booth, Kathryn A., 1957-
    Electrocardiography for healthcare professionals / Kathryn A. Booth, Thomas E. O'Brien. --
3rd ed.
      p. cm.
    Includes index.
    Rev. ed. of: Electrocardiography for health care personnel / Kathryn A. Booth, Patricia
DeiTos, Thomas O'Brien. 2nd ed. c2008.
      ISBN-13: 978-0-07-337435-2 (alk. paper)
      ISBN-10: 0-07-337435-0 (alk. paper)
    1. Electrocardiography. I. O'Brien, Thomas E. (Thomas Edward), 1959- II. Booth, Kathryn
A., 1957- Electrocardiography for health care personnel. III. Title.
    [DNLM: 1. Electrocardiography--methods--Problems and Exercises. 2. Arrhythmias,
Cardiac--diagnosis--Problems and Exercises. WG 18.2]
RC683.5.E5H256 2012
616.1'207547--dc22   2010042747

WARNING NOTICE: The clinical procedures, medicines, dosages, and other matters described in this publication are based upon research of current literature and consultation with knowledgeable persons in the field. The procedures and matters described in this text reflect currently accepted clinical practice. However, this information cannot and should not be relied upon as necessarily applicable to a given individual's case. Accordingly, each person must be separately diagnosed to discern the patient's unique circumstances. Likewise, the manufacturer's package insert for current drug product information should be consulted before administering any drug. Publisher disclaims all liability for any inaccuracies, omissions, misuse, or misunderstanding of the information contained in this publication. Publisher cautions that this publication is not intended as a substitute for the professional judgment of trained medical personnel.

The Internet addresses listed in the text were accurate at the time of publication. The inclusion of a Web site does not indicate an endorsement by the authors or McGraw-Hill, and McGraw-Hill does not guarantee the accuracy of the information presented at these sites.

www.mhhe.com

Dedication

To the students who are using this book. Thank you for choosing the field of healthcare for your career. Your skills and services are truly needed. To my kind husband who supports me with patience and love.

Kathryn Booth

I want to thank my beautiful wife Michele and our wonderful children Thomas, Robert, and Kathryn. Without their love and support, I would have nothing. They inspire me every day to make a difference in people's lives. I also want to express my sincere thanks to the faculty, staff, and students of Central Florida Institute for their encouragement and guidance. Today's students are the difference makers of tomorrow!

Thomas O'Brien

About the Authors

Kathryn A. Booth, MS, RN, RMA (AMT), RPT, CPhT is a full-time author, educator, and consultant for Total Care Programming, a multimedia software development company. Her background includes a bachelor's degree in nursing and a master's degree in education. Her 30 years of teaching, nursing, and healthcare work experience span five states. She has authored and developed multimedia software and healthcare textbooks and educational materials for McGraw-Hill Higher Education; Total Care Programming; Glencoe/McGraw-Hill; Mosby Lifeline; and Lippincott, Williams, and Wilkins. Kathy Booth has presented at numerous state, corporate, and national conventions since 1994. Her current focus is to develop up-to-date, dynamic healthcare education materials to assist educators and promote the healthcare profession. Kathy is a member of the advisory board for Globe University and Everest College. She volunteers at a local free clinic and teaches part time online for Military to Medicine. Since the last edition of this text, Kathryn has also obtained RPT and CPhT certifications.

Thomas E. O'Brien, AS, CCT, CST, CRAT is a full-time faculty member teaching Cardiovascular Basic Studies at Central Florida Institute. He is also a subject matter consultant and test writer working with Cardiovascular Credentialing International (CCI) for the Certified Cardiographic Technician and Certified Rhythm Analysis Technician Registry Examinations. His background includes over 24 years in the U.S. Air Force and U.S. Army Medical Corps. Tom O'Brien's medical career as an Air Force Independent Duty Medical Technician (IDMT) has taken him all over the United States and the world. Tom has several years experience working in the Emergency Services and Critical Care arena. He was awarded "Master Instructor" status by the U.S. Air Force in 1994 upon completion of his teaching practicum. He now has over 10 years of teaching experience; subjects include Emergency Medicine, Cardiovascular Nursing, Fundamentals of Nursing, Dysrhythmia, and 12-Lead ECG Interpretation. Tom is actively involved in book proposals, and he reviews for a number of publishers, including Glencoe/McGraw-Hill and Lippincott, Williams, and Wilkins. His current position provides challenges with the day-to-day development of curriculum to meet the ever-changing needs of the medical community and to provide first-rate education to a diverse adult education population.

Brief Contents

Preface   xii

CHAPTER 1   Role of the Electrocardiographer   1

CHAPTER 2   The Cardiovascular System   28

CHAPTER 3   The Electrocardiograph   54

CHAPTER 4   Performing an ECG   82

CHAPTER 5   Rhythm Strip Interpretation and Sinus Rhythms   122

CHAPTER 6   Atrial Dysrhythmias   148

CHAPTER 7   Junctional Dysrhythmias   168

CHAPTER 8   Heart Block Dysrhythmias   187

CHAPTER 9   Rhythms Originating from the Ventricles   205

CHAPTER 10   Pacemaker Rhythms and Bundle Branch Block   233

CHAPTER 11   Exercise Electrocardiography   252

CHAPTER 12   Ambulatory Monitoring   280

CHAPTER 13   Clinical Management of the Cardiac Patient   308

CHAPTER 14   Basic 12-Lead ECG Interpretation   337

APPENDIX A   Cardiovascular Medications   A-1

APPENDIX B   Standard and Isolation Precautions   B-1

APPENDIX **C**   **Medical Abbreviations, Acronyms, and Symbols**   **C-1**

APPENDIX **D**   **Correlation of Textbook Learning Outcomes to Certification Standards**   **D-1**

APPENDIX **E**   **Anatomical Terms**   **E-1**

APPENDIX **F**   **Pressure Measurements**   **F-1**

Glossary   **G-1**

Photo Credits   **PC-1**

Index   **I-1**

Answer Key   **Online at www.mhhe.com/boothecg3e**

Rhythm Identification/Cardiac Medication Flash Cards   **End-of-book Insert**

Contents

Preface   xii

CHAPTER 1   Role of the Electrocardiographer   1

The Electrocardiogram (ECG)   2
History of the ECG   4
Role of an Electrocardiographer   5
How ECGs Are Used   6
What You Need to Know to Perform an ECG   13
Troubleshooting   20

CHAPTER 2   The Cardiovascular System   28

Circulation and the ECG   29
Anatomy of the Heart   29
Principles of Circulation   33
The Cardiac Cycle   36
Conduction System of the Heart   38
Electrical Stimulation and the ECG Waveform   41

CHAPTER 3   The Electrocardiograph   54

Producing the ECG Waveform   54
ECG Machines   61
ECG Controls   64
Electrodes   68
ECG Graph Paper   69
Calculating Heart Rate   72

CHAPTER 4 **Performing an ECG   82**

Preparation for the ECG Procedure   83
Communicating with the Patient   85
Identifying Anatomical Landmarks   87
Applying the Electrodes and Leads   88
Safety and Infection Control   92
Operating the ECG Machine   95
Checking the ECG Tracing   95
Reporting ECG Results   100
Equipment Maintenance   101
Pediatric ECG   103
Cardiac Monitoring   104
Special Patient Considerations   105
Handling Emergencies   108
Procedure Checklist 4.1 Recording an Electrocardiogram   117
Procedure Checklist 4.2 Continuous Cardiac Monitoring   119

CHAPTER 5 **Rhythms Strip Interpretation and Sinus Rhythms   122**

Rhythm Interpretation   123
Identifying the Components of the Rhythm   123
Rhythms Originating from the Sinus Node   130
Sinus Bradycardia   133
Sinus Tachycardia   135
Sinus Dysrhythmia   136
Sinus Arrest   138

CHAPTER 6 **Atrial Dysrhythmias   148**

Introduction to Atrial Dysrhythmias   149
Premature Atrial Complexes   149
Wandering Atrial Pacemaker   151
Multifocal Atrial Tachycardia   153
Flutter   155
Atrial Fibrillation   157

CHAPTER 7   **Junctional Dysrhythmias**   **168**

Introduction to Junctional Dysrhythmias   169
Premature Junctional Complex (PJC)   169
Junctional Escape Rhythm   171
Accelerated Junctional Rhythm   173
Junctional Tachycardia Rhythm   175
Supraventricular Tachycardia (SVT)   177

CHAPTER 8   **Heart Block Dysrhythmias**   **187**

Introduction to Heart Block Dysrhythmias   187
First Degree Atrioventricular (AV) Block   188
Second Degree Atrioventricular (AV) Block, Mobitz I (Type I or Wenckebach)   189
Second Degree Atrioventricular (AV) Block, Type II (Mobitz II)   192
Third Degree Atrioventricular (AV) Block (Complete)   194

CHAPTER 9   **Rhythms Originating from the Ventricles**   **205**

Introduction to Ventricular Dysrhythmias   206
Premature Ventricular Complexes (PVCs)   207
Agonal Rhythm   210
Idioventricular Rhythm   211
Accelerated Idioventricular Rhythm   213
Ventricular Tachycardia   215
Ventricular Fibrillation   217
Asystole   219

CHAPTER 10   **Pacemaker Rhythms and Bundle Branch Block**   **233**

Introduction to Pacemaker Rhythms   233
Evaluating Pacemaker Function   235
Pacemaker Complications Relative to the ECG Tracing   240
Introduction to Bundle Branch Block Dysrhythmias   242

CHAPTER 11   **Exercise Electrocardiography**   252

What Is Exercise Electrocardiography?   253
Why Is Exercise Electrocardiography Used?   255
Variations of Exercise Electrocardiography   256
Preparing the Patient for Exercise Electrocardiography   257
Providing Safety   261
Performing Exercise Electrocardiography   263
Common Protocols   265
Following Exercise Electrocardiography   268
Procedure Checklist 11-1   Assisting with Exercise Electrocardiography (Stress Testing)   276

CHAPTER 12   **Ambulatory Monitoring**   280

What is Ambulatory Monitoring?   280
How Is Ambulatory Monitoring Used?   282
Functions and Variations   283
Educating the Patient   288
Preparing the Patient   292
Applying an Ambulatory Monitor   292
Removing an Ambulatory Monitor and Reporting Results   295
Procedure Checklist 12-1   Applying and Removing an Ambulatory (Holter) Monitor   303

CHAPTER 13   **Clinical Management of the Cardiac Patient**   308

Coronary Arteries   309
Cardiac Symptoms   311
Atypical Patient Presentation   313
Acute Coronary Syndrome   315
Heart Failure   316
Cardiac Patient Assessment and Immediate Treatment   320
Further Treatment for the Cardiac Patient   326

CHAPTER **14** **Basic 12-Lead ECG Interpretation 337**

The Views of a Standard 12-Lead ECG and Major Vessels   337
Ischemia, Injury, and Infarction   342
Electrical Axis   346
Bundle Branch Block   348
Left Ventricular Hypertrophy (LVH)   350

Appendix A   Cardiovascular Medications   A-1
Appendix B   Standard and Isolation Precautions   B-1
Appendix C   Medical Abbreviations, Acronyms, and Symbols   C-1
Appendix D   Correlation of Textbook Learning Outcomes to Certification
             Standards   D-1
Appendix E   Anatomical Terms   E-1
Appendix F   Pressure Measurements   F-1
Glossary   G-1
Photo Credits   PC-1
Index   I-1
Answer Key   Online at www.mhhe.com/boothecg3e
Rhythm Identification/Cardiac Medication Flash Cards   End-of-book Insert

Preface

Healthcare is an ever-changing and growing field. Flexibility is key to obtaining, maintaining, and improving your career. Obtaining ECG certification, whether it be in addition to your current career, or as your career, will make you a valuable employee. The third edition of ECG for Healthcare Professionals will prepare you for a national ECG certification examination. The fact that you are currently reading this book means that you are willing to acquire new skills or specialize the skills you already possess. This willingness translates into your enhanced value, job security, marketability, and mobility. Once you complete this textbook, completing the certification examination will be your next step.

This third edition of *Electrocardiography for Healthcare Professionals* was designed not just for classroom but also for independent and distance learning. Checkpoint Questions and student CD exercises correlated to the Learning Outcomes make the learning process interactive and promote increased comprehension. The variety of materials included with the program provides for multiple learning styles and ensures your success.

The text/workbook/CD is divided into 14 chapters.

- *Chapter 1 Role of the Electrocardiographer* introduces you into the field of electrocardiography and helps to promote the various roles in the field. You will also learn about the history and how ECGs are used.

- *Chapter 2 The Cardiovascular System* provides a complete introduction and review of the heart and its electrical system. The information focuses on what you "need to know" to understand and perform an ECG. Specific topics include anatomy of the heart, principles of circulation, cardiac cycle, conduction system and electrical stimulation, and the ECG waveform.

- *Chapter 3 The Electrocardiograph* creates a basic understanding of the ECG, including producing the ECG waveform, the ECG machine, electrodes, and the ECG graph paper.

- *Chapter 4 Performing an ECG* describes the procedure for performing an ECG in a simple step-by-step fashion. Each part of the procedure is explained in detail, taking into consideration the latest guidelines. The chapter is divided into the following topics: preparation, communication, anatomical landmarks, applying the electrodes and leads, safety and infection control, operating the ECG machine, checking the tracing, reporting results, and equipment maintenance. Extra sections are included regarding pediatric ECG, special patient circumstances, and emergencies. Procedure checklists are included to practice performing both an ECG and continuous monitoring.

- *Chapter 5 Rhythm Strip Interpretation and Sinus Rhythms* introduces the five-step criteria for classification approach to rhythm interpretation that will be utilized throughout Chapters 5 to 10. Updated rhythm strip figures, explanations, and checkpoint questions help the student learn to interpret the sinus rhythms, including criteria for classification, how the patient may be affected, basic patient care, and treatment.

- *Chapter 6 Atrial Dysrhythmias* provides an introduction to and interpretation of the atrial dysrhythmias, including criteria for classification, how the patient may be affected, basic patient care. and treatment.

- *Chapter 7 Junctional Dysrhythmias* provides an introduction to and interpretation of the junctional dysrhythmias, including criteria for classification, how the patient may be affected, basic patient care, and treatment.

- *Chapter 8 Heart Block Dysrhythmias* provides an introduction to and interpretation of the heart block dysrhythmias, including criteria for classification, how the patient may be affected, basic patient care, and treatment.

- *Chapter 9 Rhythms Originating from the Ventricles* provides an introduction to and interpretation of the ventricular dysrhythmias, including criteria for classification, how the patient may be affected, basic patient care, and treatment.

- *Chapter 10 Pacemaker Rhythms and Bundle Branch Block* provides an introduction to pacemaker rhythms, evaluation of pacemaker function, and complications related to the ECG tracing. An introduction to bundle branch block dysrhythmias, including criteria for classification, how the patient may be affected, basic patient care, and treatment, is also included.

- *Chapter 11 Exercise Electrocardiography* provides the information necessary to assist with the exercise electrocardiography procedure. The competency checklist provides the step-by-step procedure for practice and to develop proficiency at the skill.

- *Chapter 12 Ambulatory Monitoring* includes the latest information about various types of ambulatory monitors and includes what you need to know to apply and remove a monitor. A procedure checklist is also provided for this skill.

- *Chapter 13 Clinical Management of the Cardiac Patient* expands upon the anatomy of the coronary arteries and relates them to typical and atypical cardiac symptoms. STEMI, non-STEMI, and heart failure are introduced. The chapter finishes with assessment, immediate care, and continued treatment of the cardiac patient.

- *Chapter 14 Basic 12-Lead ECG Interpretation* provides a basic introduction to the concept of 12-lead ECG interpretation. It includes anatomic views of the coronary arteries on the 12-lead ECG, and the morphologic changes of ischemia, injury, and infarction. Axis deviation, bundle branch block, and left ventricular hypertrophy round out the chapter concepts.

New to the 3rd Edition

- Doubled the content from 7 to 14 chapters.
- Chapter 5 has been split into five chapters, introducing interpretation of sinus, atrial, junctional, heart block, ventricular, pacemaker, and bundle branch block rhythms.
- New Chapter 13 Clinical Management of the Cardiac Patient.
- New Chapter 14 Basic 12-Lead ECG Interpretation.
- Learning Outcomes for all 14 chapters are correlated to the level I headings of the chapters.
- Correlations to national ECG certification standards within the student edition book (Appendix D).
- Interpret-TIP throughout chapters 5 to 10 provides simple and easy guidelines to help students distinguish unique features of each ECG rhythm presented.
- Added Rhythm Identification and Cardiovascular Medication Flash Cards to the back of the book.
- Checkpoint and review questions are correlated to the learning outcomes and include over 35 new rhythm strips for interpretation.
- Over 25 new and updated figures throughout the textbook and student CD.

Features of the Text/Workbook/CD

- **Key Terms, Glossary, and Audio Glossary:** Key terms are identified at the beginning of each chapter. These terms are in **bold, color** type within the chapter and are defined both in the chapter and in the glossary at the end of the book. Open the student CD to hear the pronunciation of each key term, and practice learning the term with the "Key Term Quiz" and the "Key Term Concentration" game.

- **Checkpoint Questions:** At the end of each main heading in the chapter are short-answer Checkpoint Questions. Answer these questions to make sure you have learned the basic concepts presented.

- **CD Activities:** After you have finished the Checkpoint Questions, you are sent to the interactive student CD activity to further your review and practice of the concepts presented in each section. Be sure to complete the activities on the CD before you continue to the next section.

- **Troubleshooting:** The Troubleshooting feature identifies problems and situations that may arise when you are caring for patients or performing a procedure. At the end of this feature, you are asked a question to answer in your own words.

- **Safety & Infection Control:** You are responsible for providing safe care and preventing the spread of infection. This feature presents tips and techniques to help you practice these important skills relative to electrocardiography.

- **Patient Education & Communication:** Patient interaction and education and intrateam communication are integral parts of healthcare. As part of your daily duties, you must communicate effectively, both orally and in writing, and you must provide patient education. Use this feature to learn ways to perform these tasks.

- **Law & Ethics:** When working in healthcare, you must be conscious of the regulations of HIPAA (Health Insurance Portability and Accountability Act) and understand your legal responsibilities and the implications of your actions. You must perform duties within established ethical practices. This feature helps you gain insight into how HIPAA, law, and ethics relate to the performance of your duties.

- **Realistic ECG Strips:** Actual ECG rhythm strips have been provided for easy viewing and to make the task of learning the various dysrhythmias easier and more realistic. Use of these ECG rhythm strips for activities and exercises throughout the program improves student comprehension and accommodates visual learners.

- **Rhythm Strip Flash Cards and Quizzes:** Review all of the rhythm in the book using the print flash cards or student CD flash cards or flash card quizzes.

- **Chapter Summary:** Once you have completed each chapter, take time to read and review the summary table. It has been correlated to key concepts and learning outcomes within each chapter and includes handy page number references.

- **Chapter Review:** Complete the chapter review questions, which are presented in a variety of formats. These questions help you understand the content presented in each chapter. Chapters 4, 11, and 12 include Procedure Checklists for you to use to practice and apply your knowledge.

- **Get Connected and the Online Learning Center:** The Get Connected activity directs you to the Online Learning Center (OLC) that accompanies the text/workbook. The OLC provides links for you to complete research and activities related to the information presented in the chapter. You will also find other review activities and materials on the OLC to assist you in learning electrocardiography.

- **Chapter Test:** Open the student CD to take a final test of your knowledge of material in each chapter. Review the material again with the "Spin the Wheel" game, and then take the chapter test. You can print or e-mail your score to your instructor.

Connect Plus

McGraw-Hill *Connect Plus Electrocardiography for Healthcare Professionals* is a web-based assignment and assessment platform that gives students the means to better connect with their coursework, with their instructors, and with the important concepts that they will need to know for success now and in the future. With *Connect Plus Electrocardiography for Healthcare Professionals*, instructors can deliver assignments, quizzes, and tests easily online. Students can practice important skills at their own pace and on their own schedule. With *Connect Plus Electrocardiography for Healthcare Professionals*, students also get 24/7 online access to an eBook—an online edition of the text—to aid them in successfully completing their work, wherever and whenever they choose.

Guided Tour

Features to Help You Study and Learn

Chapter Outlines, Learning Outcomes, Key Terms, and an Introduction begin each chapter to introduce you to the chapter and help prepare you for the information that will be presented.

Checkpoint Questions are provided at the end of each section in the chapter to help you understand the information you just read.

CD-ROM references direct you to the interactive CD activity to further your review and practice the concepts presented in each section.

"The CD ROM is a great learning tool and is user friendly. The information on universal precautions is very important and not covered in other EKG texts." Sheri Melton, PhD, West Chester University

Troubleshooting exercises identify problems and situations that may arise on the job. You may be asked to answer a question about the situation.

Heart Block Dysrhythmias — 8

Chapter Outline
- Introduction to Heart Block Dysrhythmias (p. 187)
- First Degree Atrioventricular (AV) Block (p. 188)
- Second Degree Atrioventricular (AV) Block, Mobitz I (Type I or Wenckebach) (p. 189)
- Second Degree Atrioventricular (AV) Block, Type II (Mobitz II) (p. 192)
- Third Degree Atrioventricular (AV) Block (Complete) (p. 194)

Learning Outcomes
- 8.1 Describe the various heart block dysrhythmias.
- 8.2 Identify first degree heart block using the criteria for classification, and explain how the rhythm may affect the patient, including basic patient care and treatment.
- 8.3 Identify second degree atrioventricular (AV) block, Mobitz I, using the criteria for classification, and explain how the rhythm may affect the patient, including basic patient care and treatment.
- 8.4 Identify second degree atrioventricular (AV) block, Mobitz II, using the criteria for classification, and explain how the rhythm may affect the patient, including basic patient care and treatment.
- 8.5 Identify third degree atrioventricular (AV) block using the criteria for classification, and explain how the rhythm may affect the patient, including basic patient care and treatment.

Key Terms
blocked or nonconducted impulse
cardiac output parameters
dissociative

8.1 Introduction to Heart Block Dysrhythmias
In heart block rhythms, the electrical current has difficulty traveling along the normal conduction pathway, causing a delay in or absence of ventricular depolarization. The degree of blockage is dependent on the area affected and the cause of the delay or blockage. There are three levels of heart blocks. The P-P interval is regular with all heart blocks.

187

---

pacemaker.

Check Point Question (LO 5.4)

1. Using the criteria for classification, select the rhythm that most closely resembles sinus bradycardia rhythm.

A.

B.

Which unique feature(s) led you to make the selection?

_____

_____

RL = right leg — White / Black
LL = left leg — Green / Red
V1 to V6 = chest leads — Brown

Troubleshooting — Check the Lead Wires

Each of the lead wires is coded by color and letter. If you place the lead wires incorrectly, the ECG will not record at all or it will record the waveforms improperly. Always check and double-check the lead wires before you begin the tracing. An ECG recording produced with the lead wires attached incorrectly is not acceptable and will have to be repeated.

If you attempt to record an ECG and no tracing is seen, what should you do?

_____

_____

To understand the circuits for the first six leads (three standard and three augmented), we can use the Einthoven triangle. Einthoven is the scientist credited with developing the first ECG machine. The Einthoven triangle is formed by three of the limb electrodes: those on the right arm

Einthoven triangle
A triangle formed by three of

Patient Education & Communication boxes give you helpful information for communicating effectively—both orally and written—with patients.

"I have been examining textbooks for approximately eight years now and this ECG text provides students with the most complete and accurate information without overwhelming them." Donna Folmar, Belmont Technical College

Interpret-TIP features throughout Chapters 5-10 provide simple and easy guidelines to help students recognize each of the ECG rhythms presented.

Safety & Infection Control boxes present tips and techniques for you to apply on the job.

Law & Ethics boxes help you gain insight into necessary information related to the performance of your duties.

---

angle of Louis
anterior axillary line
dextrocardia
intercostal space (ICS)
midaxillary line
midclavicular line

posterior axillary line
seizure
somatic tremor
suprasternal notch
wandering baseline

4.1 Preparation for the ECG Procedure

Now that you understand how the ECG is used, the anatomy of the heart, and the electrocardiograph, the next step is to record an ECG. The ECG experience should be pleasant to the patient and not produce anxiety. The ECG procedure must be done correctly, and the tracing must be accurate.

Prior to performing the ECG, you will need to prepare the room. Certain conditions in the room where the ECG is to be performed should be considered. For example, electrical currents in the room can interfere with the tracing. If possible, choose a room away from other electrical equipment and x-ray machines. If possible, turn off any electrical equipment that is in the room during the tracing. The ECG machine should be placed away from other sources of electrical currents, such as wires or cords.

An ECG must be ordered by a physician or other authorized personnel, and an order form must be completed prior to the procedure. This form may be called a requisition or consult and should be placed in the patient's record. It should include why the ECG was ordered and the following identifying information:

- Patient name, identification number or medical record number, and birth date
- Location, date, and time of recording
- Patient age, sex, race, and cardiac medications the patient is currently taking
- Weight and height
- Any special condition or position of the patient during the recording

If this information is not included on the requisition or consult, you should ask the patient or find the information in the patient's record.

Many facilities have computerized systems. The ECG order is frequently entered through this system. Entering the patient identifying information into the computer will produce the order form and generate patient

Patient Education & Communication — **Cardiac Medications**
Certain cardiac medications can change the ECG tracing. Prior to the ECG procedure, determine if your patient is on any cardiac medications and, if so, inform the physician and write the names of the medications on the ECG report. See Appendix A for examples of common cardiac medications.

g an ECG   **83**

Interpret-TIP

Ventricular Fibrillation

Ventricular fibrillation is the absence of organized electrical activity. The tracing is disorganized or chaotic in appearance.

How the Patient Is Affected and What You Should Know

What appears to be ventricular fibrillation on the monitor may not be it at all. Remember to always check your patient first. Fibrillatory waveforms may be caused by a variety of different things, like poorly attached or dried out electrodes, broken lead wires, excessive patient movement, etc. If your patient is talking to you, they are *not* in ventricular fibrillation.

In true ventricular defibrillation, patients will be unresponsive when the ventricles are quivering without contracting. *This will always be a Code Blue situation, in which immediate intervention is necessary to prevent biological death.* Every patient experiencing ventricular fibrillation will be unconscious, apneic (apnea means not breathing), and pulseless. CPR and emergency measures should begin immediately. It is recommended that appropriate personnel begin the advanced cardiac life support (ACLS) to regain normal cardiac function. Rhythm strips are maintained and used as documentation in the patient's medical record.

apnea The absence of breathing.

advanced cardiac life support (ACLS) A set of clinical interventions for the urgent treatment of cardiac arrest and other life threatening medical emergencies, as well as the knowledge and skills to deploy those interventions.

Safety & Infection Control — **Crash Cart**
Emergency equipment found on the "crash cart" must be ready when a code situation occurs. It is important that the cart be well stocked and the emergency equipment functioning properly. Each facility has a policy that requires regular checking and documentation of all emergency equipment and "crash carts."

crash carts A cart or tray used during emergencies containing medication/equipment at site of medical/surgical emergency for life support.

Checkpoint Question (LO 9.7) — Using the criteria for classification, select the rhythm that most closely resembles ventricular fibrillation.

A.

(Continued)

Law & Ethics — **Scope of Practice**
Your role regarding evaluation of the rhythm strip and assessment of the patient will depend on your training and place of employment. Working outside of your scope of practice is illegal, and you could be held liable for performing tasks that are not part of your role as a healthcare professional.

without signs and symptoms of decreased cardiac output) may only complain of palpitations and state, "I'm just not feeling right" or "My heart is fluttering." When the patient's condition is *unstable*, he or she may experience any symptom of low cardiac output, which is reflective of the heart not pumping effectively to other body systems. Many patients may present initially with a stable condition and then a few minutes later experience unstable symptoms such as those presented in Table 5-2.

Observe the patient for signs and symptoms of low cardiac output. Signs, symptoms, and rhythm changes need to be communicated quickly to a licensed practitioner for appropriate medical treatment. Because tachycardia significantly increases myocardial oxygen demand, treatment should begin as early as possible. It is difficult to predict how long a patient's heart can beat at a rapid rate before it begins to affect the other body systems.

Check Point Questions (LO 7.6)

1. What are the rate and the origination point of a supraventricular tachycardia?

2. What might you be asked to do when a patient has a supraventricular dysrhythmia?

3. List common sensations described by patients experiencing SVT.

ECG Rhythm Strips make the task of learning the various dysrhythmias easier and more realistic. Over 200 strips within the textbook.

"Practice ECG rhythm strips are key tools for practicing rhythm recognition. An excellent comprehensive textbook for the Electrocardiography student." Stephen Nardozzi, Westchester Community College

Key Points correlated to the learning outcomes in the Chapter Summaries help you review what was just learned.

Chapter Reviews consist of various methods of quizzing you. True/False, Multiple Choice, Matching, and Critical Thinking questions, among others, appeal to all types of learners.

At the end of each chapter, you will be directed to visit the Internet and the student CD to experience more interactive activities about the information you just learned.

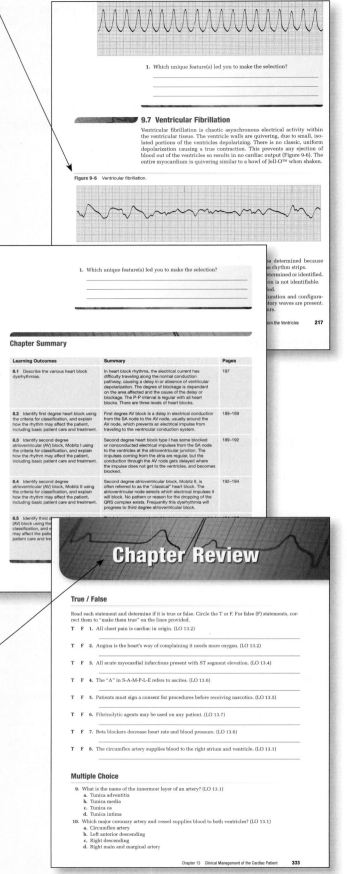

1. Which unique feature(s) led you to make the selection?

9.7 Ventricular Fibrillation

Ventricular fibrillation is chaotic asynchronous electrical activity within the ventricular tissue. The ventricle walls are quivering, due to small, isolated portions of the ventricles depolarizing. There is no classic, uniform depolarization causing a true contraction. This prevents any ejection of blood out of the ventricles so results in no cardiac output (Figure 9-6). The entire myocardium is quivering similar to a bowl of Jell-O™ when shaken.

Figure 9-6   Ventricular fibrillation.

1. Which unique feature(s) led you to make the selection?

Chapter Summary

Learning Outcomes	Summary	Pages
8.1 Describe the various heart block dysrhythmias.	In heart block rhythms, the electrical current has difficulty traveling along the normal conduction pathway, causing a delay in or absence of ventricular depolarization. The degree of blockage is dependent on the area affected and the cause of the delay or blockage. The P-P interval is regular with all heart blocks. There are three levels of heart blocks.	187
8.2 Identify first degree heart block using the criteria for classification, and explain how the rhythm may affect the patient, including basic patient care and treatment.	First degree AV block is a delay in electrical conduction from the SA node to the AV node, usually around the AV node, which prevents an electrical impulse from traveling to the ventricular conduction system.	188–189
8.3 Identify second degree atrioventricular (AV) block, Mobitz I using the criteria for classification, and explain how the rhythm may affect the patient, including basic patient care and treatment.	Second degree heart block type I has some blocked or nonconducted electrical impulses from the SA node to the ventricles at the atrioventricular junction. The impulses coming from the atria are regular, but the conduction through the AV node gets delayed where the impulse does not get to the ventricles, and becomes blocked.	189–192
8.4 Identify second degree atrioventricular (AV) block, Mobitz II using the criteria for classification, and explain how the rhythm may affect the patient, including basic patient care and treatment.	Second degree atrioventricular block, Mobitz II, is often referred to as the "classical" heart block. The atrioventricular node selects which electrical impulses it will block. No pattern or reason for the dropping of the QRS complex exists. Frequently this dysrhythmia will progress to third degree atrioventricular block.	192–194
8.5 Identify third degree atrioventricular (AV) block using the criteria for classification, and explain how the rhythm may affect the patient, including basic patient care and treatment.		

Chapter Review

True / False

Read each statement and determine if it is true or false. Circle the T or F. For false (F) statements, correct them to "make them true" on the lines provided.

T F **1.** All chest pain is cardiac in origin. (LO 13.2)

T F **2.** Angina is the heart's way of complaining it needs more oxygen. (LO 13.2)

T F **3.** All acute myocardial infarctions present with ST segment elevation. (LO 13.4)

T F **4.** The "A" in S-A-M-P-L-E refers to ascites. (LO 13.6)

T F **5.** Patients must sign a consent for procedures before receiving narcotics. (LO 13.5)

T F **6.** Fibrinolytic agents may be used on any patient. (LO 13.7)

T F **7.** Beta blockers decrease heart rate and blood pressure. (LO 13.6)

T F **8.** The circumflex artery supplies blood to the right atrium and ventricle. (LO 13.1)

Multiple Choice

9. What is the name of the innermost layer of an artery? (LO 13.1)
a. Tunica adventitia
b. Tunica media
c. Tunica os
d. Tunica intima

10. Which major coronary artery and vessel supplies blood to both ventricles? (LO 13.1)
a. Circumflex artery
b. Left anterior descending
c. Right descending
d. Right main and marginal artery

Chapter 13   Clinical Management of the Cardiac Patient   **333**

Procedure Checklists help you learn and apply the knowledge presented.

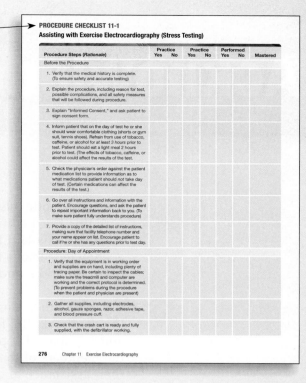

PROCEDURE CHECKLIST 11-1

Assisting with Exercise Electrocardiography (Stress Testing)

Procedure Steps (*Rationale*)	Practice Yes	No	Practice Yes	No	Performed Yes	No	Mastered
Before the Procedure							
1. Verify that the medical history is complete. (To ensure safety and accurate testing)							
2. Explain the procedure, including reason for test, possible complications, and all safety measures that will be followed during procedure.							
3. Explain "Informed Consent," and ask patient to sign consent form.							
4. Inform patient that on the day of test he or she should wear comfortable clothing (shorts or gym suit, tennis shoes). Refrain from use of tobacco, caffeine, or alcohol for at least 3 hours prior to test. Patient should eat a light meal 2 hours prior to test. (The effects of tobacco, caffeine, or alcohol could affect the results of the test.)							
5. Check the physician's order against the patient medication list to provide information as to what medications patient should *not* take day of test. (Certain medications can affect the results of the test.)							
6. Go over all instructions and information with the patient. Encourage questions, and ask the patient to repeat important information back to you. (To make sure patient fully understands procedure)							
7. Provide a copy of the detailed list of instructions, making sure that facility telephone number and your name appear on list. Encourage patient to call if he or she has any questions prior to test day.							
Procedure: Day of Appointment							
1. Verify that the equipment is in working order and supplies are on hand, including plenty of tracing paper. Be certain to inspect the cables; make sure the treadmill and computer are working and the correct protocol is determined. (To prevent problems during the procedure when the patient and physician are present)							
2. Gather all supplies, including electrodes, alcohol, gauze sponges, razor, adhesive tape, and blood pressure cuff.							
3. Check that the crash cart is ready and fully supplied, with the defibrillator working.							

276   Chapter 11   Exercise Electrocardiography

Review and Practice Rhythm Identification throughout textbook activities.

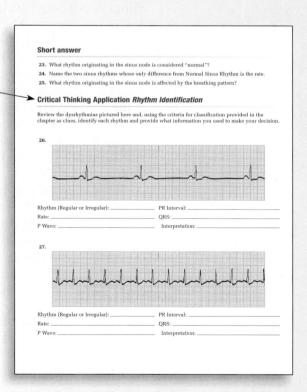

Short answer

23. What rhythm originating in the sinus node is considered "normal"?

24. Name the two sinus rhythms whose only difference from Normal Sinus Rhythm is the rate.

25. What rhythm originating in the sinus node is affected by the breathing pattern?

Critical Thinking Application *Rhythm Identification*

Review the dysrhythmias pictured here and, using the criteria for classification provided in the chapter as clues, identify each rhythm and provide what information you used to make your decision.

26.

Rhythm (Regular or Irregular): _____   PR Interval: _____
Rate: _____   QRS: _____
P Wave: _____   Interpretation: _____

27.

Rhythm (Regular or Irregular): _____   PR Interval: _____
Rate: _____   QRS: _____
P Wave: _____   Interpretation: _____

Acknowledgments

Authors

Kathryn Booth: Thanks to all the reviewers who have spent time making sure this third edition is up to date. In addition, I would like to acknowledge McGraw-Hill for supporting this book into its third edition. A special acknowledgement to Jody, Tom, Cynthia, Jennifer, and Susan for all their time, attention, and efforts in helping make this project a success.

I would like to acknowledge Patricia Dei Tos and the members of the Inova Health system, who help to create and support the development of this textbook, the Inova Learning Network, who provided encouragement and lab space for photo opportunities. Also, I would like to acknowledge the members of the Inova Heart and Vascular Institute and Inova eICU for their assistance in obtaining photographs and video selections.

Thomas O'Brien: I would like to acknowledge Mr. David Rubin, President & CEO of Aerotel Medical Systems (1998) Ltd., 5 Hazoref St., Holon 58856, Israel. I would like to express my sincere appreciation to a pair of former students and Central Florida Institute graduates, Rebecca Walton, CCT, for her contribution of Interpret-Tips and to Jamie Merritt, CCT, for "bunny branch block." I would also like to give a special thank you to the staff members of the Non-Invasive Cardiology Departments at the Pepin Heart Hospital, Morton Plant Hospital, All Children's Hospital, and Palms of Pasadena Hospital for their inputs and generous donation of their time and expertise.

Additionally I would like to thank my co-workers and the leadership at CFI: Rose Lynn Greene, Director, Susan Burnell, DOE, Steve Coleman, NCMA, Education Supervisor, Amanda L. Jones, MBA, NR-CMA, NCPT, CPC, Medical Assistant Program Director (CFI), and Nicholas R. Senger, RMA, Medical Assistant Program Instructor (CFI).

Finally, a very special thank you to my son Rob for his hours devoted to scanning many of the cardiac rhythms in this text.

Consultants

Cynthia T. Vincent, MMS, PA-C
Alderson Broaddus College,
Philippi, WV

Jennifer Childers, MS PAC
Alderson Broaddus College, Philippi, WV

Susan Hurley Findley, RN, MSN
Houston, TX

Lynn M. Egler, RMA, AHI, CPhT
St. Clair Shores, MI

Kimberly Speiring, MA
St Clair Shores, MI

Reviewers

Jesse A. Coale, PA-C
Philadelphia University
Philadelphia, PA

Stephen Coleman
Central Florida Institute
Palm Harbor, FL

Harvey Conner, AS, REMT-P
Oklahoma City Community
*   College*
Oklahoma City, OK

Grace Haines
National College
Dayton, OH

Linda Karp
Atlantic Cape Community
*   College*
Mays Landing, NJ

Deborah Kufs, MS, BSN,
    CEN, EMT-P
Hudson Valley Community College
Troy, NY

Elizabeth Laurenz
National College
Columbus, OH

Suzanne Wambold, PhD., RN,
    RDCS, FASE
The University of Toledo
Toledo, OH

Danny Webb
Milan Institute
Visalia, CA

Fran Wojculewicz, RN, BSN, MS
Maricopa Community College
Glendale, AZ

Previous Edition Reviewers

Emil P. Asdurian, MD
Bramson ORT College
Forest Hills, NY

Vanessa J. Austin, RMA, CAHI
Clarian Health Sciences Center,
*   Medical Assistant*
Indianapolis, IN

Rhonda J. Beck, NREMT-P
Central Georgia Technical College
Macon, GA

Nia Bullock, PhD
Miller-Motte Technical College
Cary, NC

Barbara S. Desch, LVN, CPC, AHI
San Joaquin Valley College Inc.
Visalia/Hanford Campus
Visalia, CA

Melissa L. Dulaney
MedVance Institute of Baton Rouge
Baton Rouge, LA

Mary Patricia English
Howard Community College
Columbia, MD

Michael Fisher, Program
    Director
Greenville Technical College
Greenville, SC

Donna L. Folmar
Belmont Technical College
St. Clairsville, OH

Anne Fox
Maric College
Carson, CA

James R. Fry, MS, PA-C
Marietta College
Marietta, OH

Michael Gallucci, MS, PT
Assistant Professor of Practice,
*   Program in Physical Therapy*
School of Public Health,
*   New York Medical College*
New York, NY

Jonathan I. Greenwald
Arapahoe Community College
Littleton, CO

Susie Laughter, BSN, RN
Cambridge Institute of Allied Health
Longwood, FL

Sheri A. Melton, PhD
West Chester University
West Chester, PA

Stephen J. Nardozzi
Westchester Community College
Valhalla, NY

David James Newton, NREMT-P
Dalton State College
Dalton, GA

R. Keith Owens
AB-Tech Community College
Asheville, NC

Douglas A. Paris, BS, NREMT-P
Greenville Technical College
Department of Emergency Medical
Technology
Greenville, SC

David Rice, AA, BA, MA
Career College of Northern Nevada
Reno, NV

Dana M. Roessler, RN, BSN
Southeastern Technical College
Glennville, GA

Wayne A. Rummings, Sr.
Lenoir Community College
Kingston, NC

David Lee Sessoms, Jr., M.Ed.,
CMA
Miller-Motte Technical College
Cary, NC

Mark A. Simpson, NREMT-P, RN,
CCEMTP
Director of EMS
Northwest-Shoals Community
College
Muscle Shoals, AL

Linda M. Thompson, MS, RRT
Madison Area Technical College
Madison, WI

Dyan Whitlow Underhill,
MHA, BS
Miller-Motte Technical College
Cary, NC

Eddy van Hunnik, PhD
Gibbs College Boston
Boston, MA

Danielle Schortzmann Wilken
Goodwin College
East Hartford, CT

Stacey F. Wilson, MT/PBT
(ASCP), CMA
Cabarrus College of Health Sciences
Concord, NC

Roger G. Wootten
Northeast Alabama Community
College
Rainsville, AL

First Edition

Civita Allard
Mohawk Valley Community
College
Utica, NY

Vicki Barclay
West Kentucky Technical College
Paducah, KY

Nina Beaman
Bryant and Stratton College
Richmond, VA

Cheryl Bell
Sanz School
Washington, DC

Lucy Della Rosa
Concorde Career Institute
Lauderdale Lakes, FL

Myrna Lanier
Tulsa Community College
Tulsa, OK

Debra Shafer
Blair College
Colorado Springs, CO

Role of the Electrocardiographer 1

Chapter Outline

- The Electrocardiogram (ECG) (p. 2)
- History of the ECG (p. 4)
- Role of an Electrocardiographer (p. 5)
- How ECGs Are Used (p. 6)
- What You Need to Know to Perform an ECG (p. 13)
- Troubleshooting (p. 20)

Learning Outcomes

1.1 Explain what an ECG is and its importance in medicine.
1.2 Discuss the history of obtaining and using the ECG.
1.3 Describe career opportunities for an electrocardiographer.
1.4 Compare the uses of the ECG in the hospital, in the doctor's office or ambulatory clinic, or outside of a healthcare facility.
1.5 Identify the skills and knowledge needed to perform an ECG.
1.6 Define troubleshooting, and explain its importance to you as a healthcare professional.

Key Terms

angioplasty
arrhythmia
automatic external defibrillator (AED)
body mechanics
cardiopulmonary resuscitation (CPR)
cardiovascular
Code Blue
coronary artery disease (CAD)
defibrillator
electrocardiogram (ECG)
electrocardiograph

electrocardiology
galvanometer
healthcare provider
Holter monitor
isolation precautions
myocardial infarction (MI) (heart attack)
pacemaker (artificial)
standard precautions
stat
technician
technologist
telemetry

1.1 The Electrocardiogram (ECG)

cardiovascular Related to the heart and blood vessels (veins and arteries).

coronary artery disease (CAD) Narrowing of the blood vessels around the heart causing reduced blood flow to the heart.

electrocardiograph An instrument used to record the electrical activity of the heart.

electrocardiogram (ECG) A tracing of the heart's electrical activity recorded by an electrocardiograph.

The number one cause of death in the United States every year since 1918 is **cardiovascular** disease, or a disease of the heart and blood vessels. Approximately 2500 Americans die every day because of **coronary artery disease (CAD)**, which is narrowing of the blood vessels surrounding the heart that causes a reduction of blood flow to the heart. Unbelievably, one out of every three American adults has some form of CAD. You may know someone who has hypertension (high blood pressure) or other heart conditions. Maybe someone you know has had an MI (myocardial infarction, or heart attack). Table 1-1 contains more information on ways to reduce or prevent heart disease, stroke, or heart attack.

An instrument known as an **electrocardiograph** allows the heart's electrical activity to be recorded and studied. It is used to produce an electrical (*electro*) tracing (*graph*) of the heart (*cardio*). This tracing is known as an **electrocardiogram,** or **ECG.** The standard ECG machine has lead wires that are attached to a patient's chest to produce the electrical tracing (Figure 1-1).

Performing the actual ECG procedure is not difficult; however, it must be performed competently. The tracing of the electrical current of the heart

TABLE 1-1 Ways to Reduce or Prevent Heart Disease, Stroke, or Heart Attack

The American Heart Association now recommends that you watch your ABCs:

A. Avoid tobacco.
   1. Stop smoking. A smoker's risk is twice that of a nonsmoker. Even exposure to environmental tobacco smoke (secondhand smoke, passive smoking) may increase the risk of heart disease.
   2. Decrease stress.
   3. Maintain healthy blood pressure. Find ways to lower blood pressure and to keep the numbers down. The goal is a blood pressure of less than 120/80 mmHg.
   4. Maintain healthy blood cholesterol. Cholesterol will cause the fat to be lodged in your arteries, which will sooner or later cause a heart attack or stoke. It is important to keep the total cholesterol less than 200 mg/dL.

B. Be more active.
   1. Increase physical activity. Goal is to increase physical activities on most days of the week to 30 to 60 minutes of physical activity. Increase in activity will decrease the following:
      a. Stress
      b. High blood pressure
      c. High blood cholesterol
      d. Obesity

C. Choose good nutrition. Maintain a well-balanced diet, which helps to decrease the following:
   1. Alcohol consumption
   2. Stress
   3. High blood pressure
   4. High blood cholesterol
   5. Diabetes
   6. Obesity

Adapted from the American Heart Association's Guidelines

must be accurate because it is used to make decisions about a patient's care. An inaccurate tracing could result in a wrong decision about the patient's medication or treatment. These decisions could result in a negative outcome for the patient.

Figure 1-1 A 12-lead ECG machine is attached to the patient's chest, arms, and legs using electrodes and leads wires. It records a tracing of the electrical activity of the heart.

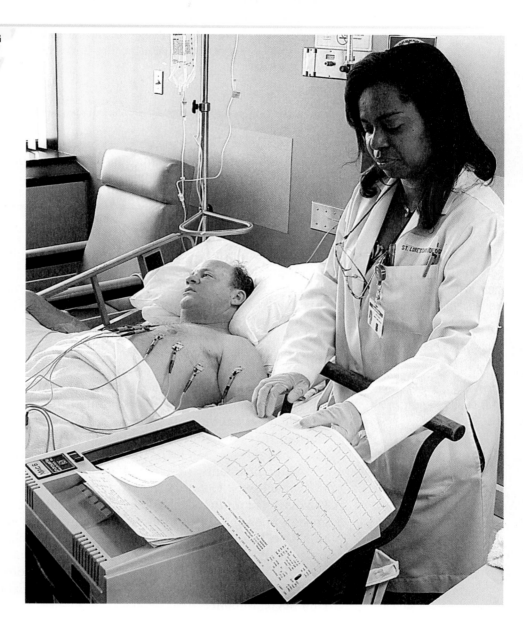

1. What is the leading cause of death in the United States?

   Cardiovascular Disease

1.2 History of the ECG

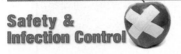

Knowing the history of obtaining electrical tracings from the heart will help you better understand the reasons ECGs are performed and their importance in medicine. As early as 1676, scientists made the discovery that animals generate electricity. In 1887, an English physician, Dr. Augustus D. Waller (1856–1922), was the first to show that electrical currents are produced during the beating of the human heart and can be recorded. Dr. Waller was credited with having performed the first electrocardiogram on a human.

Safety & Infection Control

Electricity and the ECG

An ECG does not produce electricity; it only records the electrical activity of the heart. It is a safe and harmless procedure.

galvanometer An instrument is used to detect electrocardiograph waves.

electrocardiology The study of the heart's electrical activity.

arrhythmias Abnormal heartbeats.

myocardial infarction (MI) A blockage of one or more of the coronary arteries causing lack of oxygen to the heart and damage to the muscle tissue.

Wilhelm Einthoven (1860–1927), a Dutch physiologist, continued the development of the ECG. He developed the first practical **galvanometer,** an instrument used to detect electrocardiograph waves. In 1903, Einthoven invented the first electrocardiograph. Einthoven's instrument introduced the field of **electrocardiology,** or the study of the heart's electrical activity, and he won the Nobel Prize in Physiology or Medicine in 1924 for the significance of his invention.

Other scientists extended the work of Einthoven. Sir Thomas Lewis of London (1881–1945) studied how the ECG related to cardiac **arrhythmias** (abnormal heartbeats). His work formed the basis for much of the current knowledge about the ECG. In 1918, an American physician, James B. Herrick, showed that an abnormal tracing and physical symptoms could indicate a **myocardial infarction** (MI), also known as a heart attack.

Advancements in technology have brought about today's modern ECG machines. Computer interpretation of the ECG tracing is common. Currently, computer technology continues to improve the availability and speed of computer interpretation and quickly communicates this information to a healthcare professional. An ECG machine is now as small as a wristwatch. With the use of digital information, healthcare professionals are able to monitor patients from remote locations miles away. Patients in hospitals can be monitored through cameras, ECG readings, and other vital sign measurements.

Checkpoint Question (LO 1.2)

1. Who is credited with having performed the first ECG on a human?

Dr. Augustus D. WALLER

1.3 Role of an Electrocardiographer

Electrocardiography is an expanding career field. Many healthcare professionals are trained to record or monitor the heart's electrical activity. These include physicians, nurse practitioners, physician assistants, nurses, paramedics, medical assistants, trained nursing assistants, and emergency medical technicians, though this list is not inclusive. With the changing healthcare field, other healthcare employees, such as respiratory or radiology personnel, are also learning to perform ECGs to improve healthcare delivery in a variety of healthcare settings. Healthcare professionals who perform ECGs should also be trained in **cardiopulmonary pulmonary resuscitation (CPR)**, a technique used to provide ventilations (breaths) and chest compressions (blood circulation) for a person who shows no signs of breathing or having a heartbeat.

Healthcare personnel who are proficient at recording an ECG can expect to increase their employability and advance their careers. In addition, there are career opportunities for individuals who may want to specialize in the field of electrocardiography. These include, but are not limited to, the ECG technician, the ECG monitoring technician, and the cardiovascular technologist.

An electrocardiograph (ECG) **technician** is an individual who records the ECG and prepares the report for the physician. ECG technicians should be able to determine if a tracing is accurate and recognize abnormalities caused by interference during the recording procedure. Most ECG technicians are employed in hospitals, but they may also work in medical offices, cardiac centers, cardiac rehabilitation centers, and other healthcare facilities. In some large hospitals, the ECG technician works in the home healthcare branch. He or she takes the ECG machine to the patient's home, records the ECG, and gives, sends, or telecommunicates the report to the physician for interpretation. With the development of multiple tests to evaluate the heart, the ECG technician who obtains continuing education can expect a rewarding career.

ECG monitor technicians view and evaluate the electrical tracings of patients' hearts on an oscilloscope (Figure 1-2). ECG monitor technicians are employed at hospitals or other inpatient facilities where patients are attached to continuous or **telemetry** monitors. The main responsibility of an ECG monitor technician is to view the ECG tracings and, if an abnormal heart rhythm occurs, alert the healthcare professional who can treat the abnormality. ECG monitor technicians are required to understand the various heart rhythms and recognize abnormal ones. ECG monitor technicians must be able to evaluate the ECG tracing. They may also be asked to perform other duties such as maintaining patient records and recording ECGs.

If you enjoy the field of electrocardiology and want to advance your skills or education, you may choose to be a cardiovascular **technologist**. Technologists require more extensive training than technicians. They may assist physicians with invasive cardiovascular diagnostic tests such as **angioplasty**, heart surgery, or implantation of electronic, **artificial pacemakers.** Another specialization for cardiovascular technologists is performing ultrasounds on the blood vessels. Ultrasound equipment transmits sound waves and then collects the echoes to form an image on a screen. As part of their duties, cardiovascular technologists may also perform ECGs.

cardiopulmonary resuscitation (CPR) To provide ventilations (breaths) and chest compressions (blood circulation) for a person who shows no signs of breathing or having a heartbeat.

technician An individual who has the knowledge and skills to carry out technical procedures.

telemetry The transmission of data electronically to an unattached or distant location.

technologist An individual who specializes in a field of science.

angioplasty Surgical repair of blood vessels.

pacemakers (artificial) A device that delivers a small, measured amount of electrical energy to cause myocardial depolarization. Most artificial pacemakers are electronic.

Figure 1-2 Multiple patients can be monitored on a single monitor screen. The patients being monitored may be in a hospital or at home depending upon the type of monitoring device they are using.

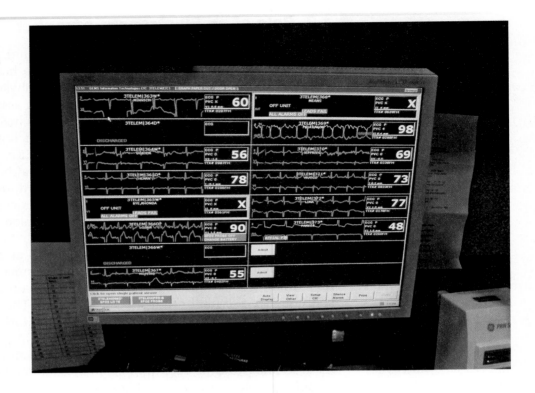

Checkpoint
Question
(LO 1.3)

1. An ECG technician's role includes the following:

_____

_____

1.4 How ECGs Are Used

healthcare providers
The scope of practice of each healthcare provider will determine the extent of the interpretation and treatment of each of the cardiac dysrhythmias or conditions. Each specific scope is determined by the licensure of each state. For example: Prescribing a medication is the responsibility of the physician. But some state practices allow nurse practitioners and physician assistants to prescribe medication under the guidance of the physician.

Healthcare providers, such as physicians, study the ECG tracing to determine many things about the patient's heart. They look for changes from the normal ECG tracing or from the first ECG tracing, which provides a baseline for comparison of subsequent ECGs performed. The American Heart Association recommends that individuals over the age of 40 have an ECG done annually as part of a complete physical. This baseline tracing assists the physician in diagnosing abnormalities of the heart. A sample of a normal tracing is shown in Figure 1-3. We discuss normal and abnormal ECG tracings in Chapter 2 and Chapter 5.

The ECG tracing is recorded using a variety of ECG machines and can be performed in a number of healthcare settings. These include acute care settings such as hospitals, ambulatory care settings such as clinics or doctors' offices, and even outside of a healthcare facility. Emergency personnel routinely perform ECGs during emergencies. An ECG tracing can also be transmitted over the telephone, mobile, or Internet from a person's home or other remote location. The type of ECG tracing produced depends upon the setting and the type of ECG machine used to record.

Figure 1-3 A normal ECG tracing is a horizontal line with upward and downward spikes or deflections that indicate electrical activity within the heart.

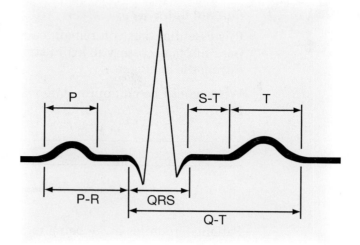

In the Hospital (Acute Care)

A 12-lead ECG is one of the most commonly used ECGs in the hospital setting. A 12-lead ECG provides a tracing of the electrical activity in the patient's heart at the exact time the ECG tracing is done. In the hospital, a 12-lead ECG is done as a routine procedure or during an emergency such as a **Code Blue.** An emergency ECG may be referred to as "stat," meaning immediately. These are done when a patient experiences chest pain or has a change in his or her cardiac rhythm. Routine ECGs are usually obtained in the early morning so they are available for the physician to review when he or she does patient rounds. Routine ECGs are also frequently done before surgery. Both routine or stat ECGs must be performed safely and with accuracy because these tracings will provide critical information about the patient. An inaccurate tracing could result in misdiagnosis, incorrect medications being administered, or other serious outcomes.

Code Blue Typically means that a patient is unresponsive and needs assistance immediately.

stat Immediately.

Another use of the ECG tracing in the hospital is in continuous monitoring. The purpose of continuous monitoring is to check the pattern of the electrical activity of the patient's heart over time. During continuous monitoring, electrodes are attached to the patient's chest and the tracing is viewed on an oscilloscope. Patients on continuous monitoring are usually in an *intensive care unit (ICU), coronary care unit or cardiac care unit (CCU), surgical intensive care unit (SICU),* or even an *emergency room (ER).* Some continuous monitors can also monitor the vital signs and the oxygen level in the blood. Continuous monitoring is also done routinely during surgery.

Another type of continuous monitoring done in a hospital is known as *telemetry monitoring.* Telemetry monitors are small boxes with electrodes and lead wires attached to the chest. The monitor is usually housed in a case and is attached to the patient so he or she can move about. The ECG tracing is transmitted to a central location for evaluation. When several patients are on a telemetry unit, the tracings of all the patients are recorded on multiple oscilloscopes at the nursing or patient care station.

New technology has allowed for evaluation and monitoring of patients and their rhythms from a remote location. This is being referred to as an *e-ICU.*

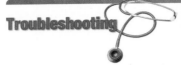

Troubleshooting

Remain Calm

It is essential that you remain calm when recording a stat ECG. Remaining calm is necessary to avoid stress to the patient and reduce confusion during the emergency.

What would be an appropriate way to tell a patient you are doing a stat ECG?

_____

_____

Patients are miles away being monitored by nurses for their heart rhythm and vital signs. This is in addition to the close monitoring done at the hospital.

Performing ECGs in Doctors' Offices and Ambulatory Care Clinics

A 12-lead ECG is a routine diagnostic test performed in almost any doctor's office or ambulatory care facility. It may be performed as part of a general or routine examination. This routine ECG provides a baseline tracing to be used for comparison if problems arise with a patient. The physician or trained expert looks for changes in a tracing that may indicate different types of health problems. Table 1-2 provides a complete list of conditions that may be diagnosed by an ECG. The procedure for performing a 12-lead ECG is discussed in Chapter 4.

Two other ECG-type tests that may be performed in an office include treadmill stress testing and the ambulatory monitor, or **Holter monitor**, testing (Figure 1-4 and Figure 1-5).

Holter monitor An instrument that records the electrical activity of the heart during a patient's normal daily activities; also known as an *ambulatory monitor*.

TABLE 1-2   Conditions Evaluated by the ECG

- Disorders in heart rate or rhythm and the conduction system
- Presence of electrolyte imbalance
- Condition of the heart prior to defibrillation
- Damage assessment during and after a myocardial infarction (heart attack)
- Symptoms related to cardiovascular disorders such as weakness, chest pain, or shortness of breath
- Diagnosis of certain drug toxicity
- Diagnosis of metabolic disorders such as hyper- or hypokalemia, hyper- or hypocalcemia, hyper- or hypothyroidism, acidosis, and alkalosis
- Heart condition prior to surgery for individuals at risk for undiagnosed or asymptomatic heart disease
- Damage assessment following blunt or penetrating chest trauma or changes after trauma or injury to the brain or spinal cord
- Assessment of the effects of cardiotoxic or antiarrhythmic therapy
- Suspicion of congenital heart disease
- Pacemaker function

Figure 1-4 This patient is performing a treadmill stress test, also known as exercise electrocardiography. During the exercise, the patient's heart, blood pressure, and oxygen use are being monitored.

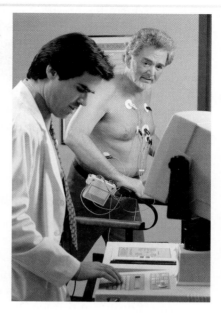

Figure 1-5 The Holter, or ambulatory, monitor allows the patient to participate in routine daily activities while the electrical activity of the heart is being recorded.

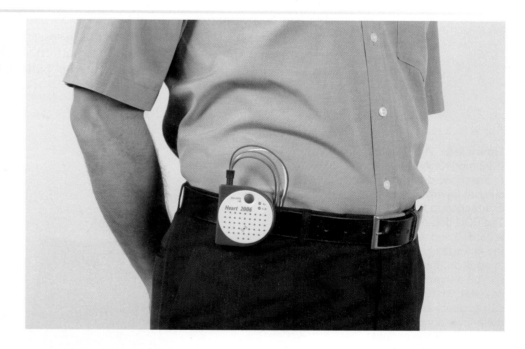

The treadmill stress test, also known as exercise electrocardiography, is done to determine if the heart gets adequate blood flow during stress or exercise. While the stress test is being performed, the patient is attached to an ECG monitor as he or she is walking on the treadmill. The speed of the treadmill can be varied to measure how this might "stress" the heart. The ECG tracing is recorded and analyzed for changes during the exercise. A physician should always be present during this procedure. The stress test is frequently ordered because it is a safe, noninvasive, inexpensive, and reliable method of measuring the heart's condition if a problem is suspected by the physician. We discuss the stress test in more detail in Chapter 6.

A Holter monitor is a small box that is strapped to a patient's waist or shoulder to monitor the heart for 24 to 48 hours or up to 30 days during a patient's normal daily activity. After the monitoring period, the patient returns to the office for the monitor to be removed. The ambulatory monitor is usually a small tape recorder or digital disc. When the recording is finished, it is examined with a special instrument called a scanner. The ECG tracing is then analyzed and interpreted by the physician. Some patients can connect these monitors to a computer where the information can be e-mailed to the physician. We discuss the ambulatory monitor in detail in Chapter 7.

Outside of a Healthcare Facility

Outside of a healthcare facility, the ECG is a valuable tool used during a cardiac emergency such as a myocardial infarction. Emergency medical technicians and paramedics are equipped with portable ECG machines that can produce an ECG tracing at the site of the emergency. Whether the patient is at home, in a car, or in a crowded football stadium, emergency personnel can monitor and trace the electrical activity of the heart. Figure 1-6 shows one example of a portable ECG machine. In an emergency setting, the tracing can be evaluated for an abnormal ECG pattern. It is either transmitted back to the physician for evaluation or assessed by the emergency medical personnel at the scene. An abnormal pattern, such as for sudden cardiac arrest, requires immediate treatment; the patient becomes unresponsive,

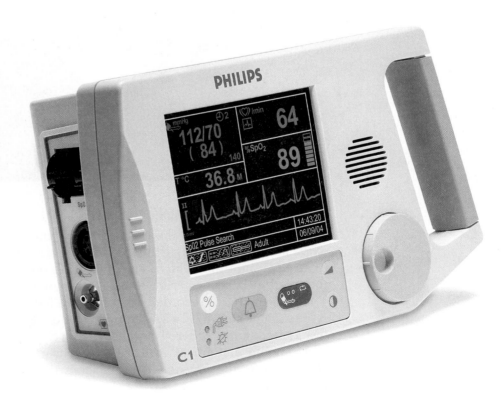

Figure 1-6 A portable ECG monitor is transported to the scene during a cardiac emergency and is attached to the patient. The ECG tracing is recorded and viewed by the emergency personnel. In addition, the tracing can be transmitted to the hospital, where a physician can evaluate and determine the necessary drugs and treatment for the patient based upon the heart rhythm viewed and the report from the emergency personnel.

which leads to death if not treated within minutes. Treatment for these abnormal rhythms includes use of a **defibrillator** and/or administration of cardiac medications. When the heart is in this chaotic rhythm of ventricular fibrillation or pulseless ventricular tachycardia, the heart must be "defibrillated" quickly. The survival rate of the victim decreases 7% to 10% for every minute a normal heartbeat is not restored. A defibrillator produces an electrical shock to the heart that is intended to correct the heart's electrical pattern. A defibrillator is commonly used in emergencies such as a Code Blue in the hospital or other care facilities or at the site of the emergency by appropriate personnel.

Automatic external defibrillators (**AEDs**) have enabled lay rescuers to help a patient with sudden cardiac arrest (Figure 1-7). AEDs are available in public and/or private places where large numbers of people gather or live or are kept by people who are at high risk for heart attacks. An AED is a lightweight, portable device that recognizes an abnormal rhythm and determines if the rhythm is considered a "shockable rhythm." The equipment is *only* placed on patients who are unresponsive (not able to be aroused) to stimulation and have no evidence of breathing or a pulse. AEDs will only shock the rhythms of ventricular fibrillation or ventricular tachycardia that do not produce a heartbeat. These rhythms are discussed in Chapter 5. When the machine recognizes other rhythms that cause the patient to be unresponsive, the AED recommends beginning CPR. Individuals using an AED should consider safety for themselves and the patient. A healthcare provider level CPR course is best for learning this technique. The patient should be checked for nitroglycerin patches, pacemakers, and metal objects that could cause burns. In addition, do not use an AED when the patient is in water.

Once the equipment is placed on the patient's bare chest, the machine will either automatically analyze or require the operator to push the "ANALYZE" button. The machine will analyze the rhythm to determine if it is a rhythm that is likely to respond to an electric shock through the chest to the heart. Once it has positively identified the abnormal rhythm, the machine will indicate that a "SHOCK IS ADVISED." All persons next to the patient

Figure 1-7 Automatic external defibrillators (AEDs) can reverse an abnormal heart rhythm and increase the survival rate of myocardial infarction victims. They can be found in public places and require minimal training to operate.

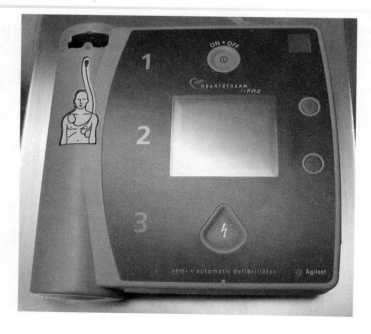

must move back and not touch the patient. One person will then announce "I'm clear, you're clear, we are all clear" and press the shock button. After the shock has been provided, the rescuers continue administering CPR until the patient wakes up, the machine indicates to defibrillate again, or specially trained healthcare professionals take over. These new machines now make it possible for laypersons to perform defibrillation safely. The AED is being viewed as a necessary piece of equipment—similar to a fire extinguisher.

Another use of the ECG tracing outside of a healthcare facility is through telemedicine. In telemedicine, ECG tracings are communicated to the physician via the telephone or digital system. *Transtelephonic monitoring* means transmitted (*trans*) over the telephone (*telephonic*). The improvements in solid-state digital technology have expanded transtelephonic transmission of ECG data and enhanced the accuracy of software-based analysis systems. Digital monitoring allows ECG data to be recorded with a personal computer and then transmitted over the Internet to the healthcare facility. Transtelephonic monitoring requires a licensed practitioner to read and evaluate the tracing, whereas the digital monitoring provides a report that is validated by the licensed practitioner.

Both of these types of monitoring evaluate the ECG tracing of a patient over time. The two types of ambulatory monitoring methods are useful for patients with symptoms of heart disease that did not occur while they were in the healthcare facility. The recorded monitoring can be accomplished with magnetic tape (transtelephonic) or digital (computerized) recordings that are used for up to 30 days. A transtelephonic monitor is placed on a telephone mouthpiece, and the ECG is transmitted to a healthcare facility on specific days throughout the monitoring period (Figure 1-8). Individuals using a transtelephonic monitor must understand when and how to record and send a transmission. A digital monitor requires the individual to be able to use a computer and understand how to send a transmission.

Figure 1-8 Transtelephonic monitoring uses a cellular phone device (circled) to transmit the patient's ECG tracing to a central location for monitoring.

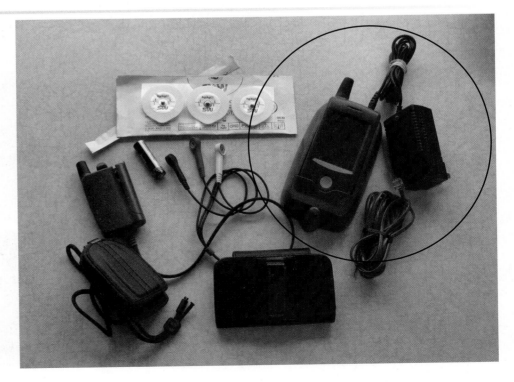

Depending upon which equipment your facility uses, you may be required to teach the patient how to use the monitor. Become familiar with the type of monitor used at your facility.

There are two specific types of telemedicine monitors. One monitors the heart continuously, and the other records the ECG tracing when the patient is having symptoms. Continuous telemedicine monitoring is programmed to record the ECG tracing constantly. It is useful to record the ECG tracing before, during, and after a patient has symptoms. These symptoms may include chest pain, shortness of breath, dizziness, or palpitations. This type of monitor is a small device that attaches to the patient's chest with two electrodes. The smallest monitor available is about the size and shape of a jump drive or a thin credit card.

Symptom-based telemedicine monitoring is in the form of either a handheld or a wristwatch device. The handheld type has electrode feet that are pressed against the patient's chest after symptoms occur. Currently, one type is as small as a credit card and can be carried in a pocket or wallet. The wristwatch type monitor is worn on the left arm at all times. The patient must turn on this type of monitor when symptoms begin.

Telemedicine monitoring is generally used to evaluate artificial pacemaker functioning. In addition, monitors are sometimes given to patients after an emergency room visit. If the patient has symptoms of cardiac problems but is not admitted to the hospital, a physician will often give the patient a monitor to record an ECG when the symptoms recur. It is less expensive to give patients a monitor to take home than to admit them to the hospital.

Checkpoint Questions (LO 1.4)

1. A 12-lead ECG can be obtained by an electrocardiographer in which healthcare venues?

_____

_____

2. An automatic external defibrillator (AED) is used to treat what conditions?

_____

_____

1.5 What You Need to Know to Perform an ECG

body mechanics Using movements that maintain proper posture and avoid muscle and bone injuries.

In order to perform an ECG, you should become familiar with the procedure and the ECG machine. You must have the ability to lift and move the patient, if necessary. This requires using proper **body mechanics** and getting assistance when needed. Body mechanics is using movements that maintain proper posture and avoid muscle and bone injuries (Table 1-3). You need to be able to transport and operate the ECG machine. In addition, you must understand basic principles of safety and infection control, patient education and professional communication, and law and ethics.

TABLE 1-3   Proper Body Mechanics

Movement	Your Action
Maintain a wide base of support	Keep your feet apart and at shoulder-width at all times.
Avoid twisting	Face the direction in which you intend to move.
Protect your back	Bend at your hips and knees, and keep your back straight at all times.
Use stronger and/or most muscles for lifting	Lift with your legs, not your back. Use both arms
Maintain body alignment	Keep your chin up and shoulders back, and avoid unnecessary reaching.

Equipment

Knowing how to use the equipment is part of performing an ECG. You must be able to transport, operate, maintain, and store the ECG equipment used at your facility. There are many different machines available to perform an ECG, and directions provided by the manufacturer are an important source of information. Many ECG machines have reference cards or instructions posted in a convenient place on or with the equipment. Refer to these printed materials when performing an ECG. Although all ECG machines are similar, you should become familiar with the particular machine you are using. You should always practice performing ECGs before using any machine on a patient. Since an ECG is noninvasive, you can practice on a volunteer, friend, co-worker, or fellow student. A procedure checklist like the one found at the end of Chapter 4 can be used for practice as well as to document your proficiency at the skill.

Safety

When performing healthcare procedures, you must always maintain the safety of yourself and the patient. General safety guidelines should be followed at all times. Certain safety precautions specific to performing the ECG procedure should also be followed. These specific precautions are discussed in more detail in Chapter 4.

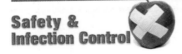

Safety & Infection Control

Guidelines

Follow safety and infection control guidelines at all times when working in a healthcare facility and performing an ECG.

Infection Control

standard precautions
Procedures, such as wearing gloves, used with all patients that are designed to prevent the spread of infection.

Preventing the spread of infection is an essential part of providing healthcare and performing an ECG. This is for your safety as well as the safety of your patients. The Centers for Disease Control and Prevention (CDC) have implemented two levels of precautions to prevent infections—**standard precautions** and **isolation precautions.**

Figure 1-9   *A*. Handwashing, especially between patients, is essential to prevent the spread of infection. *B*. The use of an alcohol-base rub on hands without visible soilage is an accepted technique for preventing infection.

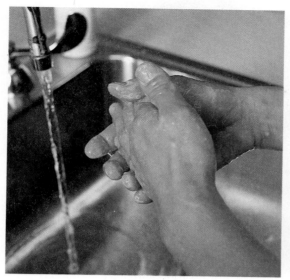

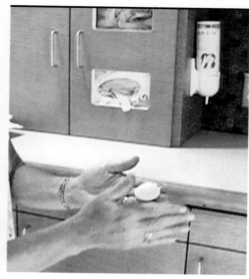

A.   B.

isolation precautions
Steps taken to prevent the spread of infection; some examples include separating the infected patient from others and using personal protective equipment.

Standard precautions include a combination of hand hygiene and wearing gloves when there is a possibility of exposure to blood and body fluids, nonintact skin, or mucous membranes (Figure 1-9). Standard precautions applies to blood, all body fluids, secretions, and excretions (except sweat), regardless of whether or not they contain visible blood, nonintact skin, and mucous membranes. Universal precautions, a subset of Standard Precautions, apply to blood and any other body fluids *only* if they contain visible blood. Standard precautions reduce the risk of transmission of microorganisms from both recognized and unrecognized sources of infection. In addition to hand hygiene and wearing gloves, practices may include the use of personal protective equipment (PPE) such as a gown, mask, and eye protection (Figure 1-10). In addition, the CDC advises that healthcare workers should not wear artificial nails, as those workers are more likely to harbor gram-negative pathogens on their fingertips than are those with natural nails, both before and after handwashing. Natural nails should be no more than one-fourth inch long.

The second level includes *isolation precautions,* which are based on how the infectious agent is transmitted. Isolation precautions are

1. airborne precautions that require special air handling, ventilation, and additional respiratory protection (HEPA or N95 respirators);
2. droplet precautions requiring mucous membrane protection (goggles and masks); and
3. contact precautions requiring gloves and gowns for direct skin-to-skin contact or for contact with contaminated linen, equipment, and so on.

Standard precautions are practiced in all employment situations in which exposure to blood or body fluids is likely. Isolation precautions are used less often and only with patients who have specific infections. When isolation precautions are in place for a patient during an ECG, you will be required to follow the specific guidelines for the type of precautions

Figure 1-10 Personal protection equipment (PPE) is used to reduce the risk of transmission of infection. PPE includes items such as gloves, mask, gown, and eye protection.

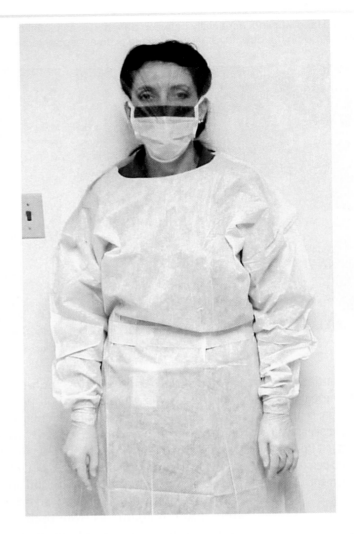

implemented. Table 1-4 provides a list of standard precautions that should be practiced when recording an ECG. See Appendix B for additional information about standard and isolation precautions.

Patient Education and Communication

Communicating with your patients is key to successfully recording an ECG. You must develop a positive relationship and atmosphere to reduce apprehension and anxiety during an ECG. You can reduce the patient's fears and make the ECG a positive experience by developing a helpful relationship with your patient and practicing effective communication techniques. Clearly explaining the procedure and answering questions are essential for good patient communication. Maintain a friendly, confident manner while interacting with your patient. Your patient will be more cooperative if he or she trusts that you are competent to perform your job.

Helping the patient understand the procedure and follow instructions is essential to performing any ECG procedure. When explaining the procedure, use simple terms and speak slowly and distinctly. Encourage the patient to ask questions and repeat the instructions. This process will help ensure patient understanding.

TABLE 1-4 Standard Precautions Related to Electrocardiography

Hand Hygiene

- Wash your hands after touching blood, body fluids, secretions, excretions, and contaminated items.
- Wash your hands before putting on gloves and after removing gloves.
- Wash your hands between patient contacts.
- Wash your hands between tasks and procedures on the same person.
- Use alcohol-based hand rub if you have no visible soilage.

Gloves

- Wear gloves when touching blood, body fluids, secretions, excretions, and contaminated items.
- Wear gloves when touching mucous membranes and nonintact skin.
- Change gloves between procedures and patients.
- Change gloves after contacting materials that are highly contaminated.
- Remove gloves promptly after use.
- Remove gloves before touching uncontaminated surfaces or items.
- Wash your hands immediately after glove removal.

Masks, Eye Protection, and Face Shields

- Masks, eye protection, and face shields protect the mucous membranes of the mouth, eyes, and nose from splashes and sprays.
- Wear mask, eye protection, and face shields during procedures and tasks that are likely to cause splashes or sprays of blood, body fluids, secretions, and excretions.

Gowns

- Gowns protect the skin and clothing.
- Wear a gown during procedures and activities that are likely to cause splashes or sprays of blood, body fluids, secretions, or excretions.
- Remove a soiled gown promptly.
- Wash your hands immediately after gown removal.

Equipment

- Equipment may be soiled with blood, body fluids, secretions, and excretions.
- Handle used equipment carefully.
- Prevent skin and mucous membrane exposure and clothing contamination.
- Reusable equipment must be cleaned, disinfected, or sterilized before it is used on another person.
- Discard single-use equipment promptly.

Environmental Control

- Follow facility procedures for the routine care, cleaning, and disinfection of surfaces. This includes environmental surfaces, nonmovable equipment, and other frequently touched surfaces.

Occupational Health and Bloodborne Pathogens

- Use resuscitation devices for mouth-to-barrier resuscitation.

In addition, in your role as a healthcare professional, you will need to be able to work in a variety of situations as a team member and be able to resolve conflicts. As with any job, you should continue to improve in your performance through further education and practice.

Hand Hygiene

Proper hand hygiene is the single most important thing you can do to prevent the spread of infection. Handwashing or the use of an alcohol-based rub on hands without visible soilage should be practiced between patients and procedures and before and after the use of gloves. **Note:** Certain types of infections, such as *Clostridium difficile,* require handwashing because the use of alcohol-based hand rubs is not sufficient to kill all the infectious organisms. Always use the method of hand hygiene that is most appropriate for the condition of the patient.

Legal and Ethical Issues

As a healthcare professional, you must understand some legal and ethical considerations of patient care. Laws are rules of conduct that are enforced by a controlling authority such as the government. An unlawful act can result in loss of your job, a fine, or other penalty such as time in jail. Ethics are concerned with standards of behavior and concepts of right and wrong. They are based upon moral values that are formed through the influence of the family, culture, and society. Unethical acts result in poor job evaluations or job loss. When comparing law and ethics, you should understand that illegal acts are always unethical but unethical acts are not always illegal.

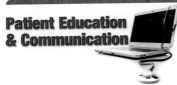

Improving Communication

When speaking to a patient who is hard of hearing, look directly at the patient and speak slowly and distinctly. The patient may be able to read your lips. When your patient speaks another language, you may want to ask an interpreter or family member to assist you with communication, thus reducing apprehension and anxiety.

Protecting Patient Information: HIPAA

Patient information has always been considered to be confidential or private. In 1996, the Health Insurance Portability and Accountability Act (HIPAA) was established in response to information that was being transferred electronically for medical transactions. This act establishes a national standard for electronic healthcare transactions and also for providers, health plans, and employers. It was to ensure that the widespread use of electronic data was limited and secured. The patient can specify who is able to see information and what information is protected. A patient's information can only be sent and viewed when specific to insurance payments and further medical treatment with a consulting healthcare professional. A patient's information cannot be shared among healthcare professionals unless it is for the patient's treatment.

Practicing Ethics

Many professions have a code of ethics. These are standards of behavior or conduct as defined by the professional group. As a healthcare professional, you must follow the standards of behavior or code of ethics set forth by your profession and place of employment. The following are some basic ethics you should practice.

Confidentiality is an essential part of patient care. You may collect information about a patient for use during his or her care and treatment; however, this information should not be made public. Confidentiality is a basic right of every patient. You should not speak about your patient or allow information about your patient to be heard or seen by anyone other than those caring for them. A breach in confidentiality is unethical, illegal, and a violation of HIPAA.

Patients should be treated with respect and dignity. You should respect the privacy of patients at all times. Avoid exposing your patient's body when performing any procedure by closing the door, pulling the curtain, and/or draping the patient. In some cases, it may be necessary for a male healthcare professional to have a third person present when performing an ECG on a female. Check the policies at the facility where you are employed.

Practicing ethics also includes professionalism, respect, and cooperation. You should maintain professionalism by continuing your education training in order to provide the highest level of care for your patients. You should respect your patients' beliefs, values, and morals; and you should work cooperatively with your co-workers and supervisors at all times.

Legal Issues You Should Know

Medical professional liability means that a healthcare professional is legally responsible for his or her performance. Healthcare professionals can be held accountable for performing unlawful acts, performing legal acts improperly, or simply failing to perform an act when they should. For example, if you find a patient's wallet after he or she leaves and you decide to keep it, this is an illegal act. While you are assisting with a treadmill stress test, if you report the blood pressure results incorrectly, resulting in the patient having a severe heart attack, this is performing a legal act improperly. If you decide to take a break when you are supposed to be monitoring a patient's heart rhythm and during the time you are gone the patient experiences an abnormal heart rhythm resulting in death from lack of prompt treatment, you have failed to perform your duties as required.

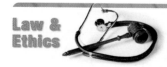

Law & Ethics

Keep Information Private

The patient's chart or computer screen with patient data should not be left out or open in an area where other patients or visitors may be able to view it. This is a breach of confidentiality and HIPAA.

You will be speaking and writing about patients as part of your job as an electrocardiographer. You should never speak defamatory words about patients even when they upset you. Making derogatory remarks about a

TABLE 1-5   Required Entries for Medical Records Related to ECG

- Patient identification, including full name, social security number, birth date, full address and telephone number, marital status, and place of employment, if applicable
- Patient's medical history
- Dates and times of all appointments, admissions, discharge, and diagnostic tests (such as an ECG)
- Diagnostic test results
- Information regarding symptoms and reason for appointment, diagnostic test, or admission
- Physician examinations and record of results, including patient instructions
- Medications and prescriptions given, including refills
- Documentation of informed consent when required
- Legal guardian or representative, if patient is unable to give informed consent

patient—or anyone else—that jeopardizes his or her reputation or means of livelihood is called *slander.* Slander is an illegal and unethical act that could cause you to lose your job. If you write defamatory words, this is known as *libel,* which is also illegal and unethical.

Medical care and treatment must be documented as part of the medical record. The medical record can be used in court as evidence in a medical professional liability case. To protect yourself legally and provide continuity of patient care, you should include complete information in the medical record. Table 1-5 contains a complete list of the necessary information to document on the medical record.

Whatever ECG procedure you are performing, the patient must agree or consent to having the procedure done. Implied consent is between the patient and healthcare professional, such as a physician in an office. For example, when a patient requests care and comes to the physician's office, he or she is agreeing to be treated by the physician. This is *implied* consent. When a patient agrees to the ECG procedure, this is also implied consent.

Certain diagnostic procedures, including a treadmill stress test, require *informed* consent. The patient must understand the procedure and its associated risks, alternative procedures and their risks, and the potential risks to the patient if he or she refuses treatment. Informed consent requires the patient to sign a consent form.

Checkpoint Question (LO 1.5)

1. What measures would you use to prevent the spread of infection to you and your patients?

_____

_____

1.6 Troubleshooting

Being able to troubleshoot situations that arise during the ECG procedure is essential. Troubleshooting requires critical thinking. Critical thinking is the process of thinking through the situation or problem and making a decision to solve it. The problem-solving process includes the following steps:

1. Identify and define the problem.
2. Identify possible solutions.
3. Select the best solution.
4. Implement the selected solution.
5. Evaluate the results.

When caring for patients and recording an ECG, you may experience a variety of problems. These problems may stem from the patient's condition, patient communication, equipment failure, or other complications. While performing an ECG, you may need to troubleshoot actual or potential complications during the procedure using the steps of the problem-solving process.

Let us say that you are about to perform an ECG, and the patient refuses to let you attach the lead wires. As part of troubleshooting, you ask the patient why he or she is refusing. The patient states, "I do not want that electricity going through me!" In a calm manner, you explain that the machine does not produce or generate electricity, and it is not harmful. After your explanation, the patient agrees to have the ECG. You have performed successful troubleshooting. This example, as you can see, is a problem with communication, however, other problems can occur with the equipment or tracing produced and troubleshooting will be necessary. Throughout this text the Troubleshooting Boxes will provide a variety of problems or situations you may encounter and then ask for your solution. Use your critical thinking and problem-solving skills to answer each question. In each chapter, review the "What Should You Do?" questions to check your ability to think critically and troubleshoot.

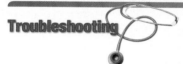

Consent

When a patient who cannot read or write is required to sign a consent form, you will need to explain the procedure to a family member and have that person sign and the patient sign unless he or she has been determined to be incompetent. If this is not possible, explain the procedure to the patient with a witness present and have the witness sign, along with having the patient place an *X* on the form.

Who should sign the consent form if a patient cannot read or write?

_____

_____

Checkpoint Question (LO 1.6)

1. Explain how you would employ the steps of the problem-solving process if a patient refuses to have an ECG.

_____

_____

Chapter Summary

Learning Outcomes	Summary	Pages
1.1 Explain what an ECG is and its importance in medicine.	An ECG is the tracing of the heart's electrical activity using an electrocardiograph. It is used to diagnosis cardiovascular disease, which is the number one cause of death in America.	2-3
1.2 Discuss the history of obtaining and using the ECG.	The heart's electricity was discovered as early as 1676. In 1903, Wilhelm Einthoven is credited with developing the first electrocardiograph and introducing the field of electrocardiography.	4
1.3 Describe career opportunities for an electrocardiographer.	Careers in electrocardiography are expanding and include such careers as ECG technician, ECG monitor technician, and cardiovascular technologist.	5-6
1.4 Compare the uses of the ECG in the hospital, in the doctor's office or ambulatory clinic, and outside of a healthcare facility.	The ECG is used routinely in the hospital before surgery, during emergencies, and as part of continuous monitoring. In a clinic, an ECG is part of an exam or is used during a treadmill stress test or Holter monitoring. Outside the healthcare facility, the ECG is used for evaluation during emergencies.	6-13
1.5 Identify the skills and knowledge needed to perform an ECG.	To perform an ECG you should know the procedure and equipment and have the ability to communicate and to lift and move patients.	13-20
1.6 Define troubleshooting, and explain its importance to you as a healthcare professional.	Troubleshooting is the process of critical thinking or thinking through the situation, then making a decision to try to solve it. Troubleshooting is a necessary part of performing ECGs.	20-21

Chapter Review

Matching

Match these terms with the correct definition. Place the appropriate letter on the line to the left of each term.

_____ 1. cardiovascular (LO 1.1)

_____ 2. electrocardiogram (LO 1.1)

_____ 3. arrhythmia (LO 1.2)

_____ 4. electrocardiology (LO 1.1)

_____ 5. electrocardiograph (LO 1.1)

_____ 6. defibrillator (LO 1.3)

_____ 7. AED (LO 1.3)

a. an instrument used to record the electrical activity of the heart

b. a tracing of the signal produced by the heart's electrical activity and used for diagnostic evaluation of the heart

c. the study of the heart's electrical activity

d. abnormal or absence of normal heartbeat, also known as dysrhythmia

e. used to analyze the heart rhythm and produce a shock if necessary

f. related to the heart and blood vessels (veins and arteries)

g. a machine that produces and sends an electrical shock to the heart that is intended to correct the abnormal electrical pattern of the heart

True/False

Read each statement and determine if it is true or false. Circle the T or F. For false (F) statements, correct them on the line provided to "make them true."

T   F   8. An ECG machine produces and records the electrical activity of the heart. (LO 1.1)

_____

T   F   9. Standard precautions are guidelines written for healthcare providers to help prevent the spread of infection. (LO 1.5)

_____

T   F   10. When performing an ECG, you should know the equipment, infection control principles, communication techniques, and safety guidelines. (LO 1.5)

_____

T   F   11. A transtelephonic monitor transmits an ECG over the Internet. (LO 1.4)

_____

Multiple Choice

Circle the correct answer.

12. Which of the following is a reason that an ECG is performed? (LO 1.4)
    a. To determine if the electrolyte balance is normal.
    b. To determine pacemaker function.
    c. To determine cardiac output.
    d. To predict the possibility of an MI.

13. Which physician invented an instrument to detect electrograph waves? (LO 1.2)
    a. Sir Thomas Lewis
    b. William Einthoven
    c. Augustus Walker
    d. Joseph Electrocardiograph

14. The first ECG machine was developed in _____ by _____. (LO 1.2) He won the Nobel Prize for this invention.
    a. 1903, Wilhelm Einthoven
    b. 1918, James B. Herrick
    c. 1876, Augustus D. Waller
    d. 1945, Sir Thomas Lewis

15. The main responsibility of an ECG monitor technician is to (LO 1.3)
    a. Determine whether an abnormal heart rhythm occurs.
    b. View the ECG tracing.
    c. Alert the healthcare professional.
    d. All of the above.

16. Which of the following is *not* a reason for performing an ECG? (LO 1.4)
    a. To evaluate heart conditions
    b. To check for problems with the flow of electricity through the heart
    c. To see how well the heart is contracting and pumping
    d. To evaluate the rate and rhythm of breathing

17. A defibrillator can be used (LO 1.1)
    a. to treat an abnormal heart rhythm.
    b. without training.
    c. to produce an electrical rhythm.
    d. to record only ECG rhythms.

18. Transtelephonic monitoring allows for information to be (LO 1.4)
    a. reviewed immediately by a physician.
    b. transmitted over a telephone.
    c. submitted for billing purposes only.
    d. recorded by a computerized device.

19. A continuous ECG monitor is used most commonly in a(n) (LO 1.4)
    a. physician's office.
    b. hospital.
    c. assisted-living center.
    d. clinic.

20. Which of the following is most commonly performed in a clinic or hospital? (LO 1.4)
- **a.** Transtelephonic monitoring
- **b.** Ambulatory monitoring
- **c.** 12-lead ECG
- **d.** Defibrillation

21. To write derogatory words about a patient is known as (LO 1.5)
- **a.** slander.
- **b.** libel.
- **c.** ethical.
- **d.** unethical.

22. Your most important duties include monitoring an ECG tracing and notifying the physician of abnormalities. You are most likely a(n) (LO 1.5)
- **a.** ECG monitoring technician.
- **b.** cardiovascular technologist.
- **c.** ECG technician or medical assistant.
- **d.** physician's assistant.

23. Which of the following measures help ensure that your patients' information is protected? (LO 1.5)
- **a.** Standard precautions
- **b.** Isolation procedures
- **c.** Patient precautions
- **d.** HIPAA

24. _____ is the key to successful recording of an ECG. (LO 1.5)
- **a.** Hand hygiene
- **b.** Communication
- **c.** Patient education
- **d.** HIPAA

25. What is the single most important procedure you can perform to prevent the spread of infection? (LO 1.5)
- **a.** Use of standard precautions
- **b.** Hand hygiene
- **c.** Patient education
- **d.** Communication

26. When speaking to a person who is hard of hearing, it is important that you (LO 1.5)
- **a.** look directly at the patient.
- **b.** speak slowly and distinctly.
- **c.** speak into the hearing aid if the patient has one.
- **d.** all of the above.

27. When caring for patients and recording an ECG, you may encounter many situations that require you to (LO 1.5)
- **a.** critically think about the situation.
- **b.** always follow the same steps each time.
- **c.** not worry about what the patient tells you.
- **d.** not prepare for what may possibly be asked of you during the procedure.

Critical Thinking Application *What Should You Do?*

Read the following situations and use critical thinking skills to determine how you would handle each. Write your answer in detail in the space provided.

28. You have been performing ECGs at a local clinic for about six months. Your favorite uncle says to you, "Since I just turned 40, your Aunt Beth thinks I should have an ECG. Will you do one on me if I come by where you work?" What would you say or do for your uncle? Consider the following: (LO 1.6)

    Should your uncle have an ECG? _____

    Should you do the ECG if he stops by your office? Why or why not? _____

    _____

    _____

    _____

29. Mr. Smith has been having some mild chest pain. During his ECG, he says, "How does it look? Is there anything wrong?" What would be your best response? (LO 1.6)

    _____

    _____

    _____

30. You walk by a room where a co-worker is performing an ECG on a female patient. The door is open, and the patient is not covered. What would you do? (LO 1.6)

    _____

    _____

    _____

31. You are responsible for monitoring the heart rhythms on six patients at a local hospital when you begin to feel ill. You are in desperate need to go to the restroom, and you really want to go home. What should you do? (LO 1.6)

    _____

    _____

    _____

    _____

Get Connected *Internet Activity*

Visit the McGraw-Hill Higher Education Online Learning Center *Electrocardiography for Healthcare Professionals* Web site at **www.mhhe.com/boothecg3e** to complete the following activities.

1. History of the ECG. If you would like to learn more about the history of the ECG, visit the ECG Library: A brief history of electrocardiography.
2. Career Exploration. If you would like to obtain more information about a career as a cardiovascular technologist or technician, visit the Bureau of Labor Statistics Occupational Outlook Handbook.

3. **Automatic External Defibrillators.** To learn more about automatic external defibrillators, visit the American Heart Association's Web site and search for the keyword *AED* or *automatic external defibrillator.*

4. **Risk Factors.** Go to the American Heart Association's Web site. Identify at least five cardiovascular facts related to a specific cultural group and/or identify five risk factors for cardiovascular disease and what can be done to reduce the risk of disease for males or females.

 ## Using the Student CD

Now that your have completed the material in the chapter text, return to the student CD and complete any chapter activities you have not yet done. Practice your terminology with the "Key Term Concentration" game. Review the chapter material with the "Challenge" and "Spin the Wheel" games. Take the final chapter test; complete the troubleshooting question, and email or print your results to document your proficiency for this chapter.

2 The Cardiovascular System

Chapter Outline

- Circulation and the ECG (p. 29)
- Anatomy of the Heart (p. 29)
- Principles of Circulation (p. 33)
- The Cardiac Cycle (p. 36)
- Conduction System of the Heart (p. 38)
- Electrical Stimulation and the ECG Waveform (p. 41)

Learning Outcomes

2.1 Describe circulation as it relates to the ECG.

2.2 Recall the structures of the heart, including valves, chambers, and vessels.

2.3 Differentiate between pulmonary, systemic, and coronary circulation.

2.4 Explain the cardiac cycle, and relate the difference between systole and diastole.

2.5a Describe the parts and function of the conduction system.

2.5b Recall the unique qualities of the heart and their relationship to the cardiac conduction system.

2.5c Explain the conduction system as it relates to the ECG.

2.6a Identify each part of the ECG waveform.

2.6b Describe the heart activity that produces the ECG waveform.

Key Terms

action potential
aorta
aortic semilunar valve
atrioventricular (AV) node
atrium (pl. atria)
automaticity
bundle branches
bundle of His (AV bundle)
cardiac cycle
complexes
conductivity
contractility

coronary circulation
deoxygenated blood
depolarization
diastole
excitability
interval
interventricular septum
ischemia
left atrium
left ventricle
mitral (bicuspid) valve
myocardial

oxygenated blood
pericardium
polarization
pulmonary artery
pulmonary circulation
pulmonary semilunar valve
pulmonary vein
Purkinje fibers
Purkinje network
repolarization

right atrium
right ventricle
segment
semilunar valve
sinoatrial (SA) node
systemic circulation
systole
tricuspid valve
vena cava (pl. venae cavae)

2.1 Circulation and the ECG

The function of the heart is to pump blood to and from all the tissues of the body. Blood supplies the tissues with nutrients and oxygen and removes carbon dioxide and waste products. The process of transporting blood to and from the body tissues is known as circulation. The heart's powerful muscular pump performs the task of circulation. Circulation of the blood is dependent upon the heart and its ability to contract or beat. Each electrical activity of the heart is recorded on the ECG. Knowledge of the heart, its functions, and what produces the ECG tracing will provide you with a clear understanding of the tasks you will be performing as an ECG healthcare professional.

Checkpoint Questions (LO 2.1)

1. What is circulation?

    _____

    _____

2. What is recorded on the ECG strip?

    _____

    _____

2.2 Anatomy of the Heart

The heart lies near the center of the chest, under the sternum, and in between the lungs. Two-thirds of it lies to the left of the sternum. The heart varies in size and weight depending upon a person's weight, physical condition, and gender. The average heart is approximately the size of your fist and weighs about 10.6 ounces or 300 grams (Figure 2-1).

The heart is a powerful muscular pump that beats an average of 72 times per minute, 100,000 times per day, and 22.5 billion times in the average lifetime. The heart pumps about 140 mL of blood per beat, for a total output of 5 liters per minute. Each day the heart pumps approximately 7250 liters or 1800 gallons of blood. This is enough to fill an average size bathtub about 36 times.

The entire heart is enclosed in a sac of tissue called the **pericardium.** This sac consists of two layers: the tough, outer layer is called the parietal

pericardium A two-layered sac of tissue enclosing the heart.

Figure 2-1 The heart is tipped to the left side of the body with about two-thirds of it is located on the left side of the chest.

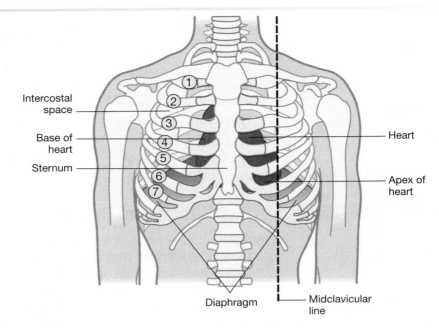

Intercostal space

Base of heart

Sternum

Heart

Apex of heart

Diaphragm

Midclavicular line

layer, and the inner layer is called the visceral layer. The visceral pericardium adheres closely to the heart. It is also referred to as the epicardium, the outermost layer of the heart. The purpose of the pericardium is to protect the heart from infection and trauma. The space between the two layers is called the pericardial space. It contains about 10 to 20 mL (about ½ ounce) of fluid, which serves to cushion the heart against blows and decreases friction between the layers created by the pumping heart.

The heart consists of three layers: the endocardium, the myocardium, and the epicardium (or visceral pericardium). The epicardium, the outermost layer, is thin and contains the coronary arteries. The myocardium is the middle muscular layer that contracts the heart. The endocardium is the innermost layer, which lines the inner surfaces of the heart chambers and the valves. The Purkinje fibers are located just below this innermost layer (Table 2-1 and Figure 2-2).

TABLE 2-1 Heart Layers

Layer	Location and Function
Endocardium	Inner layer of the heart that lines the chambers and valves. The Purkinje fibers are located just below this layer.
Myocardium	Middle, thickest muscular layer, responsible for heart contraction
Epicardium (also called the visceral pericardium)	Outside, thin layer of the heart that contains the coronary arteries; it is also known as the inner layer of the pericardium
Pericardium (made up of the visceral pericardium and the parietal pericardium)	A double-layer sac that encloses the heart. The inner layer, or visceral pericardium, is also called the epicardium; the outer layer is the parietal pericardium.

Figure 2-2 Three distinct layers can be identified on the heart. A sac called the pericardium protects it.

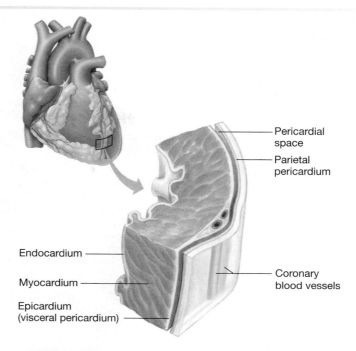

Pericardial space
Parietal pericardium
Endocardium
Myocardium
Epicardium (visceral pericardium)
Coronary blood vessels

right atrium The right upper chamber of the heart, which receives blood from the body.

left atrium The left upper chamber of the heart, which receives blood from the lungs.

right ventricle The right lower chamber of the heart, which pumps deoxygenated blood to the lungs.

left ventricle The left lower chamber of the heart, which pumps oxygenated blood through the body. It is the biggest and strongest chamber, known as the workhorse of the heart.

interventricular septum A partition or wall (septum) that divides the right and left ventricles.

tricuspid valve Valve located between the right atrium and right ventricle; it prevents backflow of blood into the right atrium.

mitral (bicuspid) valve Valve with two cusps or leaflets located between the left atrium and left ventricle; it prevents backflow of blood into the left atrium.

pulmonary artery Large artery that transports deoxygenated blood from the right ventricle to the lungs. This is the only artery in the body that carries deoxygenated blood.

aorta The largest artery of the body, which transports oxygenated blood from the left ventricle of the heart to the entire body.

Chambers and Valves

The heart is divided into four chambers. The top chambers are the **right atrium** and **left atrium**. The bottom chambers are the **right ventricle** and **left ventricle**.

Between the right and left ventricles is a partition known as the **interventricular septum**. The myocardium varies in thickness between chambers. It is thin in the atria, thick in the right ventricle, and thickest in the left ventricle. The thicker the myocardium of a chamber is, the stronger the muscular contraction of that chamber. The left ventricle is sometimes known as the "workhorse of the heart" because of its thick myocardium and powerful muscular contraction.

Between the right atrium and right ventricle is the **tricuspid valve**. Between the left atrium and left ventricle is the **mitral (bicuspid) valve**. These two valves are known as atrioventricular (AV) valves because they divide the atria from the ventricles. The **pulmonary artery** and the **aorta** each have a **semilunar valve**. They are called semilunar because the valve flaps look like a half (*semi*) moon (*lunar*). These valves are called the **aortic semilunar valve** and the **pulmonary semilunar valve** (Table 2-2 and Figure 2-3). The semilunar valves separate the ventricles from the arteries leading to the lungs or body.

TABLE 2-2 Heart Valves and Their Locations

Name	Valve Type	Location
Aortic	Semilunar	Between left ventricle and aorta
Pulmonary	Semilunar	Between right ventricle and pulmonary artery
Tricuspid	Atrioventricular	Separates right atrium and right ventricle
Mitral (bicuspid)	Atrioventricular	Separates left atrium and left ventricle

Figure 2-3 Heart chambers, valves, and vessels.

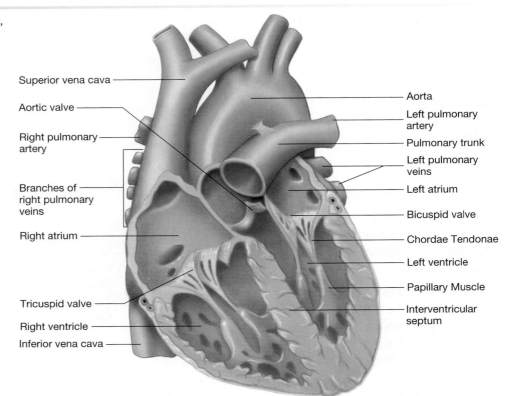

Superior vena cava

Aortic valve

Right pulmonary artery

Branches of right pulmonary veins

Right atrium

Tricuspid valve

Right ventricle

Inferior vena cava

Aorta

Left pulmonary artery

Pulmonary trunk

Left pulmonary veins

Left atrium

Bicuspid valve

Chordae Tendonae

Left ventricle

Papillary Muscle

Interventricular septum

semilunar valve A valve with half-moon-shaped cusps that open and close, allowing blood to travel only one way; located in the pulmonary artery and the aorta.

aortic semilunar valve Valve located in the aorta that prevents the backflow of blood into the left ventricle.

pulmonary semilunar valve A valve found in the pulmonary artery that prevents backflow of blood into the right ventricle.

atrium Top two chambers of the heart.

The one-way valves in the heart keep the blood flow headed in the right direction. The flaps or "cusps" open to allow the blood to flow then close to prevent the backflow of blood. The mitral and tricuspid valves separate the atria and ventricles and prevent the blood from flowing back from the ventricles to the **atrium** (pl. atria). The semilunar valves in the pulmonary artery and the aorta prevent the backflow of blood into the ventricles (Figure 2-4). When the AV valves are open, the semilunar valves are closed; and when the semilunar valves are open, the AV valves are closed.

Figure 2-4 Valves viewed from a cross section of the heart.

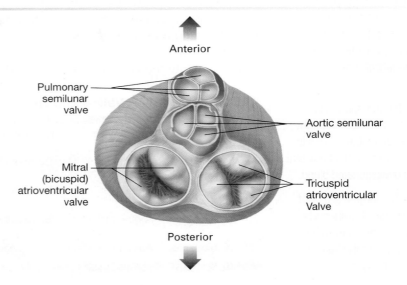

Anterior

Pulmonary semilunar valve

Mitral (bicuspid) atrioventricular valve

Aortic semilunar valve

Tricuspid atrioventricular Valve

Posterior

vena cava Largest vein in the body, which provides a pathway for deoxygenated blood to return to the heart; its upper portion, the superior vena cava, transports blood from the head, arms, and upper body; and its lower portion, the inferior vena cava, transports blood from the lower body and legs.

deoxygenated blood Blood that has little or minimal oxygen (oxygen-poor blood).

pulmonary veins Transports oxygenated blood back into the left atrium of the heart. These are the only veins that carry oxygenated blood.

The Major Vessels of the Heart

Blood vessels are the veins and arteries that transport blood all over the body. The major blood vessels that transport blood to and from the heart are the venae cavae, pulmonary artery, pulmonary veins, and the aorta.

Blood travels from the body tissue through the veins toward the heart. The blood is returned through the largest veins of the body, the **vena cava** (pl. venae cavae), to the right atrium. The superior vena cava transports blood from the head, arms, and upper body. The inferior vena cava transports blood from the lower body and legs.

When the heart contracts, the right ventricle pumps **deoxygenated blood** (blood that has little or minimal oxygen) to the lungs via the pulmonary artery. In the lungs, the exchange of carbon dioxide and oxygen occurs to enrich the blood with oxygen. The **pulmonary veins** transport **oxygenated blood** (blood containing oxygen) back to the heart into the left atrium. Transporting blood to the entire body is the function of the aorta. When the left ventricle contracts, the blood is pumped into the aorta. The first vessels to branch off the aorta are the coronary arteries. Coronary arteries are part of the **coronary circulation,** which supplies blood to the muscular heart pump (Figure 2-5).

Checkpoint Questions (LO 2.2)

1. What is the name of the middle layer of the heart (the muscular layer)?

   _____

   _____

2. Which valve is located between the left atrium and left ventricle?

   _____

   _____

---

oxygenated blood Blood having oxygen (oxygen-rich blood).

coronary circulation The circulation of blood to and from the heart muscle.

pulmonary circulation The transportation of blood to and from the lungs; blood is oxygenated in the lungs during pulmonary circulation.

systemic circulation The pathways for pumping blood throughout the body and back to the heart.

2.3 Principles of Circulation

The heart is actually a two-sided pump. The left side of the heart is a high-pressure pump that pumps oxygenated blood to the body tissue. The right side of the heart is a low-pressure pump that pumps deoxygenated blood to the lungs. Think of the heart like this:

left side → high pressure → oxygen

right side → low pressure → no oxygen

The pathways for pumping blood to and from the lungs are known as **pulmonary circulation.** The pathways for pumping blood throughout the body and back to the heart are known as **systemic circulation.** The circulation of blood to and from the heart muscle is known as **coronary circulation.**

Pulmonary Circulation: The Heart and Lung Connection

Deoxygenated blood enters the right atrium through the superior and inferior venae cavae. Blood travels through the tricuspid valve into the right ventricle. The right ventricle pumps the blood through the pulmonary

Figure 2-5 Pathways for blood through the heart.

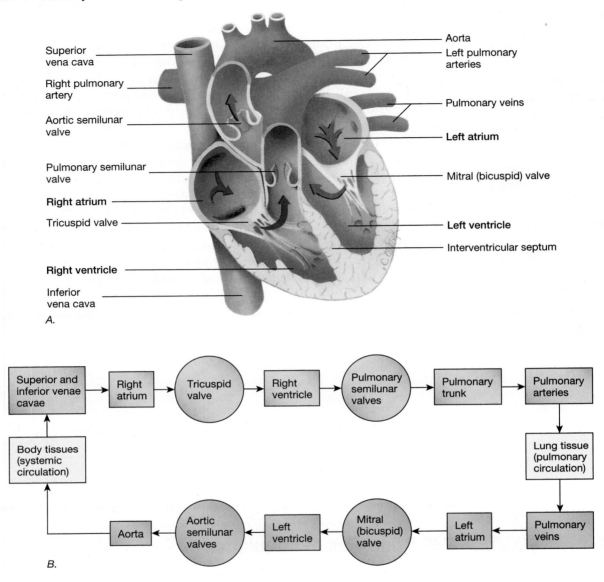

A.

Superior vena cava
Right pulmonary artery
Aortic semilunar valve
Pulmonary semilunar valve
Right atrium
Tricuspid valve
Right ventricle
Inferior vena cava

Aorta
Left pulmonary arteries
Pulmonary veins
Left atrium
Mitral (bicuspid) valve
Left ventricle
Interventricular septum

B.

Superior and inferior venae cavae → Right atrium → Tricuspid valve → Right ventricle → Pulmonary semilunar valves → Pulmonary trunk → Pulmonary arteries → Lung tissue (pulmonary circulation) → Pulmonary veins → Left atrium → Mitral (bicuspid) valve → Left ventricle → Aortic semilunar valves → Aorta → Body tissues (systemic circulation) → Superior and inferior venae cavae

coronary circulation The circulation of blood to and from the heart muscle.

semilunar valve into the pulmonary artery, then into the lungs. In the lungs, the blood is oxygenated. The blood returns to the heart through the pulmonary veins into the left atrium. The left atrium is the last step of pulmonary circulation.

Systemic Circulation: The Heart and Body Connection

Oxygenated blood enters the left atrium and travels through the mitral valve into the left ventricle. The left ventricle pumps the blood through the aortic semilunar valve into the aorta. The aorta provides the pathway for the blood to circulate through the body. In the body, the oxygen in the blood is exchanged with carbon dioxide. After traveling through the body, the deoxygenated blood returns to the heart through the superior and inferior vena cava (Figure 2-6).

Figure 2-6 Pulmonary and systemic circulation.

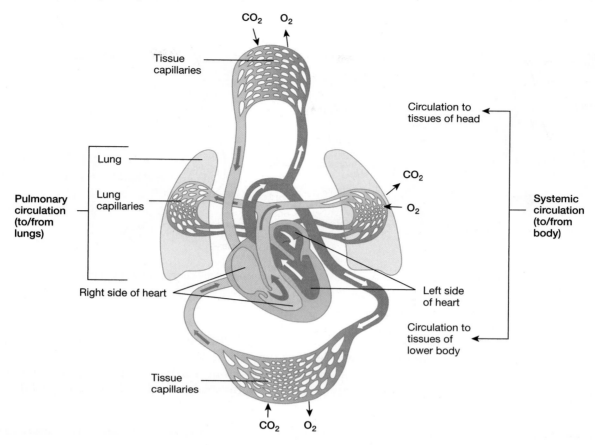

Coronary Circulation: The Heart's Blood Supply

Oxygenated blood from the left ventricle travels through the aorta to the coronary arteries. There are two main coronary arteries, the left main coronary artery and the right main coronary artery. These arteries branch to supply oxygenated blood to the entire heart. The left main artery has more branches than the right because the left side of the heart is more muscular and requires more blood supply. The deoxygenated blood travels through the coronary veins and is collected in the coronary sinus, which empties the blood directly into the right atrium (Figure 2-7).

The Heart as a Pump

The heart is an amazing pump that distributes blood throughout the body. The average heart beats 72 times a minute. Each ventricle pumps 70 milliliters (mL) of blood during contraction. This volume of blood ejected with each contraction is referred to as *stroke volume.* This amount can vary depending upon things such as a person's gender, level of physical fitness, disease state, or genetics. The volume of blood pumped each minute is referred to as *cardiac output.* The average cardiac output is approximately 5 liters (L) per minute. When the volume of blood decreases, the heart rate decreases; similarly, if the contractile force of the heart decreases,

Figure 2-7 Coronary circulation.

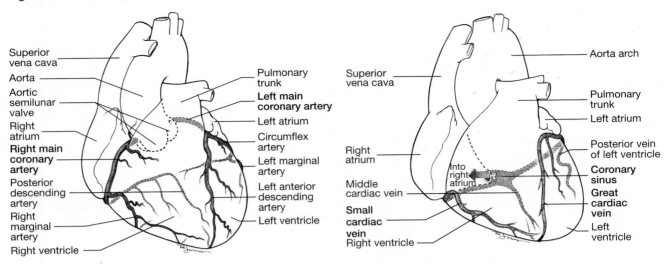

A. Branches of the coronary arteries supply blood to the heart tissue.

B. Branches of the cardiac veins drain blood from the heart tissue.

the cardiac output is decreased. In such cases, patients show signs of decreased or low cardiac output, including pallor, confusion, low blood pressure, nausea, and dizziness. The cardiac output of a patient is estimated by multiplying heart rate by stroke volume (HR × SV = CO).

Checkpoint Questions (LO 2.3)

1. What are the first vessels to branch off the aorta known as?

   _____

   _____

2. Describe the three types of circulation.

   _____

   _____

   _____

3. What is cardiac output?

   _____

   _____

2.4 The Cardiac Cycle

cardiac cycle The contraction and relaxation of the heart.

Each beat of the heart has two phases that indicate the contraction and the relaxation periods of the heart. The contraction and relaxation of the heart together make up the **cardiac cycle.** When the heart contracts, it is squeezing blood out to the body. As the heart relaxes, it is expanding and refilling.

diastole The phase of the cardiac cycle when the heart is expanding and refilling; also known as the relaxation phase.

systole The contraction phase of the cardiac cycle, during which the heart is pumping blood out to the body.

The relaxation phase of the heart is known as **diastole**. The contraction phase is known as **systole**.

Diastole: Relaxation of the Heart

During diastole the heart chambers are relaxing and filling. Blood from the upper body returns to the heart via the superior vena cava, and blood from the lower body returns via the inferior vena cava. The right atrium fills with blood, pushing open the tricuspid valve. This allows blood to flow into the right ventricle. At the same time, blood is returning from the lungs via the pulmonary veins to the left atrium. This blood fills the left atrium and forces the mitral valve open to allow blood to flow into the left ventricle.

Systole: Contraction of the Heart

During the systolic phase, the heart muscle contracts, creating pressure to open the pulmonary and aortic valves. Blood from the right ventricle is pushed into the lungs to exchange oxygen and carbon dioxide. Blood from the left ventricle is pushed through the aorta to be distributed throughout the body to provide oxygen for tissues and remove carbon dioxide.

In adults, the average heart beats approximately 60 to 100 times per minute. In general, women have a faster heartbeat than men. Children's heart rates are usually faster than an adult's heart rate and depend upon the age and size of the child. If you listen to the heart with a stethoscope, you will hear two sounds: "lubb" and "dupp." These sounds are made by the opening and closing of the heart valves, which is caused by the contraction of the heart. The "lubb" you hear is the sound made during the systolic phase by the contraction of the ventricles and the closing of the mitral and tricuspid valves. The "dupp" sound is made during the diastolic phase. It is shorter and occurs during the beginning of ventricular relaxation. This sound is from the closure of the pulmonary and aortic valves. Each complete "lubb-dupp" you hear is actually one beat of the heart (Figure 2-8).

Figure 2-8 Diastole and systole.

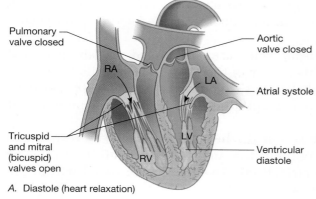

A. Diastole (heart relaxation)

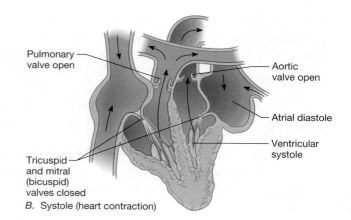

B. Systole (heart contraction)

1. What is the cardiac cycle?

   _____

   _____

2. How are diastole and systole the same?

   _____

   _____

2.5 Conduction System of the Heart

The pumping cycle is controlled by electrical impulses: electrical impulses stimulate contraction of heart muscle, and the absence of electrical impulses allow the heart muscle to relax. These electrical impulses are initiated by specialized pacemaker cells in the heart. The electrical impulses are transferred through the heart by the electrical conduction system. Once the working cells of the heart receive these impulses, they respond by shortening, causing cardiac contraction and blood to flow. The conduction system is necessary for the heart to pump continuously and rhythmically.

Unique Qualities of the Heart

The conduction system is a network of conducting tissue that creates the heartbeat and establishes a pattern for the electrical activity of the heart. The conducting tissue of the heart has several unique qualities that control the beat of the heart and produce the electrical wave. They include automaticity, conductivity, contractility, and excitability.

Automaticity is the ability of the heart to initiate an electrical impulse without being stimulated by a source outside the heart. Automaticity is a form of the word *automatic,* which is exactly how the heart beats—automatically. The heart tissue has its own innate ability to initiate an electrical impulse.

The heartbeat relies on the ability of the **myocardial** cells to conduct electrical impulses. **Conductivity** is the ability of the heart cells to receive and transmit an electrical impulse. The electrical impulse is initiated by automaticity and then travels through the rest of the heart due to the conductivity of the heart cells.

When the heart muscle cells are stimulated by an electrical impulse, they contract. This ability of the heart muscle cells to shorten in response to an electrical stimulus is known as **contractility.** The contraction of the heart muscle cells produces the heartbeat or pumping of the heart.

Excitability is the ability of the heart muscle cells to respond to an impulse or stimulus. Without the quality of excitability, the heart would not react to the electrical impulses that are initiated within the heart.

automaticity The ability of the heart to initiate an electrical impulse without being stimulated by another or independent source.

myocardial Pertaining to the heart (*cardi*) muscle (*myo*).

conductivity The ability of the heart cells to receive and transmit an electrical impulse.

contractility The ability of the heart muscle cells to shorten in response to an electrical stimulus.

excitability The ability of the heart muscle cells to respond to an impulse or stimulus.

As you can see, the heart's unique qualities are essential to the rhythmic contraction of the heart muscle and the circulation of blood through the body. Without these qualities, the heart would not beat.

Regulation of the Heart

In addition to automaticity, the heartbeat is controlled by the *autonomic nervous system (ANS)*. Like the unique qualities of the heart, the ANS is involuntary. This means you have no conscious control over its functions. The *sympathetic* branch of the ANS increases the heart rate by secreting norepinephrine. This happens automatically when you are under stress or become frightened. You can think of the automaticity of the heart as the cruise control in your car. In a normal heart, automaticity sets the rate of the heart to 60 to 100 beats a minute. When the sympathetic branch of the ANS is stimulated, it speeds up the heart. When you let your foot off the accelerator (remove the stimulation to the sympathetic branch of the ANS), the heart rate coasts down to the cruise control speed of 60 to 100.

The *parasympathetic* branch of the ANS exerts a depressant effect on the heart by secretion of acetylcholine. The vagus nerve is the major nerve of the parasympathetic system and exerts an effect on many of the body organs. It is widespread throughout the body. Stimulation of the vagus nerve slows the heart, acting like a brake to the heart rate. When a patient is experiencing an abnormally fast heart rate, stimulation of the vagus nerve is used to bring the heart back to its normal cruise control rate.

Other factors can affect the heart. For example, exercise, stress, or a fever can increase the heart rate. The cardiac control center, located in the brain, sends impulses to decrease the heart rate when the blood pressure rises. When the blood pressure falls, it sends impulses to increase the heart rate. The levels of the electrolytes potassium and calcium play a role in the control of the heart. When there is a low concentration of potassium ions in the blood, the heart rate decreases; but a high concentration causes an abnormal heart rate or rhythm. A low concentration of calcium ions in the blood depresses heart actions, but a high concentration of calcium causes heart contractions that are longer than normal heart contractions.

Pathways for Conduction

The conduction system consists of the sinoatrial (SA) node, atrioventricular (AV) node, bundle of His (AV bundle), bundle branches, and the Purkinje fibers in the ventricles. The SA and AV nodes are small, round structures that consist of many specialized cardiac cells. The **sinoatrial (SA) node** is located in the upper portion of the right atrium. It is the pacemaker of the heart and initiates the heartbeat. The automaticity of the fibers in the SA node produces the contraction of the right and left atria. The SA node fires at about 60 to100 times per minute. Normal conduction in the heart begins with the SA node.

On the floor of the right atrium is another mass of specialized cardiac cells known as the **atrioventricular (AV) node.** Impulses travel to the AV node because of the unique quality of conductivity through a specialized pathway through the atria. The AV node itself causes a delay (slowdown)

sinoatrial (SA) node An area of specialized cells in the upper right atrium that initiates the heartbeat.

atrioventricular (AV) node Delays the electrical impulse to allow the atria to complete their contraction.

in the electrical impulse. This process is important for two reasons. First, it provides time for additional blood to travel from the atria to the ventricles before they contract. This additional blood is known as the atrial kick. The atrial kick increases the cardiac output or the amount of blood that is pumped out of the heart into the body with each contraction. Second, the delay in the electrical impulse reduces the number of electrical impulses transmitted to the ventricles. This is important when the atria are firing too fast. It prevents an excessive rate of electrical impulses from reaching the ventricles. A third benefit to the delay in contraction of the atria is that it allows the ventricles to contract from the bottom up to avoid conflicting contractions between atria and ventricles. The delay aids in coordinated contraction of the heart. The AV node can also act as the pacemaker if the SA node is not working. It will fire at a rate of 40 to 60 times per minute. This is known as the inherent rate of the AV node.

The **bundle of His (AV bundle)**, located next to the AV node, provides the transfer of the electrical impulse from the atria to the ventricles. When the impulse reaches the ventricles, it is divided into the bundle branches. The **bundle branches** are located along the left and right side of the interventricular septum. The electrical impulse travels through the right and left bundle branches to the right and left ventricles. The bundle branches are like a fork in the road, and the electrical impulse splits and travels down both sides.

The right and left bundle branches are pathways down the interventricular septum, where the impulses travel to activate the myocardial tissue to contract. Impulses traveling down the left bundle branch will stimulate the interventricular septum to contract in a left-to-right pattern. The ventricles receive their electrical impulses from the bundle branches.

Purkinje fibers form a network, the **Purkinje network**, that spreads the electrical impulse throughout the ventricles." These fibers provide an electrical pathway for each of the cardiac cells. The electrical impulses accelerate and activate the right and left ventricles at the same time to cause the ventricles to contract. The electrical impulse produces an electrical wave (Table 2-3 and Figure 2-9).

bundle of His (AV bundle) Located next to the AV node; provides the transfer of the electrical impulse from the atria to the ventricles.

bundle branches Left and right branches of the bundle of His that conduct impulses down either side of the interventricular septum to the left and right ventricles.

Purkinje fibers The fibers within the heart that distribute electrical impulses from cell to cell throughout the ventricles.

Purkinje network Spreads the electrical impulse throughout the ventricles by means of the Purkinje fibers.

TABLE 2-3 Parts of the Conduction System

Part	Function
Sinoatrial (SA) node (pacemaker)	Electrical impulses occur at a rate of 60 to 100 beats per minute
Atrioventricular (AV) node	Delays the electrical impulse to allow for the atria to complete their contraction and ventricles to fill before the next contraction
Bundle of His (AV bundle)	Conducts electrical impulses from the atria to the ventricles
Bundle branches	Conducts impulses down both sides of the interventricular septum
Purkinje fibers (network)	Distributes the electrical impulses through the right and left ventricles

Figure 2-9 Conduction pathways.

1. The heartbeat originates in the sinoatrial (SA) node and travels across the wall of the atrium to the atrioventricular (AV) node.
2. The impulse passes through the AV node into the AV bundle or bundle of His to the interventricular septum.
3. The impulse is divided between the right and left bundle branches and travels to the apex of the heart through the interventricular septum via the bundle branches.
4. The Purkinje fibers carry the impulse through the right and left ventricles, causing them to contract.

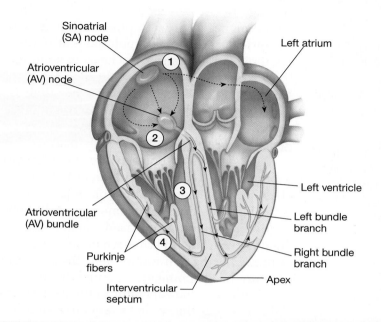

Checkpoint Questions (LO 2.5a, b, c)

1. List the parts of the conduction system in the order the electrical impulse travels.

   _____

   _____

2. The ability of the heart muscle cell to respond to a stimulus is called

   _____

   _____

3. Where does the electrical impulse get delayed to allow all the blood to leave the atria before the ventricles contract?

   _____

   _____

2.6 Electrical Stimulation and the ECG Waveform

Polarization is the state during which the heart cells are at their peak resting energy. During this portion of the cycle, the cells (in their resting state) are electrically polarized. This means the inside of the cardiac cell is

polarization The state of cellular rest in which the inside is negatively charged and the outside is positively charged.

depolarization The electrical activation of the cells of the heart that initiates contraction of the heart muscle.

action potential The change in the electrical potential of the heart muscle when it is stimulated; depolarization followed by repolarization.

repolarization When heart muscle cells return to their resting electrical state and the heart muscle relaxes.

isoelectric The period when the electrical tracing of the ECG is at zero or a straight line, no positive or negative deflections are seen.

interval The period of time between two activities within the heart.

segment A portion or part of the electrical tracing produced by the heart.

complexes Atrial or ventricular contractions as they appear on the ECG; complete ECG waveforms.

negatively charged in relation to the outside of the cell. This is much like the opposite ends of a battery. One is negative and one is positive. This state of cellular rest, polarization, is the ready phase of the heart.

Depolarization, on the other hand, is a state of cellular stimulation, which precedes contraction. It is the electrical activation of the cells of the heart when the electrical charge is reversed across the cell membrane so the interior becomes positively charged. This rapid change in polarization is known as **action potential.** The action potential is brought on by a rapid change in the cell membrane permeability to certain ions (they lose their internal negativity). Depolarization moves from cell to cell through the electrical pathways. Depolarization is the most important electrical event in the heart—it causes the heart to contract and pump blood to the body.

Repolarization is a state of cellular recovery, which follows each contraction. The cardiac cells return to their resting phase of internal negativity. After depolarization, the cardiac cells return to this state in order to prepare for another depolarization. During repolarization, the heart relaxes and allows the chambers of the heart to refill.

The cycle of polarization, depolarization and repolarization is often compared to a camera with an automatic flash. When the little light on the back of the camera is lit, this is just the same as polarity or peak resting energy. Once this light comes on and the button is pressed when you take a picture, energy is released, causing the light to flash. This is the same as depolarization and the wave of energy that spreads throughout the myocardium, causing contraction and the pumping action of the heart. After the picture has been taken, you may have noticed a quiet sound as the energy is building in the capacitor in the camera as it prepares for the next picture. This event is the same as repolarization or the resting, reenergizing phase of action potential.

The ECG waveform is recorded from the electrical activity produced during depolarization and repolarization of the heart. The waveform on the electrocardiogram is a series of up-and-down deflections off a straight line known as an **isoelectric** line. The isoelectric line represents the period when no electrical activity is occurring in the heart and is known as a baseline. Deflections, which appear as waves on the ECG tracing, indicate electrical activity in the heart. The deflections that go up are positive; the deflections that go down are negative.

When the waveform was first discovered, Einthoven labeled the waves of the electrocardiogram as P, Q, R, S, and T. Legend holds that he chose the letters from the center of the alphabet because he did not know what the waves meant or whether other waves preceding the P wave or following the T wave would be discovered. The U wave was added after Einthoven's discovery. Each of these waves indicates specific activity in the heart.

In addition to the waves, the ECG waveform contains **intervals, segments,** and **complexes.** Each of these elements indicates specific activity within the heart. The elements include the QRS complex, the ST segment, the PR interval, and the QT interval (Table 2-4).

What Each Part of the Waveform Represents

The first deflection is positive and is known as the P wave. This P wave is seen when the atria depolarize. The P wave is small (compared to the other waves of the ECG), rounded, and is the first wave of the normal complex.

TABLE 2-4   ECG Components

Component	Appearance	Heart Activity
P wave	Upward small curve	Atrial depolarization with resulting atrial contraction
QRS complex	Q, R, and S waves	Ventricular depolarization and resulting ventricular contraction (larger than the P wave); atrial repolarization occurs (not seen)
T wave	Small upward sloping curve	Ventricular repolarization
U wave	Small upward curve	Repolarization of the bundle of His and Purkinje fibers (not always seen) *Electrolyte imbalance = low Balance*
PR interval	P wave and baseline prior to QRS complex	Beginning of atrial depolarization to the beginning of ventricular depolarization
QT interval	QRS complex, ST segment, and T wave	Period of time from the start of ventricular depolarization to the end of ventricular repolarization
ST segment	End of QRS complex to the beginning of T wave	Time between ventricular depolarization and the beginning of ventricular repolarization

During the delay of conduction that occurs at the atrioventricular node, a small baseline segment is seen on the waveform. There is no electrical activity occurring (depolarization or repolarization); thus, no wave or deflection is seen. It is during this time that atrial kick occurs. Atrial kick occurs when the blood is ejected into the ventricles by the atria.

The next three waves occur together as the QRS complex representing ventricular depolarizations. The Q wave represents the conduction of the impulse down the interventricular septum. It is a negative deflection before the R wave. It is not unusual or abnormal for a QRS complex not to have a Q wave. A normal Q wave is less than one-fourth of the height of the R wave. The R wave is the first positive wave of the QRS complex. It represents the conduction of electrical impulse to the left ventricle. It is usually the easiest wave to locate on the ECG tracing. The S wave is the first negative deflection after the R wave. It represents the conduction of the electrical impulse through both ventricles. The QRS waves together form the QRS complex. The QRS complex represents ventricular depolarization. It is reflective of the time it takes for the impulses to depolarize the interventricular septum down through the ventricular myocardium causing the ventricles to contract (Figure 2-10).

The ST segment is measured from the end of the S wave to the beginning of the T wave. This segment should normally be on the isoelectric line. It indicates the end of ventricular depolarization and the beginning of ventricular repolarization. The reason this segment is studied in a 12-lead ECG recording is to determine whether there is any ischemia or myocardial (heart) damage. **Ischemia,** which is lack of blood causing reduced oxygen to the heart muscle, can result in a change in the ST segment. The ST segment will elevate or become depressed, depending upon the extent of the ischemia and the amount of damage to the cardiac cells. A change in the ST segment typically indicates some form of injury to the heart muscle. These changes are studied when interpreting an ECG. More information about interpreting an ECG is included in Chapter 5.

ischemia Lack of blood supply to an area of tissue due to a blockage in the circulation to that area.

Figure 2-10 Electrical activity in the heart.

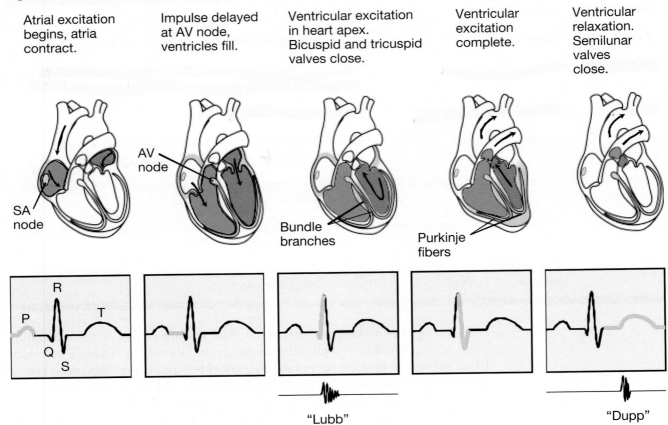

Atrial excitation begins, atria contract.

Impulse delayed at AV node, ventricles fill.

Ventricular excitation in heart apex. Bicuspid and tricuspid valves close.

Ventricular excitation complete.

Ventricular relaxation. Semilunar valves close.

SA node

AV node

Bundle branches

Purkinje fibers

R

P

T

Q

S

"Lubb"

"Dupp"

The T wave represents ventricular repolarization. As repolarization occurs, the ventricular muscles relax. Normal T waves are in the same direction as the QRS complex and the P wave. A normal T wave peaks toward the end instead of the middle. Unlike the symmetrical mountain shape of the P wave, the T wave looks like a small mountain with one sloping side.

The U wave follows the T wave. The U wave represents repolarization of the bundle of His and Purkinje fibers. The U wave does not always show up on the ECG; however, its presence can indicate an electrolyte imbalance.

The PR interval is measured from the beginning of the P wave to the beginning of the QRS complex. The normal length of time for the PR interval is 0.12 to 0.20 second. The PR interval on a normal ECG should be consistent. This time interval represents the time the electrical impulse is initiated until the ventricles are stimulated by the impulse to start the contraction.

The QT interval is the time required for ventricular depolarization and repolarization to take place. It begins at the beginning of the QRS complex and ends at the end of the T wave. It includes the QRS complex, ST segment, and the T wave.

Many variables, such as the heart rate, coronary artery disease, electrolyte imbalance, and antidysrhythmic medications affect QT interval. A longer-than-normal QT interval may indicate that the patient is at an increased risk for certain ventricular dysrhythmias and sudden cardiac death. When the heart rate exceeds 100 beats per minute (bpm), the QT interval is of little clinical significance due to the intervals closing as a result of the increased heart rate.

The R-R interval is the
complex in a rhythm to the
are readily seen on the EC
regular rhythm. We discus
    The junction of the
This represents the end
tion. The J point is imp
plex and interpreting t
0.1 second (Figure 2-11

Figure 2-11 The ECG waveform and heart activity.

Chapter Summary

Learning Outcomes

2.1 Describe circulatio
the ECG.

2.2 Recall t
heart, incl
vessels,

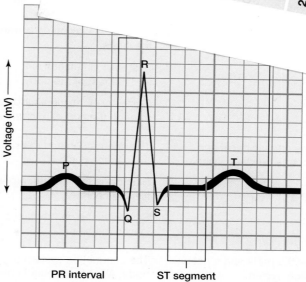

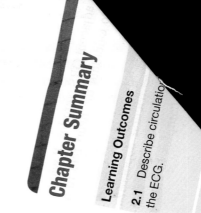

**Checkpoint
Questions
(LO 2.6a, b, c)**

1. Which electrical event is represented by the cardiac contraction of the heart?

   _____

   _____

2. Which wave represents the atrial depolarization? Ventricle repolarization?

   _____

   _____

3. What is ischemia?

   _____

   _____

	Summary	Pages
...n as it relates to	The heart action creates circulation; circulation provides nutrients and oxygen to the tissues and removes waste and carbon dioxide; the ECG waveform is a measurement of the heart actions.	29
...he structures of the ...ding valves, chambers, and	The heart consists of four chambers (two atria and two ventricles), four major valves (mitral/bicuspid, tricuspid, and two semilunar valves). The major vessels of the heart include the venae cavae, pulmonary artery and veins, and the aorta.	29–33
2.3 Differentiate between pulmonary, systemic, and coronary circulation.	Pulmonary circulation is transportation of the blood to and from the lungs. Systemic circulation is transportation of blood between the heart and the rest of the body, excluding the lungs. Coronary circulation supplies blood to and from the heart through the coronary arteries and coronary sinus.	33–36
2.4 Explain the cardiac cycle and relate the difference between systole and diastole.	The contraction and relaxation period of the heart together make the cardiac cycle. Diastole is the relaxation phase of the cardiac cycle when blood fills the heart. Systole is the contraction phase of the cardiac cycle when blood leaves the heart.	36–38
2.5a Describe the parts and function of the conduction system.	The conduction system of the heart includes the SA node, AV node, AV bundle, bundle branches, and Purkinje fibers, which together create and maintain the electrical activity of the heart.	39–41
2.5b Recall the unique qualities of the heart and their relationship to the cardiac conduction system.	The conducting tissue of the conduction system has qualities that control the beat of the heart, including automaticity, conductivity, contractility, and excitability.	38–39
2.5c Explain the conduction system as it relates to the ECG.	The conduction system of the heart creates the electrical activity and thus creates the ECG waveform.	39–41
2.6a Identify each part of the ECG waveform.	The ECG waveform includes the P wave, QRS complex, T wave, U wave (not always seen), PR interval, QT interval, and the ST segment.	42–45
2.6b Describe the heart activity that produces the ECG waveform.	The parts of the ECG waveform are created by the various heart activities of the conduction system, including atrial and ventricular depolarization and repolarization.	41–42

Chapter Review

Matching I

Match the valves, vessels, and chambers of the heart to their definitions. Place the correct letter on the line provided. (LO 2.2)

_____ 1. left ventricle

_____ 2. tricuspid valve

_____ 3. left atrium

_____ 4. aorta

_____ 5. pulmonary artery

_____ 6. right atrium

_____ 7. right ventricle

_____ 8. semilunar valve

_____ 9. pulmonary vein

_____ 10. mitral valve

a. artery that transports blood to the entire body

b. type of valve located in the aorta and the pulmonary artery

c. atrioventricular valve between the left atrium and left ventricle

d. heart chamber that pumps blood to the body, known as the workhorse of the heart

e. heart chamber that receives blood from the lungs

f. chamber of the heart that receives blood from the body

g. chamber of the heart that pumps blood to the lungs

h. blood vessel that transports blood from the lungs to the left atrium

i. valve located between the right atrium and right ventricle

j. blood vessel that provides a pathway for deoxygenated blood to return to the lungs

Matching II

Match the conduction system parts and unique qualities of the heart to their definitions. Place the correct letter on the line provided. (LO 2.5a, b)

_____ 11. excitability

_____ 12. automaticity

_____ 13. bundle branches

_____ 14. SA node

_____ 15. contractility

_____ 16. depolarization

_____ 17. AV node

_____ 18. Purkinje fibers

a. delays the electrical conduction through the heart

b. ability of the heart to initiate an electrical impulse

c. branches off the bundle of His that conduct impulses to the left and right ventricles

d. ability of the heart cells to receive and transmit an electrical impulse

e. an electrical current that initiates the contraction of the heart muscle

f. ability of the heart muscle cells to shorten in response to an electrical stimulus

g. ability of the heart muscle cells to respond to an impulse or stimulus

_____ 19. repolarization

_____ 20. conductivity

h. heart muscle cells return to their resting electrical state and the heart muscle relaxes

i. initiates the heartbeat

j. distribute electrical impulses from cell to cell throughout the ventricles

Multiple Choice

Circle the correct answer.

21. The PR interval is usually (LO 2.6c)
    a. 0.06 to 0.10 second.
    b. 0.12 to 0.20 second.
    c. greater than 0.20 second.
    d. less than 0.06 second.

22. What part of the ECG tracing represents the repolarization of the Purkinje fibers? (LO 2.6b)
    a. T wave
    b. PR interval
    c. U wave
    d. P wave

23. What part of the ECG tracing represents the time from the start of the atrial activity to the start of ventricular activity? (LO 2.6b)
    a. WRS complex
    b. J point
    c. QT interval
    d. PR interval

24. What part of the ECG tracing is measured from the end of the S wave to the beginning of the T wave and is normally on the isoelectric line? (LO 2.6b)
    a. ST segment
    b. QT segment
    c. U wave
    d. QRS complex

25. What wave on the ECG tracing is not always seen and sometimes, when seen, can indicate an electrolyte imbalance? (LO 2.6b)
    a. U wave
    b. P wave
    c. Q wave
    d. R wave

26. The heart's ability to create its own electrical impulse is known as (LO 2.5b)
    a. conductivity.
    b. contractility.
    c. automaticity.
    d. excitability.

27. When stimulated, sympathetic system of the body causes the heart rate to (LO 2.5b)
    a. increase.
    b. decrease.
    c. remain the same.
    d. none of the above.

28. Which vessel of the body contains the highest concentration of oxygen? (LO 2.2)
    a. Aorta
    b. Pulmonary artery
    c. Pulmonary vein
    d. Vena cava

29. The heart is contained inside a sac also known as the (LO 2.2)
    a. endocardium.
    b. pericardial sac.
    c. myocardium sac.
    d. fluid sac.

30. Which of the following would have the *least* effect on the heart rate? (LO 2.5c)
    a. Stress, exercise, and fever
    b. ANS
    c. Potassium and calcium
    d. Respiratory rate

Matching III

Match the information about circulation and the cardiac cycle to the definitions. Place the correct letter on the line provided.

_____ 31. deoxygenated blood (LO 2.2)

_____ 32. cardiac cycle (LO 2.4)

_____ 33. systole (LO 2.4)

_____ 34. coronary circulation (LO 2.3)

_____ 35. systemic circulation (LO 2.3)

_____ 36. oxygenated blood (LO 2.2)

_____ 37. diastole (LO 2.4)

_____ 38. pulmonary circulation (LO 2.3)

a. period between the beginning of one beat of the heart to the next

b. circulation of blood through the heart and heart muscle

c. blood that has little or no oxygen

d. phase of the cardiac cycle when the heart is expanding and refilling; also known as the relaxation phase

e. blood having oxygen

f. circulation between the heart and the entire body, excluding the lungs

g. transportation of blood to and from the lungs

h. contraction phase of the cardiac cycle, when the heart is pumping blood out to the body

Label the Parts

39. a.–p. Label the vessels, valves, and chambers of the heart by using the letters of the terms. (LO 2.2)

- **a.** Right atrium
- **b.** Aorta
- **c.** Right ventricle
- **d.** Right pulmonary veins
- **e.** Left atrium
- **f.** Left ventricle
- **g.** Superior vena cava
- **h.** Pulmonary trunk
- **i.** Aortic valve
- **j.** Tricuspid valve
- **k.** Right pulmonary artery
- **l.** Mitral (bicuspid) valve
- **m.** Inferior vena cava
- **n.** Left pulmonary veins
- **o.** Left pulmonary artery
- **p.** Interventricular septum
- **q.** chordae tendonae
- **r.** papillary muscle

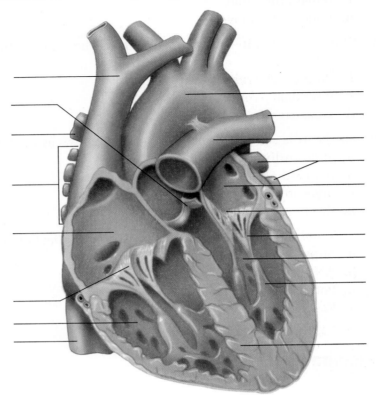

40. a.–m. Label the following diagram representing the flow of blood through the heart. Write the letters of the terms in the appropriate circle or box. (LO 2.3)

- **a.** Superior and inferior venae cavae
- **b.** Right atrium
- **c.** Aorta
- **d.** Right ventricle
- **e.** Pulmonary semilunar valves
- **f.** Left atrium
- **g.** Mitral (bicuspid) valve
- **h.** Pulmonary trunk
- **i.** Pulmonary veins
- **j.** Tricuspid valve
- **k.** Left ventricle
- **l.** Aortic semilunar valve
- **m.** Pulmonary arteries

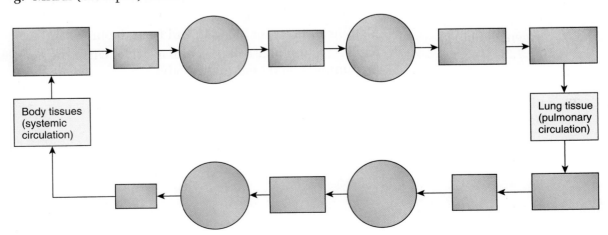

41. a.–h. Label the parts of the conduction system. Write the lette

    a. Interventricular septum
    b. Left bundle branch
    c. Purkinje fibers
    d. AV node
    e. SA node
    f. AV bundle
    g. Right bundle branch
    h. Apex

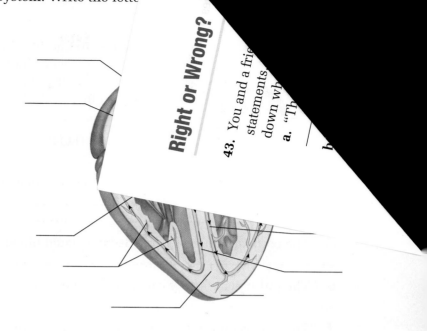

Right or Wrong?

43. You and a fri
statements
down wh
a. "Th

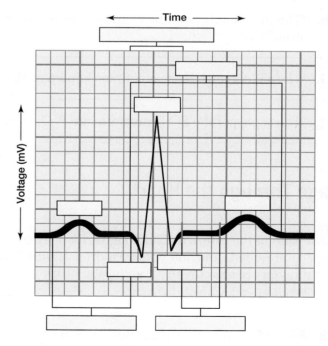

42. a.–i. Label the waves, complexes, intervals, and segments of the ECG waveform. Write the letter of the terms in the appropriate box. (LO 2.6c)

    a. S wave
    b. R wave
    c. P wave
    d. T wave
    e. Q wave
    f. QT interval
    g. ST segment
    h. QRS complex
    i. PR interval

nd have just finished studying this chapter. Your friend makes the following
Are his or her statements correct or incorrect? If the statement is incorrect, write
at you would say to correct your friend.
e valves between the atria and the ventricles are semilunar." (LO 2.2) _____

b. "The atria always pump the blood." (LO 2.2) _____

c. "The heart is a two-sided pump that produces pulmonary circulation and systemic circulation." (LO 2.4) _____

d. "The coronary arteries carry deoxygenated blood." (LO 2.2) _____

e. "The pulmonary artery carries oxygenated blood." (LO 2.2) _____

f. "The waves on the ECG waveform are positive when they are up and negative when they are down." (LO 2.6a) _____

g. "If you are a man, you will have a faster heartbeat." (LO 2.5b) _____

h. "The top chambers of the heart are the ventricles, and the bottom chambers of the heart are the atria." (LO 2.2) _____

i. "The right ventricle is sometimes known as the workhorse of the heart." (LO 2.2) _____

j. "The waves of the ECG waveform are P, Q, R, S, T, and sometimes a U." (LO 2.6b) _____

Voyage Through the Heart

44. For each of the following statements, identify the vessel or structure you are in. Write only in the space provided. Imagine you are a drop of blood traveling through the heart. Returning from the brain, you are about ready to enter the heart. (LO 2.3)
   a. What vessel are you in? _____

   b. After you enter the right atrium, you have to go through a door in order to enter the right ventricle. What is the name of this door? _____

   c. You have made it to the lungs successfully and are traveling back to the heart. What vessels are you in? _____

d. When you get to the heart, where will you be? _____

e. You have finally made it to the last chamber of the heart. The left ventricle pumps you into the entire body. After entering the aorta, what are the very first vessels you will travel into?

Critical Thinking Application *What Should You Do?*

Read the following situations, and use your critical thinking skills to determine how you would handle each. Write your answer in detail in the space provided.

45. When the atria outside of the SA node stimulates the atria to beat too fast, this is known as atrial flutter or atrial fibrillation. When these heart rhythms occur, the ventricles do not beat at the same rate as the atria. What part of the conduction system prevents the ventricles from beating as fast as the atria, and how does it occur? (LO 2.5a)

46. You are working in the emergency room recording an ECG when the electricity goes out. There is a short period of darkness followed by a very loud noise. When you regain power, the hearts of both you and your patient are beating extremely fast. What part of the cardiovascular system is responsible for this increased heart rate? Should you continue recording the ECG now or later, and why? (LO 2.5b)

Get Connected *Internet Activity*

Visit the McGraw-Hill Higher Education Online Learning Center *Electrocardiography for Healthcare Professionals* Web site at **www.mhhe.com/boothecg3e** to complete the following activities.

1. Visit the National Heart, Lung, and Blood Institute's Web site for Web link for OLC information about coronary heart disease. Create a patient education brochure called, "How to Prevent Coronary Heart Disease" from what you learn.

2. Visit the Web site "Get Body Smart," and review information about the heart to prepare for the chapter test. Visit the Web site "Oracle ThinkQuest Education Foundation" and search for action potential. A better understanding of the action potential of the heart will help you interpret an ECG.

Using the Student CD

Now that you have completed the material in the chapter text, return to the student CD and complete any chapter activities you have not yet done. Practice your terminology with the "Key Term Concentration" game. Review the chapter material with the "Challenge" and "Spin the Wheel" games. Take the final chapter test and complete the troubleshooting question and email or print your results to document your proficiency for this chapter.

3 The Electrocardiograph

Chapter Outline

- Producing the ECG Waveform (p. 54)
- ECG Machines (p. 61)
- ECG Controls (p. 64)
- Electrodes (p. 68)
- ECG Graph Paper (p. 69)
- Calculating Heart Rate (p. 72)

Learning Outcomes

3.1 Identify the three types of leads, and explain how each is recorded.

3.2 Identify the functions of common ECG machines.

3.3 Explain how each ECG machine control is used.

3.4 Recognize common electrodes.

3.5 Describe the ECG graph paper.

3.6 Calculate heart rates using an ECG tracing.

Key Terms

artifact
augmented
bipolar
bradycardia
Einthoven triangle
electrodes
gain
input
lead
limb

mm (millimeter)
multichannel recorder
mV (millivolt)
output display
precordial
signal processing
speed
tachycardia
unipolar

3.1 Producing the ECG Waveform

In Chapter 2, you learned about the heart's conduction system and how the ECG waveform is produced. In this chapter, we discuss the electrocardiograph and the equipment needed to perform an ECG and record the ECG waveform. You will discover how the 12-lead system works and what the measurements are on the ECG graph paper. Learning the equipment and lead system thoroughly and correctly will prepare you to record your first ECG.

The electrical impulse that is produced by the heart's conduction system is measured with the ECG machine. The ECG machine interprets the impulse and produces the ECG waveform. The waveform indicates how the heart is functioning electrically. Since the heart is three dimensional, it is necessary to view the electrical impulse and heart functioning from different sides. A single heart rhythm tracing views the heart from one angle. A 12-lead ECG is a complete picture of the heart's electrical activity, looking at it from 12 different angles as you might look at a sculpture. It records the heart's electrical activity in 12 different views at slightly different angles. The 12-lead ECG records the electrical impulses produced in the heart. It is not a picture of the heart structure; it is a recording of the electrical activity within the heart. The 12 views provide information about how the electrical impulses travel through various parts of the heart.

A 12-lead ECG is actually recorded by only 10 lead wires, which, when attached to the chest and the **limbs** (arms and legs), provide the 12 different views for the 12-lead tracing. Six of these leads attach to the chest electrodes, and the other four attach to the electrodes on the arms and legs or shoulders and lower abdomen. **Electrodes** are small sensors placed on the skin to receive the electrical activity from the heart, and **leads** are covered wires that conduct the electrical impulse from the electrodes to the ECG machine. The lead wires are identified by color and are labeled with letters to match the correct position on the patient's body (Table 3-1 and Figure 3-1). The term *lead* also refers to the view on the ECG tracing as well as the physical location the electrode is placed on the patient. For example, Lead V2 refers to the labeled cable, the second intercostal space, right sternal margin and the V2 tracing on the printed ECG. Context is the clue to dealing with terms that have different meanings.

The 10 lead wires produce 12 different lead circuits consisting of one or more wires from the electrodes to the electrocardiograph. The 12 circuits produce 12 different tracings or views of the heart. The electrodes, or a combination of electrodes, identify each of the 12 leads. The 12 leads are made up of three different types of leads: three standard limb leads, three augmented leads, and six chest leads.

limb An arm or a leg.

electrodes Small sensors placed on the skin to detect the electrical activity from the heart.

leads Covered wires that conduct the electrical impulse from the electrodes to the ECG machine.

TABLE 3-1   Lead Identification

Identifying Letters	Designated Color	Lead Wire Placement
RA	White	Right arm
LA	Black	Left arm
RL	Green	Right leg
LL	Red	Left leg
V1–V6	Brown*	Chest leads

* V1 to V6 lead colors may vary.

Figure 3-1 When attaching the lead wires, check carefully for the correct color- and letter-coded wire.

Identifying Lead Wires

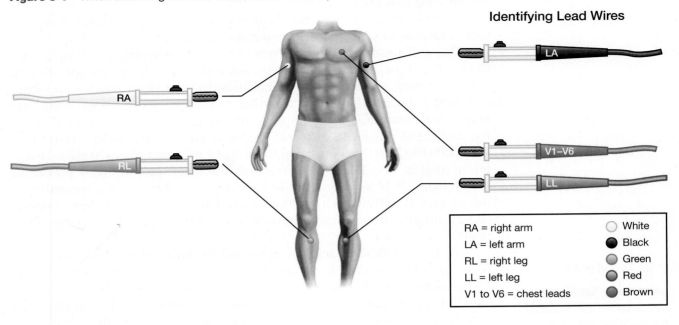

RA = right arm	○ White
LA = left arm	● Black
RL = right leg	◐ Green
LL = left leg	◐ Red
V1 to V6 = chest leads	◐ Brown

Remember the lead placements

Troubleshooting

10 electrodes

12-lead - shows 12 different views of the heart.

Check the Lead Wires

Each of the lead wires is coded by color and letter. If you place the lead wires incorrectly, the ECG will not record at all or it will record the waveforms improperly. Always check and double-check the lead wires before you begin the tracing. An ECG recording produced with the lead wires attached incorrectly is not acceptable and will have to be repeated.

If you attempt to record an ECG and no tracing is seen, what should you do?

_____

_____

Einthoven triangle
A triangle formed by three of the limb electrodes—the left arm, the right arm, and the left leg; it is used to determine the first six leads of the 12-lead ECG.

To understand the circuits for the first six leads (three standard and three augmented), we can use the Einthoven triangle. Einthoven is the scientist credited with developing the first ECG machine. The **Einthoven triangle** is formed by three of the limb electrodes: those on the right arm, the left arm, and the left leg. The right leg is used only as a ground or reference electrode (Figure 3-2).

The electrical current created by the heart is measured between the positive and negative electrodes placed on the body. If no current is flowing, the waveform is flat, or isoelectric. If the current moves toward the positive electrode, the ECG waveform will be positive, (above the isoelectric baseline). If the current moves away from the positive electrode/toward the negative electrode, the ECG waveform will be negative (downward, below the isoelectric baseline).

Figure 3-2 The Einthoven triangle helps us understand the reference points for the 12-lead ECG.

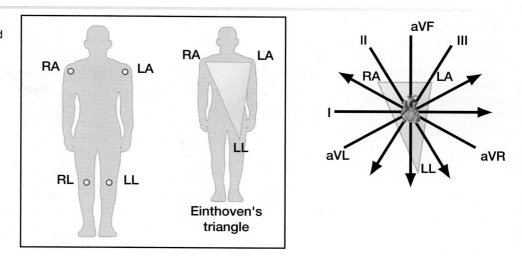

Einthoven's triangle

Figure 3-3 Leads I, II, and III are standard limb leads and are recorded from these reference points on the Einthoven triangle, producing a positive deflection.

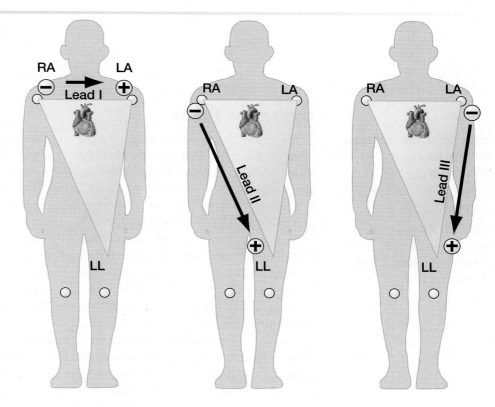

Standard Limb Leads

The first three leads are known as standard limb leads. They are also known as **bipolar** leads because they measure the flow of electrical current in two directions at the same time. These first three leads are called lead I, lead II, and lead III. In the Einthoven triangle, leads I, II, and III are positioned at the same distance from the heart's electrical activity. Lead I records the tracing from the right arm (−) to the left arm (+); lead II records the tracing from the right arm (−) to the left leg (+); and lead III records the electrical activity from the left arm (−) to the left leg (+) (Figure 3-3). All three leads produce positive deflections.

bipolar A type of ECG lead that measures the flow of electrical current in two directions at the same time.

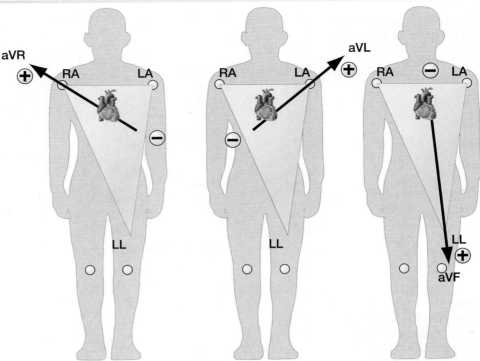

Figure 3-4 The augmented leads aVR, aVL, and aVF are recorded from midway between two points on the Einthoven triangle. Because of the lead reference points, their tracings are normally small but are augmented (enlarged) by the ECG machine.

Augmented Leads

augmented Normally small ECG lead tracings that are increased in size by the ECG machine in order to be interpreted.

unipolar A type of ECG lead that measures the flow of electrical current in one direction only.

The second three leads are known as **augmented** leads because their tracings are increased in size by the ECG machine in order to be interpreted. They are also known as **unipolar** leads because they measure toward one electrode on the body. They are called aVR, aVL, and aVF. The R, L, and F refer to the direction the lead is measuring: R is right arm, L is left arm, and F is foot (left leg/foot) (Figure 3-4). Lead aVR records electrical activity from the heart to the right arm. Lead aVR is usually a negative deflection. If it does not produce a negative deflection, you might have the electrodes or lead wires placed incorrectly. To ensure accuracy of electrodes and lead wire placement, check the aVR tracing produced when recording the 12-lead ECG; if it is not a negative deflection, verify the placement of the electrodes and lead wires to correct it.

Lead aVL records electrical activity from the heart to the left arm. Lead aVF records electrical activity from the heart to the left leg. The voltage is very low with the augmented leads because of the angle of measurement; therefore, the ECG waveform will be very small. The ECG machine must increase (augment) the size of the waveforms for these leads to be readable on the ECG tracing.

Chest Leads

precordial A type of lead placed on the chest in front of the heart; known as a V lead.

The last six leads are the chest leads. Also known as **precordial** leads, these leads are located in front of (*pre*) the heart (*cor*). The chest leads are unipolar because they are measured in one direction only. They are placed on specific sites on the chest. Each of the chest leads begins with the letter V and is numbered from V1 to V6. These leads record activity between six points on the chest and within the heart. You can view the placements in Figure 3-5. The procedure for placing electrodes is discussed in Chapter 4, "Performing an ECG."

Figure 3-5 Front and cross-sectional view of chest lead placement.

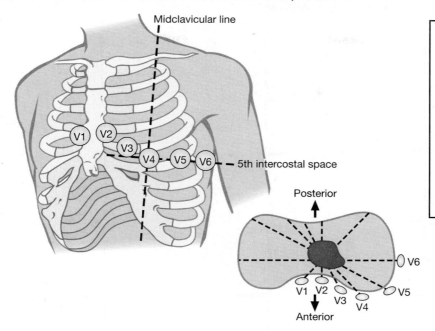

V1 — Fourth intercostal space, right sternal border

V2 — Fourth intercostal space, left sternal border

V3 — Halfway between V2 and V4

V4 — Fifth intercostal space at the midclavicular line

V5 — On the same horizontal level with V4, at the anterior axillary line

V6 — On the same horizontal level with V4 and V5, at the midaxillary line

The 12-lead ECG tracings can be interpreted separately or in conjunction with each other. When an ECG is being recorded, each of the 12 leads must be identified on the tracing. Older machines required that the ECG tracing strip be coded with identifying marks manually. Most machines identify each lead tracing automatically. Each lead tracing looks slightly different and presents a different picture of the heart. This allows the physician to determine damage or problems in specific areas of the heart (Figure 3-6).

Checkpoint Questions (LO 3.1)

1. What will you need to know to prepare yourself for recording your first ECG?

_____

_____

2. How many lead wires are used to obtain a 12-lead ECG tracing?

_____

_____

3. Name three augmented leads.

_____

_____

Figure 3-6 A 12-lead ECG produced on a multichannel ECG machine. Each lead is identified on the printout. Note that each lead tracing (I, II, III, aVR, aVL, aVF, and V1 to V6) look different.

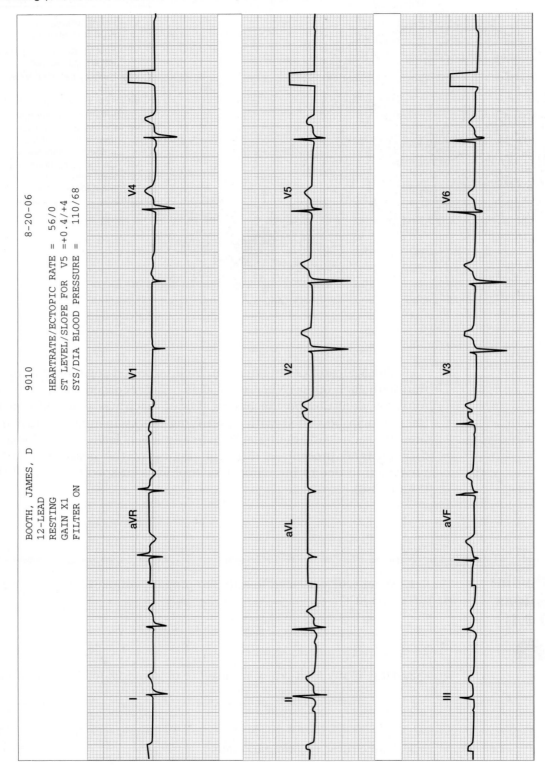

BOOTH, JAMES, D   9010   8-20-06

12-LEAD
RESTING   HEARTRATE/ECTOPIC RATE =   56/0
GAIN X1   ST LEVEL/SLOPE FOR V5 =+0.4/+4
FILTER ON   SYS/DIA BLOOD PRESSURE =   110/68

3.2 ECG Machines

Machines used today to measure an ECG weigh less than 10 pounds; some are as small as a credit card. All ECG machines vary slightly, but most have the same basic parts. The typical ECG machine sits on a small cart that can be pushed to the person requiring the ECG. You should become familiar with the type of machine you will be using by reading the manufacturer's instructions.

multichannel recorder An ECG machine that monitors all 12 leads but records three leads at once and switches automatically, recording each of the four sets of three leads.

The **multichannel**, three-channel ECG **recorder** monitors all 12 leads but records three leads at once and switches automatically, recording each of the four sets of three leads (Figure 3-7). It produces a full sheet of paper showing all 12 lead tracings. The actual recording time for this machine is approximately 10 seconds. This tracing may need to be attached to a thicker backing or copied when filed permanently with the healthcare provider's interpretation. Also available are multichannel ECG machines that can record up to six lead tracings at one time. With advancing technology, electronic copies of 12-lead tracings and interpretations are being stored and transmitted electronically via telecommunications, which is discussed later.

Functions

There are three basic functions of the electrocardiograph: input, signal processing, and output display. Sensors in the ECG machine serve as receiving devices for the electrical activity of the heart. Electrodes placed on the

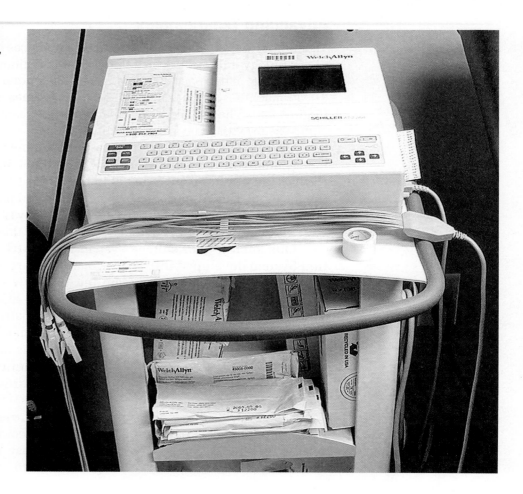

Figure 3-7 A multichannel ECG machine records three, four, or six leads at a time on a large sheet of ECG graph paper.

patient's skin direct the impulses to the ECG instrument, providing the **input** for the ECG machine.

Signal processing occurs inside the ECG machine. It amplifies the electrical impulse and converts it into mechanical actions on the display. A complex collection of transistors, resistors, and circuitry amplify and prepare the signal for transfer to the output display.

The **output display** is the result of the ECG tracing. Commonly, this is the printed report or computerized data report. The output can also appear on a screen known as an oscilloscope. An oscilloscope is frequently found on a cardiac monitor or a defibrillator. For a 12-lead ECG, the printed format is an important output display since it provides a hard copy of the information. However, electronic output is quickly becoming the most common choice for the ECG tracing.

ECG machines also perform other functions as well, including computerized measurement and analysis, storage, and communication. Computerized measurement and analysis provide a machine interpretation of the ECG. This interpretation is not meant to replace the physician's interpretation. However, the computer interpretation can distinguish between a normal and abnormal recording quickly and may provide a second opinion. All computerized interpretation should be validated.

Some ECG machines store ECG results, which then can be recalled and printed later. ECG machines are also equipped to transmit results over the telephone, fax, or Internet.

Advancing Technologies

Technology has advanced all around us. Advances have impacted the fields of cardiology and electrocardiology. ECG machines have undergone many advances over the past 30 years. They have gone from single-channel to 3-lead machines, to our current 12-lead machines and wireless technology (Figure 3.8). The 12-Lead ECG machines 30 years ago seem primitive by comparison with today's equipment.

One of the more recent advances in medicine is the area of digital technology. Many ECG machines are now able to not only acquire and store the tracings but also transmit a digital image of the 12-lead for storage in a central location. This is particularly beneficial when patients are seen in hospitals other than the one where the 12-lead ECG was obtained. Access to this vital information is much more readily available than at any time in the past.

One such digital storage system is the MUSE Cardiology Information System developed by GE Healthcare (Figure 3-9). This system is able to integrate, manage, and streamline the flow of cardiac information, such as resting 12-lead ECG, exercise stress ECG, and Holter devices. This system provides faster data delivery, distribution of information, and analysis. The MUSE digital storage system allows the provider easy access to patient information. Devices like this make the healthcare system more efficient due to its ability to communicate between the hospital information system, electronic health records, and the ECG devices themselves.

This system allows you to retrieve the current ECG and older ECGs for serial (obtained over a period of time) comparison. The retrieved 12-lead on the computer screen will look just like the printed record (Figure 3-9). The screen has a simple toolbar to make accessing common features quick and clear. These features will help with viewing and printing the ECG. The ability to view serial ECGs is important when looking to detect subtle changes that may indicate myocardial abnormalities (such as ischemia, injury, or infarction).

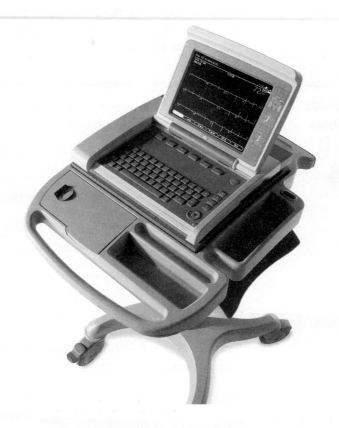

Figure 3-8 The MAC 5500 resting ECG analysis system can easily analyze, transmit, store, and retrieve ECG information quick and easily.

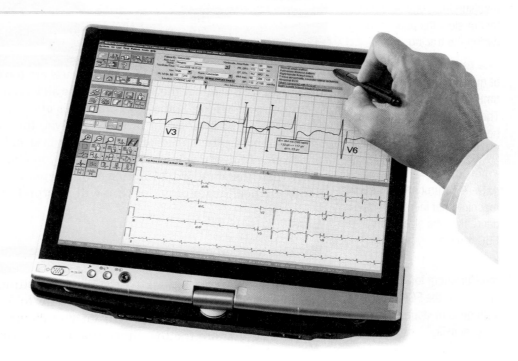

Figure 3-9 The MUSE Cardiology Information System by GE Healthcare retrieved ECG looks just like the printed record on the screen.

Systems such as the MUSE support the progressive paperless electronic health record initiative. Computer advances in medicine improve efficiency, billing accuracy, and time from test to diagnosis, and they reduce manpower demands. Ultimately, the use of MUSE and electronic health records improve the speed and quality of medical care, where quick access to critical cardiac information is the name of the game. Every second can count in reducing the long-term damage that can result from heart trauma. As technology advances, it is essential to stay current with any equipment you will be using.

Checkpoint Questions (LO 3.2)

1. A multichannel ECG monitors all 12 leads but usually records how many leads at one time?

   _____

   _____

2. What are the three basic functions of an ECG?

   _____

   _____

3.3 ECG Controls

The three most important controls on the electrocardiograph include the speed, gain, and artifact filter.

Speed

speed up because of kids

speed A control on the ECG machine that regulates how fast or slow the paper runs during the tracing.

mm (millimeter) A unit of measurement to indicate time on the ECG tracing. The time is measured on the horizontal axis.

The **speed** control regulates how fast or slow the paper or data run during the ECG procedure. *The most commonly used paper speed is 25 millimeters per second (written as 25 mm/sec).* In some cases, you may want to increase the speed to 50 mm/sec, which is twice as fast. You would do this if the patient has an unusually rapid heart rate so that the complexes are farther apart. It may also be done if the ECG waveform parts are too close together. Increasing the speed would allow the waveform to be analyzed more easily because they would appear wider. Some ECG machines allow you to reduce the speed to 5 mm/sec or 10 mm/sec in order to analyze the ECG recording more carefully. Changing the speed of the recorder is usually done at the request or preference of the physician. Remember, if you change the speed to anything other than the standard 25 mm/sec, you must note this on the tracing and notify the healthcare provider who will interpret the tracing, if possible.

Gain

gain A control on the ECG machine that increases or decreases the size of the ECG tracing.

mV (millivolt) A unit of measurement to indicate voltage on the ECG tracing. Voltage is measured on the vertical axis.

The **gain** control regulates the output or height of the ECG waveform. The normal setting is 10 mm/mV (millivolts are the units of measurement used to indicate voltage on the ECG tracing). By setting the gain to 20 mm/mV, you can double the size; by setting the gain to 5 mm/mV, you reduce the size by half. Some machines will let you change the gain, depending on which lead you are tracing. Since the tracing size can vary between leads,

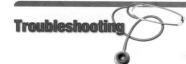 Troubleshooting

Changing the ECG Tracing Speed

When the patient's heart rate is very fast, it will be difficult to read the ECG tracing because the waveform parts will be close together. Set the speed control at 50 mm/sec to widen the complexes so the ECG can be interpreted more easily. *Circle or note the speed setting and, when possible, verbally tell the healthcare provider who will be interpreting the results about the change in speed.* This notification is essential to avoid misinterpretation of the ECG; for example, a normal ECG set to double speed can sometimes look like an abnormal rhythm known as a heart block.

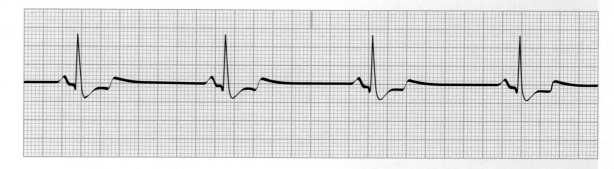

This ECG tracing was produced at a speed of 50 mm/sec. What should you do?

_____

_____

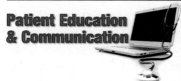 Patient Education & Communication

Know Your ECG Machine

Become familiar with the ECG machine you will be using before performing an ECG. Your uncertainty could cause anxiety or nervousness in the patient who is having the ECG performed.

setting the gain will allow the ECG waveform to be readable for any lead tracing. If you change the gain setting during any lead tracing, you must record this change on the ECG report. Digital machines standardize the wave output height automatically. A calibration or standardization mark may be seen on the tracing (Figure 3-10).

Artifact Filter *normal setting is 40 Hz*

artifact Unwanted marks on the ECG tracing caused by activity other than the heart's electrical activity.

The ECG machine you are using may have an artifact filter selection. The usual setting is between 40 and 150 Hz (hertz, a unit of frequency that indicates per second). Forty Hz is normally used to reduce **artifact** or abnormal marks on the ECG tracing due to muscle tremor and slight patient movement. We discuss artifact in more detail in Chapter 4. Remember that the

Figure 3-10 The calibration mark on the ECG tracing must be verified to ensure accuracy. The first square waveform on the ECG tracing is indicating the standardization of the machine for the recorded ECG.

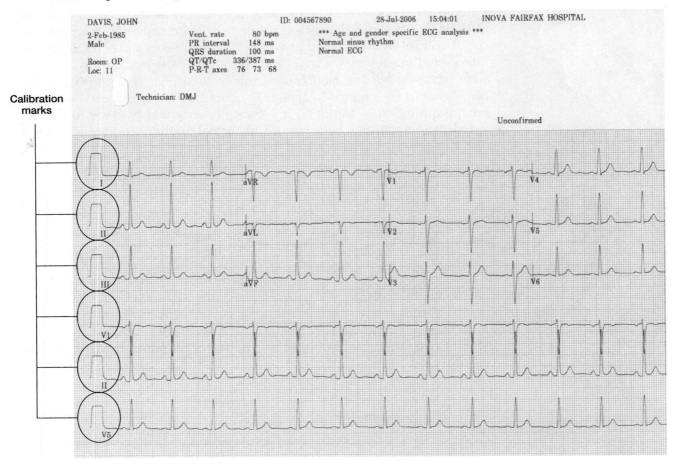

artifact filter will correct only the printed output. If the computer performs interpretation, it will interpret the results from the actual nonfiltered information from the patient, not what is printed or viewed on the screen. This could cause inaccurate interpretation by the computer, which is why it is essential that a physician as well as the computer interpret all ECGs. Some filtering of artifact will prohibit the view of pacemaker spikes. It is important to know how to modify the filter to allow for pacemaker spikes to be seen.

LCD Display

There are various other controls on the ECG machine that the user can set or use to enter information. For example, the user can enter data about the patient to be included on the printout along with the ECG results. This data can also be entered electronically by using a scanner on the patient's identification band (Figure 3-11). This information would be entered into the LCD (liquid crystal diode) display. This is the area of the machine where you can view the patient information you have entered. It is also where information from the ECG's computer is displayed. For example, some machines can detect if the arm leads or chest leads are reversed, and it will display this information in the LCD panel.

Figure 3-11 (*A.*) The ECG tracing and the patient data can be viewed when performing an ECG. (*B.*) Some machines include a bar code scanner to identify the patient and to automatically enter the patient information onto the tracing.

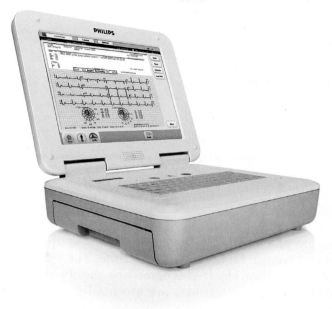

A.

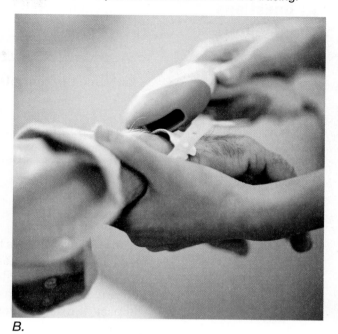

B.

Heart Rate Limits

If the ECG machine has computer interpretation, the user may be able to set the heart rate limits. In other words, the operator can set the heart rate that the machine will interpret as too slow—**bradycardia**—or too fast—**tachycardia**. If the heart rate is above or below the number set, the machine will indicate this by sounding an alarm and marking on the tracing.

Lead Selector

Most 12-lead ECG machines record each of the leads automatically. However, a lead selector is used to run each lead individually in case one or more leads needs to be repeated.

bradycardia A slow heart rate, usually less than 60 beats per minute.

tachycardia A fast heart rate, usually greater than 100 beats per minute.

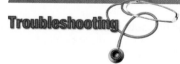

Changing the Gain

When the deflections on the ECG tracing are too short or tall, you will need to correct the gain. Be certain the machine is standardized correctly, and then adjust the gain control if necessary.

When recording an ECG and the deflections or spikes of the tracing are not large enough, what should you do?

_____

_____

Checkpoint Questions (LO 3.3)

1. What are some reasons that you may change the speed of the ECG tracing?

   _____

   _____

2. Name the controls of the ECG machine.

   _____

   _____

3.4 Electrodes

Electrodes are sensors that are placed on a person's skin to pick up the electrical activity of the heart and conduct it to the ECG machine. The standard 12-lead ECG uses 10 electrodes. These electrodes come in a variety of types and are usually disposable. Reusable electrodes are essentially a thing of the past. If used, however, they do require care and maintenance.

Disposable Electrodes

Disposable electrodes are used because they reduce the possibility of cross-contamination and can be simply removed and discarded for easier cleanup (Figure 3-12). The self-adhesive types stick easily to the patient's body. The gel is already applied so the electrodes will properly conduct the electrical impulses.

Safety & Infection Control

Do Not Mix Electrodes

You should never mix two different types of electrodes. This could cause an inaccurate tracing, which could result in incorrect treatment for the patient.

Figure 3-12 (*A.*) Disposable electrodes come in various shapes and sizes. Electrolyte gel or paste is not necessary since it is already contained on these electrodes. (*B.*) Standard resting tab electrodes are inexpensive, disposable, and easy to use for a routine ECG.

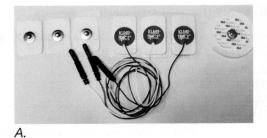

A.

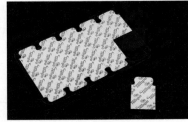

B.

Each disposable electrode is normally used for only one ECG. The only exception occurs when a second ECG is performed on the same patient immediately after the first and the electrodes are not disturbed. For example, if you are transferring a patient from an outpatient facility to a hospital, you should leave the electrodes in place for the emergency medical personnel. They will be recording one or more ECGs on the way to the hospital. If the electrodes stay on the patient's skin any longer than two sequential readings, the gel will dry out, resulting in inaccurate ECG tracings.

For hospitalized patients, longer-lasting silver electrodes are available. These electrodes are used for patients who require multiple and frequent ECGs (serial ECGs). When serial ECGs are required, it is important to ensure the same lead placement for each. A slight change often causes a change in the tracing. The silver electrodes are kept on the patient and checked daily.

No matter what type of electrodes are used, they must be handled and stored correctly. If a package contains more electrodes than needed, the remaining electrodes must be kept in a sealed plastic bag so the gel will not dry out. Always check the expiration date on the package before use. Make sure the electrode gel has not dried out on any electrode. Even new electrodes should be checked before placement.

Checkpoint Question (LO 3.4)

1. Which type of electrode is used when monitoring a patient who will be having serial ECGs done?

_____

_____

3.5 ECG Graph Paper

The ECG machine records an image of the heart's electrical activity onto graph paper. This image is the ECG waveform, or a series of waves and complexes recorded from the activity in the heart. The graph paper provides increments to measure the electrical activity produced on the tracing. Understanding the ECG paper is a necessary part of performing an ECG and is essential to interpreting the ECG (Figure 3-13).

The two most commonly used type of paper are standard grid and dot matrix. Both are heat and pressure sensitive. Because the paper is pressure sensitive, you should handle it carefully to avoid marking it. Marks on the paper could make the tracing difficult to read or inaccurate. In addition, certain substances such as alcohol, plastic, sunlight, and x-ray film can erase the tracing. Once the ECG is completed, it should be stored away from these substances. Some companies offer recording paper that requires no special handling or storage. This paper guarantees that the tracing will last for up to 50 years.

Dot matrix paper has some advantages over standard grid paper. Dot matrix reports require less ink, are easier to read, and produce sharper photocopies, yet it is much less commonly used. One advantage of standard grid paper is that it is slightly less expensive (Figure 3-14).

Figure 3-13 Choose the right size and type of graph paper for the ECG machine you will be using.

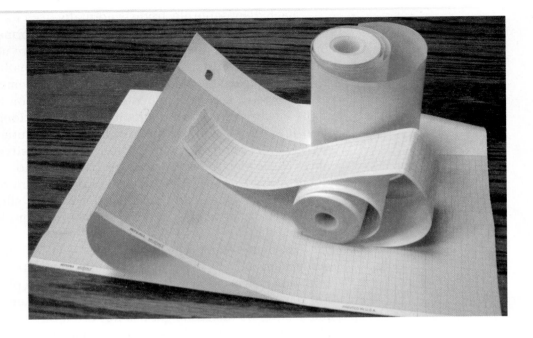

Figure 3-14 Comparison of ECG graph paper: dot matrix paper (*A.*) requires less ink, is easier to read, and produces sharper photocopies, whereas standard grid paper (*B.*) is slightly less expensive.

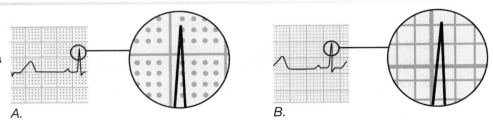

A.

B.

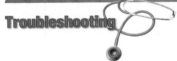

Handle the ECG Report with Care

Handle and store the ECG report with care. It can be damaged easily; and, if damaged, it cannot be interpreted by the physician.

The physician places a stack of charts on top of an ECG report you just placed on his desk. What should you do?

_____

_____

The standard paper speed for the ECG machine is 25 mm/sec. Be sure your ECG machine is set at this speed unless ordered otherwise. If you run the machine at any speed other than 25 mm/sec, be certain to note this on the ECG results. Prior to performing an ECG, make sure the machine has enough paper to record the results. Each machine has a paper loading procedure that you should become familiar with. Many of the machines warn you when the paper is nearly gone by making a red mark across the bottom of the tracing (Figure 3-15). Read the manufacturer's directions for specific instructions on how to change the ECG machine paper. Keep a supply of paper on the ECG cart in case you run out of paper in the patient's room or examination room.

Figure 3-15 While performing an ECG, a thick red line at the bottom of the graph paper indicates that the paper needs to be changed.

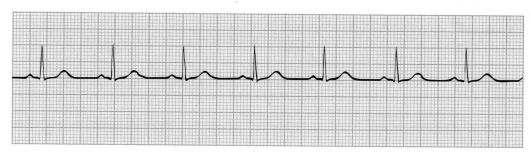

Figure 3-16 The ECG paper will provide measurement for both time and voltage. Note that each small box is either 0.1 mV in voltage or 0.04 seconds in time.

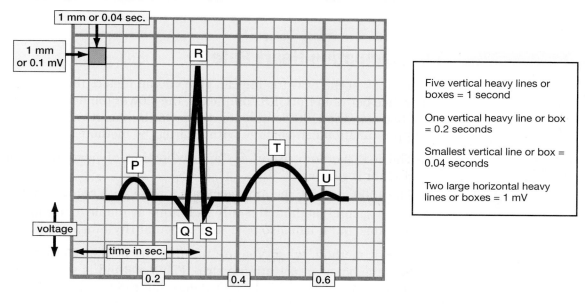

Five vertical heavy lines or boxes = 1 second

One vertical heavy line or box = 0.2 seconds

Smallest vertical line or box = 0.04 seconds

Two large horizontal heavy lines or boxes = 1 mV

Measurements

The ECG graph paper consists of precisely spaced horizontal and vertical lines. The horizontal readings represent time, measured in millimeters (mm). The vertical readings measure voltage, indicated in millivolts (mV). The heavy lines form boxes that are 5 mm by 5 mm in size. At the standard paper speed of 25 mm/sec, the paper grid can be translated into specific numerical values. The smallest box on the graph paper represents 0.04 second in time and 1 mm or 0.1 mV in voltage. One second equals 25 mm, or five heavy lines. Therefore, each vertical heavy line represents 0.20 second. Two large boxes represent 10 mm, which equals 1 centimeter (cm) for vertical measurement. ECG machines must be calibrated so that 1 cm = 1 mV. Each horizontal heavy line represents 5 mm or .5 mV (Figure 3-16). A calibration mark should always be verified on the left-hand side of the ECG before printing.

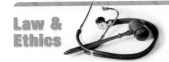

Law & Ethics

Maintaining Patient Records

Handling the ECG paper and report correctly is essential because the ECG report is part of a patient's medical records and must be maintained for at least seven years.

Checkpoint Question (LO 3.5)

1. When the paper speed is 25 mm/sec, there are how many small boxes per minute?

_____

_____

3.6 Calculating Heart Rate

A quick look at the ECG tracing can give you an idea of the heart rate. The more space between the QRS complexes, the slower the heart rate. The less space between the QRS complexes, the faster the heart rate. A more accurate approximation can be done with a variety of methods:

1. The R-R method: useful for approximation of heart rate when the rhythm is regular
2. The 1500 method: the most accurate for use with regular rhythms
3. The 6-second method: the only technique available to use for irregular rhythms, but it can also be used for regular rhythms.

For the R-R method, when you are running the ECG at 25 mm/sec, there are 300 large boxes in a 1-minute strip. (This method is sometimes called the 300 method.) You need to first determine the number of large boxes between two R waves on the ECG tracing. This number should be divided into 300. For example, if there were five boxes between the R waves, the heart rate would be 300 divided by 5, which equals 60 beats per minute. Table 3-2 provides the approximate heart rates based on this method of calculation. Figure 3-17 illustrates the process for calculating heart rates using the R-R wave method.

The most accurate method for determining the rate of a regular rhythm is by the 1500 method, named such because in a 1-minute interval there are 1500 small squares. To use this method, you should count the number of small squares between two consecutive R waves and then divide that number into 1500. For example, if you count 25 small squares between two R waves, you will divide that by 1500 ($1500 \div 25 = 60$). The heart rate would be 60 beats per minute (Figure 3-18). This technique allows you to measure up to a minimum distance of 0.5 mm. When dividing the small squares counted into 1500, it has by far the smallest margin for heart rate error. *Note:* When using the 1500 technique, remember to round the heart rate down if the heart rate has a decimal point less than 0.5 or round up if you get 0.5 or more. For example, 86.4 = 86 and 76.7 = 77.

TABLE 3-2 Calculating Heart Rates with Measurement of the R-R Interval

Large Boxes Between Two R Waves	Seconds Between Beats	Heart Beats per Minute
1	0.2	300
2	0.4	150
3	0.6	100
4	0.8	75
5	1.0	60
6	1.2	50

Figure 3-17 To estimate the heart rate with the R-R wave method, count the number of large boxes between two R waves and divide into 300. In this figure there are four full boxes between the R waves for an estimated rate of 75.

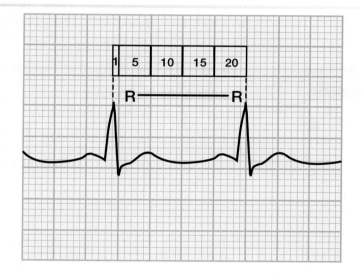

Figure 3-18 Using the 1500 method, count the number of small boxes between two R waves and divide into 1500. In this example there are 38 small boxes. 1500 ÷ 38 = 40 beats per minute.

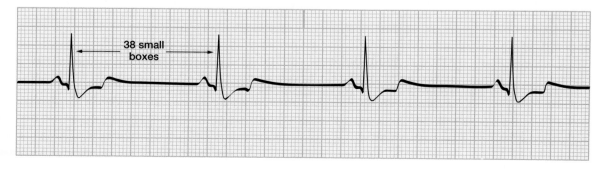

Figure 3-19 To estimate the heart rate with the six-second method, locate a six-second section of the ECG rhythm strip (each small black line or heavy red mark at the top of the strip indicates 15 boxes or three seconds), count the number of complete complexes in this section, then multiply the number of complexes by 10. In this figure, eight complete complexes equal an estimated heart rate of 70. Complex number 8 cannot be counted because it is not completely within the 6-second strip.

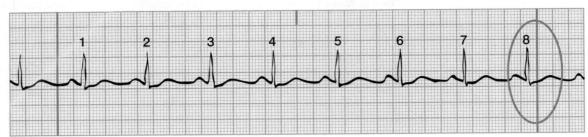

The third method (*and the only one to be used for approximating irregular heart rhythms*) is called the 6-second method. First, identify a 6-second section of the tracing. The ECG paper is usually marked at 3-second intervals on the top or bottom of the strip with a vertical line. You will need to view two sections or 30 boxes, horizontally. Second, count the number of complete complexes seen in one 6-second interval. Each complex must include the P, QRS, and T waves. The complex should not be counted unless complete. Third, multiply the number of complexes by 10 to determine the estimated heart rate (Figure 3-19 and "Troubleshooting—Counting the Heart Rate").

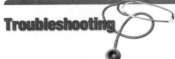

Troubleshooting

Counting the Heart Rate

When calculating the heart rate by counting the complexes in the 6-second interval, count the complete complexes only. If there is a portion of a complex at each end of the 6-second section you are using, find another section on the tracing to view. Never count incomplete complexes; this will make your results inaccurate.

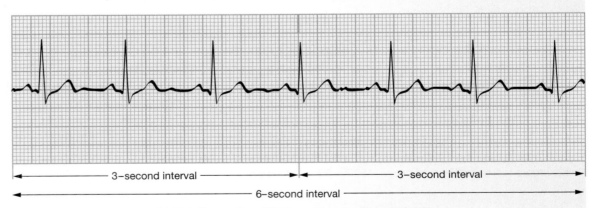

←——— 3–second interval ———→←——— 3–second interval ———→

←————————————— 6–second interval —————————————→

Multiply the number of QRS complexes or P waves by 10

What is the number of complexes in the above 6-second interval? What is the heart rate?

_____

_____

1. Calculate the heart rate for this ECG strip using the 1500 method.

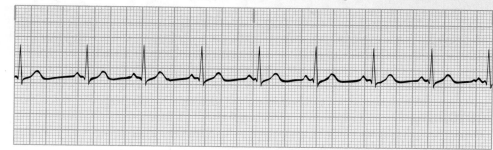

2. Estimate the heart rate for this ECG strip.

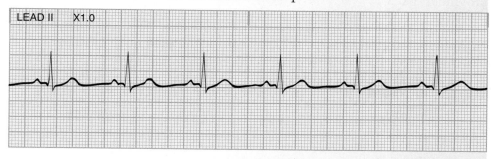

LEAD II   X1.0

Chapter Summary

Learning Outcomes	Summary	Pages
3.1 Identify the three types of leads and explain how each is recorded.	Three types of leads are used to produce the ECG: standard, augmented, and chest leads. Standard leads are bipolar, meaning they measure electricity in two directions. Augmented leads are unipolar because they measure toward one electrode on the body. Chest leads record activity between six points on the chest and within the heart.	54–59
3.2 Identify the functions of common ECG machines.	The ECG machine has three basic functions: input, signal processing, and output display.	61–62
3.3 Explain how each ECG machine control is used.	The controls for the ECG machine include the speed, gain, artifact filter, LCD display, heart rate limits, standardization, and the lead selector.	64–68
3.4 Recognize common electrodes.	Various types of disposable electrodes are used, depending upon the equipment and type of ECG being recorded.	68–69
3.5 Describe the ECG graph paper.	ECG graph paper has boxes that are 5 mm by 5 mm and indicate 0.04 second in time horizontally and 0.1 mV in voltage vertically.	69–71
3.6 Calculate heart rates using an ECG tracing.	There are three common ways to calculate the heart rate including the R-R (300) method, the 6-second method, and the 1500 method.	72–75

Chapter Review

Matching I

Match the name of each of the following leads with their lead type. Place the correct letter on the line provided. (LO 3.1)

_____ 1. V1

_____ 2. aVR

_____ 3. lead I

_____ 4. lead II

_____ 5. aVL

_____ 6. V3

_____ 7. V4

_____ 8. V6

_____ 9. aVF

_____ 10. lead III

_____ 11. V2

_____ 12. V5

a. standard limb lead

b. augmented lead

c. precordial lead

Matching II

Match these terms related to the ECG with their definitions. Place the correct letter on the line provided.

_____ 13. single-channel (LO 3.2)

_____ 14. speed (LO 3.3)

_____ 15. input (LO 3.3)

_____ 16. gain (LO 3.3)

_____ 17. lead (LO 3.1)

_____ 18. multichannel (LO 3.2)

_____ 19. mV (LO 3.5)

_____ 20. mm (LO 3.5)

_____ 21. signal processing (LO 3.2)

_____ 22. electrode (LO 3.4)

_____ 23. output display (LO 3.3)

a. disposable sensors that receive the electrical activity of the heart

b. changes the size of the ECG tracing

c. data that is entered into an ECG machine

d. indicates time on the ECG tracing

e. conductor wire attached to the ECG machine

f. ability to record more than one lead tracing at a time

g. indicates voltage on the ECG tracing

h. displays the tracing for the electrical activity of the heart

i. amplifies the electrical impulse and converts to mechanical action

j. records one lead tracing at a time

k. controls the speed of the paper during an ECG tracing

Multiple Choice

Circle the correct answer.

24. ECG machines have three basic functions. They are (LO 3.2)
  a. input, signal processing, and output display.
  b. input, standardization, and output display.
  c. multichannel, single-channel, and signal processing.
  d. standardization, input display, and output display.

25. To perform an ECG with accuracy, the best source to obtain specific information about the machine is (LO 3.2)
  a. the policy and procedure manual.
  b. the manufacturer's directions.
  c. your supervisor.
  d. your textbook.

26. The type of electrodes most commonly used is _____ and used _____. (LO 3.4)
  a. disposable, more than once
  b. reusable, more than once
  c. disposable, once
  d. reusable, once

27. "Bipolar leads" means that (LO 3.1)
  a. One electrode is placed on the chest and the machine arbitrarily places one behind the person.
  b. Both positive and negative electrodes are placed on the patient's body.
  c. Einthoven's triangle is not used.
  d. One of the leg limbs is used while the machine augments the rhythm.

28. What is the purpose of the LCD display? (LO 3.3)
  a. To allow entry and display of patient information
  b. To show the results of the ECG
  c. To sound alarms and errors
  d. To assist the patient to understand the procedure

29. The "multichannel ECG" indicates that (LO 3.2)
  a. you enter all the data into the machine prior to running a tracing.
  b. three or more leads are recorded at one time.
  c. you do not have to mount each lead separately.
  d. all of the above.

30. What is the standard paper speed? (LO 3.3)
  a. 25 mm/sec
  b. 50 mm/sec
  c. 0.25 mm/sec
  d. 0.50 mm/sec

31. Which of the following is not a type of lead? (LO 3.1)
  a. Standard
  b. Augmented
  c. Input
  d. Precordial

32. An artifact filter helps obtain a clear ECG tracing by (LO 3.3)
    a. reducing artifact or abnormal marks on the ECG tracing.
    b. always ensuring accurate readings by the computer.
    c. always recognizing that the patient has a pacemaker.
    d. all of the above.

33. Computerized interpretation (LO 3.3)
    a. can be used for actual diagnostic interpretation.
    b. never has to be validated by a physician.
    c. must always be validated by a physician.
    d. none of the above.

34. The horizontal reading on the ECG paper represents _____, and the vertical readings represent _____. (LO 3.5)
    a. voltage, time
    b. time, height
    c. time, voltage
    d. voltage, millivolts

35. Which lead tracing must be augmented by the ECG machine to be able to see the different ECG waveforms? (LO 3.1)
    a. Lead I
    b. Lead II
    c. Lead V6
    d. Lead aVF

36. The Einthoven triangle is formed by using which of the following placement sites? (LO 3.1)
    a. Right arm, left arm, left leg
    b. Right arm, left leg, right leg
    c. Right arm, middle of chest, left leg
    d. None of the above

Matching III

Match the size of the line with the time on the tracing at 25 mm/sec paper speed. Place your answer in the space provided. Note: a heavy line or box is 5 small boxes. (LO 3.5)

_____ 37. five heavy lines or boxes
_____ 38. one vertical heavy line or box
_____ 39. smallest vertical line or box

a. 1 second
b. 0.04 second
c. 0.2 second

Matching IV

Match the lead wire and its color. Place your answer in the space provided. (LO 3.1)

_____ 40. left leg (LL)
_____ 41. right arm (RA)
_____ 42. right leg (RL)
_____ 43. left arm (LA)

a. green
b. white
c. black
d. red

Label the Parts

44. Label the lead tracings that produce the Einthoven triangle. (LO 3.1)

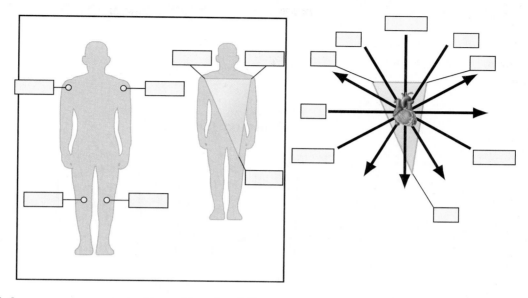

45. Label the measurements indicated on the following figure. (LO 3.5)

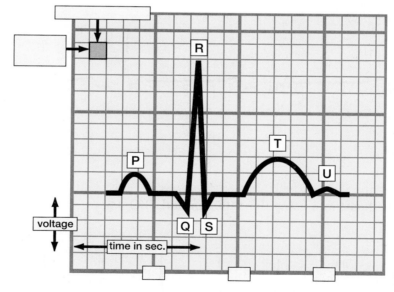

46–47. Estimate the heart rate using the R-R wave method. (LO 3.6)

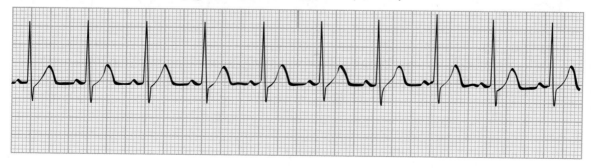

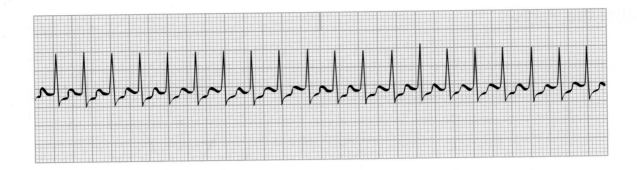

48–49. Estimate the heart rate using the 6-second method. (LO 3.6)

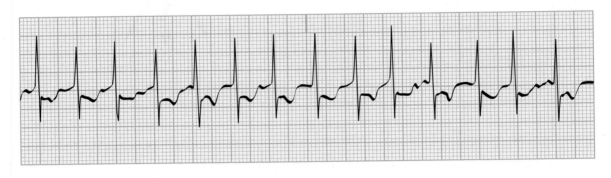

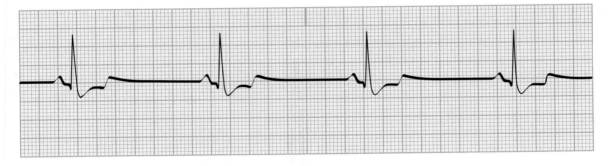

50–51. Determine the heart rate using the 1500 method. (LO 3.6)

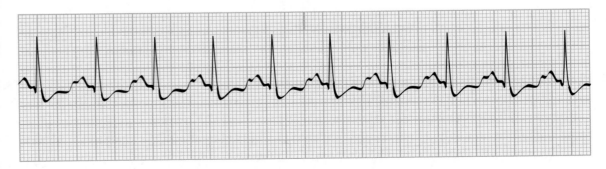

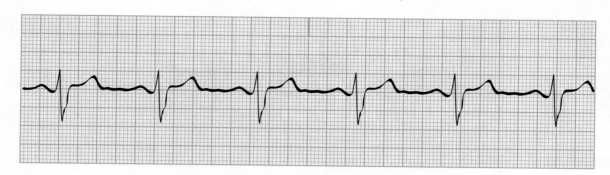

Critical Thinking Application *What Should You Do?*

Read the following situations, and use your critical thinking skills to determine how you would handle each. Write your answer in detail in the space provided.

52. When you start to perform an ECG on a patient, you notice a red line along the bottom of the ECG paper. What should you do? (LO 3.5)

_____

_____

53. When preparing to do an ECG, you find an open package of disposable electrodes on top of the ECG cart. Would you use these electrodes? Why or why not? (LO 3.4)

_____

_____

54. You are preparing to attach the electrodes and lead wires for a 12-lead ECG. You are unable to read the letters on each of the lead wires. You place the electrodes and lead wires, but when you run the tracing it looks like a bunch of scratches. What do you think the problem is and how would you solve it? (LO 3.1)

_____

_____

55. When performing a 12-lead ECG, you notice that the tracing line is very thick and hard to view. In addition, one of the leads does not record properly. What would you do? (LO 3.3)

_____

_____

Get Connected *Internet Activity*

Visit the McGraw-Hill Higher Education Online Learning Center *Electrocardiography for Healthcare Professionals* Web site at **www.mhhe.com/boothecg3e** to complete the following activity.

1. The Merck Manual online provides additional details about electrocardiography. Visit this site at www.merck.com and search for *ECG*. Review the standard ECG components, and create a chart from the information you have found.

Using the Student CD

Now that your have completed the material in the chapter text, return to the student CD and complete any chapter activities you have not yet done. Practice your terminology with the "Key Term Concentration" game. Review the chapter material with the "Spin the Wheel" game. Take the final chapter test, and complete the troubleshooting question; email or print your results to document your proficiency for this chapter.

4 Performing an ECG

Chapter Outline

- Preparation for the ECG Procedure (p. 83)
- Communicating with the Patient (p. 85)
- Identifying Anatomical Landmarks (p. 87)
- Applying the Electrodes and Leads (p. 88)
- Safety and Infection Control (p. 92)
- Operating the ECG Machine (p. 95)
- Checking the ECG Tracing (p. 95)
- Reporting ECG Results (p. 100)
- Equipment Maintenance (p. 101)
- Pediatric ECG (p. 103)
- Cardiac Monitoring (p. 104)
- Special Patient Considerations (p. 105)
- Handling Emergencies (p. 108)

Learning Outcomes

4.1 Prepare the patient, room, and equipment for an ECG.

4.2 Describe the communication needed during the ECG procedure, including the actions to take if a patient refuses to allow an ECG to be performed.

4.3 Identify the anatomical landmarks that are used to apply the ECG chest electrodes to the correct locations.

4.4 Demonstrate the procedure for applying the electrodes and lead wires for a 12-lead ECG and cardiac monitoring.

4.5 Identify at least three ways to prevent infection and provide for safety during the ECG procedure.

4.6 Describe the procedure for recording a 12-lead ECG.

4.7 Identify types of artifact and how to prevent or correct them.

4.8 Describe how to report the ECG results.

4.9 Identify the steps for cleaning and caring for the ECG equipment.

4.10 Explain variations for a pediatric ECG procedure.

4.11 Distinguish between a routine ECG and cardiac monitoring.

4.12 Summarize special patient circumstances when performing an ECG.

4.13 Recall the steps for handling an emergency during the ECG.

Key Terms

alternating current (AC) interference
angle of Louis
anterior axillary line
dextrocardia
intercostal space (ICS)
midaxillary line
midclavicular line

midscapular line
paraspinous line
posterior axillary line
seizure
somatic tremor
suprasternal notch
wandering baseline

4.1 Preparation for the ECG Procedure

Now that you understand how the ECG is used, the anatomy of the heart, and the electrocardiograph, the next step is to record an ECG. The ECG experience should be pleasant to the patient and not produce anxiety. The ECG procedure must be done correctly, and the tracing must be accurate.

Prior to performing the ECG, you will need to prepare the room. Certain conditions in the room where the ECG is to be performed should be considered. For example, electrical currents in the room can interfere with the tracing. If possible, choose a room away from other electrical equipment and x-ray machines. If possible, turn off any electrical equipment that is in the room during the tracing. The ECG machine should be placed away from other sources of electrical currents, such as wires or cords.

An ECG must be ordered by a physician or other authorized personnel, and an order form must be completed prior to the procedure. This form may be called a requisition or consult and should be placed in the patient's record. It should include why the ECG was ordered and the following identifying information:

- Patient name, identification number or medical record number, and birth date
- Location, date, and time of recording
- Patient age, sex, race, and cardiac medications the patient is currently taking
- Weight and height
- Any special condition or position of the patient during the recording

If this information is not included on the requisition or consult, you should ask the patient or find the information in the patient's record.

Many facilities have computerized systems. The ECG order is frequently entered through this system. Entering the patient identifying information into the computer will produce the order form and generate patient

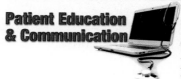

Patient Education & Communication

Cardiac Medications

Certain cardiac medications can change the ECG tracing. Prior to the ECG procedure, determine if your patient is on any cardiac medications and, if so, inform the physician and write the names of the medications on the ECG report. See Appendix A for examples of common cardiac medications.

Figure 4-1 Make sure the ECG paper is properly loaded and aligned before recording an ECG.

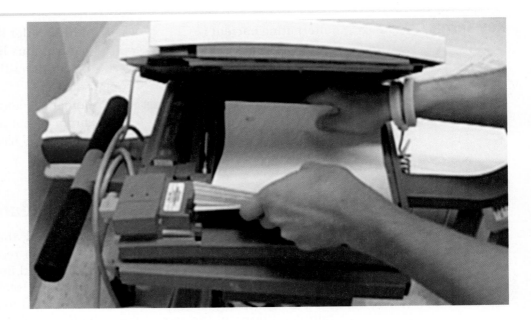

charges. Without a computer system, the information should be handwritten on the order form, consult, or requisition, whichever your facility uses.

The patient's identifying information should also be entered through the LCD panel on the ECG machine prior to the recording. If the ECG machine does not allow you to enter the information or there isn't time due to an emergency situation, you should write it on the completed ECG. Most importantly, all information should be written or entered accurately no matter what type of ECG machine or order system you are using.

Before beginning the procedure, make sure the ECG machine has a good supply of paper loaded in it. If a red line is seen across the bottom of the last tracing, you should replace the paper in the ECG machine before beginning. This should be done prior to taking the ECG machine to the room where the patient is located. Review the operator's manual or consult with your supervisor if you are unsure how to insert the new ream of paper. Most ECG machines will have a release button or lever that will open the ECG equipment for the paper to be inserted. Place the paper inside the machine correctly. Thread it through the roller to the outside of the machine and align. Close the paper-loading compartment, and run the machine to check for proper functioning and alignment (Figure 4-1).

**Checkpoint
Questions
(LO 4.1)**

1. Name four important aspects of preparing for the ECG procedure.

_____

_____

2. What information must be included on the ECG requisition?

_____

_____

4.2 Communicating with the Patient

Prior to performing any procedure, always ensure that you are performing the procedure on the correct patient. Correctly identifying the patient is the first step in ensuring that you are providing patient safety. You should always identify the name, verify the name with some form of identification, and ensure that it is the right patient for the procedure. The Joint Commission (TJC), formerly the Joint Commission on Accreditation of Healthcare Organizations (JCAHO), has stated that every patient must be identified by two forms of identification. This can be a photo ID, the patient stating his or her name, a medical record number, and/or verification of the patient's birth date with the patient statement. If the patient's information is incorrect, verify with your immediate supervisor for the next steps.

Introduce yourself by stating your name and job title. Ask the patient to state his or her name. Check the name on the patient identification band or patient's chart to verify the information. To ensure it is the correct patient, ask the patient to state his or her birth date. Often patients have similar names, but their birth dates and medical record numbers will distinguish the correct patient.

After you verify that you have the correct patient, explain what you are about to do. State "I am going to perform an electrocardiogram on you today. Have you ever had an ECG done before?" Stating both ECG and electrocardiogram helps the patient relate that they are the same. If the patient has not had an ECG, explain the procedure in more detail. Assure the patient that the procedure is harmless and painless. Avoid using words that may frighten the patient such as *electricity* or *wires*. Patients, particularly children, who have not had an ECG before may be afraid of the machine and wires. The patient should be relaxed and comfortable. Maintaining a calm, competent manner and answering the patient's questions will help the patient relax.

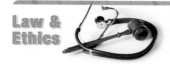

Law & Ethics

Legal Record

The ECG is part of the medical record. Enter the patient information thoroughly and accurately. Remember, the patient's medical record can be used as part of a medical professional liability case.

If the patient refuses an ECG, determine the cause of the refusal. Some people may have fear or concern about the procedure. Provide any information or reassurance the patient may need. Frequently, patients see the wires and think the machine will shock them. Be sure you explain carefully that you are only going to measure the electricity that is already inside their body. If the patient still refuses, notify your supervisor and/or the ordering physician; the patient's reason for refusal must be documented.

In preparing for an ECG, provide the patient with privacy by pulling a curtain around the bed or closing the examination room door. Because many patients are fearful and/or feel they lack privacy, inform them that closing the door or curtain is for their privacy. The patient should remove any clothing above the waist. Provide the patient with a drape, such as a sheet or blanket. The patient may also wear a hospital-type gown with the opening in the front. The patient should remove any jewelry or items that would interfere with the electrode placement or touch the electrodes. This may include necklaces, watches, bracelets, belt buckles, or ankle bracelets. In addition, all electronic devices need to be turned off and removed from the patient. These include things such as cell phones, PDAs, MP3 players, or beepers.

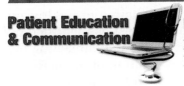

Patient Education & Communication

Explain the Procedure

Remember, even if a patient is not able to respond, he or she may still hear you. Always explain the procedure before beginning the ECG.

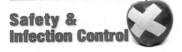

Safety & Infection Control

Proper Patient Identification

You must always check the patient's name and medical record or patient identification number and verify it with the patient's birth date prior to performing any procedure on a patient.

The patient should be positioned as comfortably as possible on his or her back and should remain relaxed and still throughout the procedure. To ensure comfort, place a small pillow under the patient's head and an extra pillow under the knees, if preferred.

The position of the patient is important during an ECG. Expose the patient's chest and extremities where you will be placing the leads. If possible, work from the left side of the bed or exam table, since most of the electrodes and leads are placed on the left side of the chest. Ensure that the arms and legs are supported on the exam table or bed. Take care to provide for privacy by using the blanket or sheet to drape the patient. It is especially important to drape a female patient's breasts for comfort and to prevent embarrassment. A sheet or blanket will also keep the patient warm and prevent chills. Chills may produce shivers that could interfere with the tracing. Make sure that the bed or exam table is not touching the wall or any electrical equipment and that the patient is not touching any metal. If the exam table is especially narrow or the patient is large, you may use blankets, sheets, or pillows to prevent direct contact with the rails, thus reducing the potential for artifact.

Checkpoint Questions (LO 4.2)

1. What should you indicate to the patient when closing the door or pulling the curtain before performing an ECG?

_____

_____

2. What should you do if a patient refuses an ECG?

_____

_____

4.3 Identifying Anatomical Landmarks

midclavicular line An imaginary line on the chest that runs vertically through the center of the clavicle.

anterior axillary line An imaginary vertical line starting at the front axilla (armpit) that extends down the left side of the chest.

midaxillary line An imaginary vertical line that starts at the middle of the axilla (armpit) and extends down the side of the chest.

intercostal space (ICS) The space between two ribs.

suprasternal notch The dip you feel at the anterior base of the neck just above the manubrium where the clavicle attaches to the sternum.

angle of Louis A ridge about an inch or so below the suprasternal notch where the main part of the sternum and the top of the sternum, known as the manubrium, are attached.

Once you have properly positioned the patient on the bed or exam table, you will need to place the electrodes on the chest and limbs. In order to place the chest electrodes for the ECG, you must have an understanding of the anatomy and certain landmarks on the chest. Each chest lead, V1 to V6, must be placed on the correct site on the chest. These sites can be identified by knowing the underlying bones and a set of imaginary lines on the exterior of the chest.

The bones of the chest include the clavicle, the sternum, and the ribs. The imaginary lines include the midclavicular line, the midaxillary line, and the anterior axillary line. On most patients, the **midclavicular line** starts in the center of the clavicle and passes vertically either through the nipple line or just medial to the nipple line. The **anterior axillary line** starts in the front of the axilla (armpit) and runs down the left side of the chest. The **midaxillary line** starts in the middle of the axilla and runs down the side of the chest.

Other sites on the chest you must be able to locate include the intercostal spaces, suprasternal notch, and the angle of Louis. To feel the **intercostal space (ICS),** or space between two ribs, locate the sternum. Press your fingers to the edge of the sternum on the left or right side. The outer edge of the sternum is known as the sternal border. Between each connected rib you should feel a dip or dent. Feeling as close to the sternal border as possible will make it easier. The **suprasternal notch** is the dip you feel at the anterior base of the neck just above the manubrium (top of the sternum), where the clavicle attaches to the sternum. The **angle of Louis** is a ridge about an inch or so below the suprasternal notch. It is where the main part of the sternum and the manubrium attach. To the right and left of the angle of Louis are the second ribs. Below each rib is the corresponding ICS (Figure 4-2).

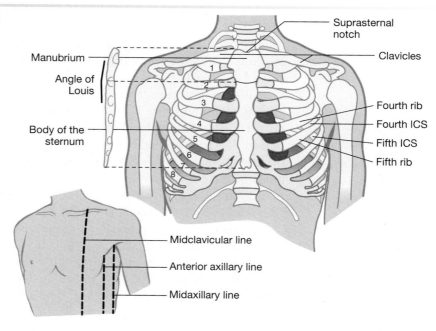

Figure 4-2 Anatomical landmarks for chest lead placement.

1. Which anatomical landmark starts in the middle of the axilla and runs down the side of the chest?

_____

_____

2. Where is the angle of Louis?

_____

_____

4.4 Applying the Electrodes and Leads

The limb electrodes are placed on the forearm or upper arms and the inside of the lower legs. You should pick a fleshy area with the least amount of hair. If the placement of the arm leads on the patient's forearm is not possible due to injury, amputation, IV placement, casts, or otherwise, you should chose a different site. The alternate site of placement for arm leads is on the deltoids (shoulders). The leads should be placed on the same site on each arm so that the placements are mirror images of each other. For example, if a patient has a cast or an IV on the left forearm, you will need to move *both* left and right electrodes to the shoulders.

When placement of the leg leads on the patient's lower legs or ankles is not possible, the alternate site for placement is on the upper legs. They should be placed as close to the trunk as possible. This may be necessary when the patient is an amputee or has an injury or bandage on one of the lower legs. The leads should be placed at the same site on each leg: if you place one lead above the knee on the left, then the right leg lead should also be placed above the knee. Attach the limb leads first since machines will not run at all without the limb leads being attached. However, the ECG machine will run if the limb leads are attached and the chest leads are not. This is important in the event that a patient is having a cardiac crisis. A tracing from the frontal plain is better than nothing. The physician could be looking at this tracing while you connect the precordial leads and run the full 12-lead ECG.

Before applying the electrodes on the chest, make sure the skin at the sites is clean and dry. Remove any lotion or oil from the skin with alcohol wipes or soap and water. You may use electrolyte pads to prep the skin. If the patient has a great deal of chest hair, you may also need to shave small areas of the chest so the electrodes will adhere to the skin properly. Small areas of the chest may be shaved, but it is preferred to clip the hair instead of shaving. This prevents the patient from scratching the electrode site as the hair grows in (Table 4-1).

Start by applying the V1 electrode. First locate the angle of Louis; then locate the second rib, which is adjacent to this landmark. Each intercostal space is felt between the ribs with the corresponding intercostal space below the rib location. The fourth intercostal space is the dent you feel between the fourth and fifth ribs. Chest lead V1 is placed at the right sternal border at this location. V2 should be placed at the fourth intercostal space on the left sternal border. Skip V3 and place V4 next. V4 is placed at the fifth intercostal space on the left midclavicular line. Locate the site of the intersection between the fifth intercostal space and the midclavicular line. In young people, this site is directly below the nipple. Now place V3 midway between V2 and V4. Continuing in the fifth intercostal space on the same horizontal level as V4, and place V5 at the anterior axillary line. Place V6 at the midaxillary line on the same horizontal line as V4 (Table 4-2 and Figure 4-3). (Another method of placement for V5 and V6 is to place V6 first then place V5 midway between V4 and V6.) The anatomical

TABLE 4-1 Applying Leads Correctly

- Choose a flat, nonmuscular area.
- Use the forearms and ankles for the limb leads if at all possible.
- Alternate sites include the upper arms near the shoulders (deltoids) and upper legs.
- Prep the skin with an electrolyte pad, if available.
- When necessary, cleanse the electrode sites with an alcohol pad, mild soap and water, or electrolyte pad.
- Dry the skin completely before applying the electrodes.
- If the patient is diaphoretic (sweaty) consider using antiperspirant, tincture of benzoin, or mastisol to help pads remain adhered to the patient's skin.
- Shave the hair from the site only if necessary such as during an emergency.
- Clip hair, instead of shaving. Use tape to remove cut hairs.

TABLE 4-2 Chest Lead Placement

V1 Fourth intercostal space, right sternal border
V2 Fourth intercostal space, left sternal border
V3 Halfway between V2 and V4
V4 Fifth intercostal space at the midclavicular line
V5 At the anterior axillary line on the same horizontal level as V4
V6 At the midaxillary line on the same horizontal level as V4

Figure 4-3   Chest lead placement.

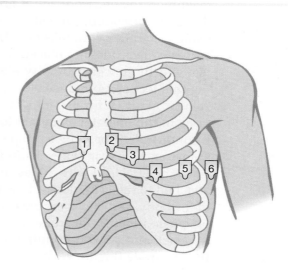

landmarks should always located when placing chest electrodes. Do not place them visually.

The procedure is the same when placing the chest electrodes on a female. If the patient has large breasts, you can ask the patient to move her own breasts (if able); or, using the back of your hand, simply lift the left breast and place the electrodes in the closest position possible. The breast may sit on top of the electrode, but not the other way around. Leads V3, V4, and V5 will be the most affected by breast tissue. Electrodes should be placed as close as possible to the proper placement without placing the electrodes directly on the breast tissue because breast tissue is a poor conductor of electricity. In the event of large breasts, V3 may not be perfectly in line, but should be as close as possible to the midpoint halfway between V2 and V4.

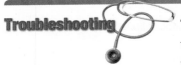

Troubleshooting

The Midclavicular Line

When locating the midclavicular line for chest lead placement, keep in mind that the midclavicular line does not always run directly through the nipple line. This is most often the case with obese patients or females with large breasts.

When applying the V4 electrode to a patient who weighs 326 pounds, you have difficulty finding the midclavicular line. What should you do?

_____

_____

After all of the electrodes have been properly positioned, you must attach the lead cable wires. Identify the correct cable for each electrode based on color and letter abbreviations. For example, the chest leads are marked V1 to V6 (Figure 4-4). The correct cable must be attached to the corresponding electrode to ensure an accurate tracing. With some ECG machines, the electrode wires are placed with the wire connection toward the same direction, typically away from the direction of the feet. When using electrodes with tabs on which the alligator-type clips are used, chest and arm electrodes are placed with the tabs pointing downward toward the feet and the lower extremity electrodes pointing toward the head. Utilizing this technique reduces tension on the electrodes and provides a more "clean" or artifact-free tracing. Ultimately, refer to the manufacturer's directions in the operator's manual for the most optimum placement technique recommended for your equipment. In all cases, the electrodes should be secure and the lead wires should be supported.

The ECG lead wire cables should follow the contours of the body when attached to the ECG electrodes. Avoid crossing or looping the wires outside of the body, and check each wire once it is connected to ensure that there is no tension on the electrodes or leads. Individual loops may be used to take up slack and prevent looping outside the body, thus reducing tension on the electrode (Figure 4-5).

Figure 4-4 Color and letter coding identify the lead wires for an ECG machine.

Identifying Lead Wires

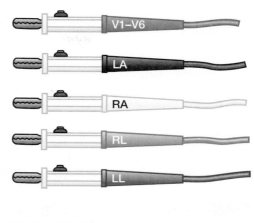

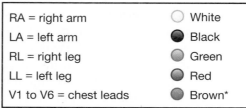

RA = right arm	○ White
LA = left arm	● Black
RL = right leg	◐ Green
LL = left leg	● Red
V1 to V6 = chest leads	● Brown*

*Check lead label V1 to V6 are not always brown.

Figure 4-5 Correct (*A.*) and incorrect (*B.*) lead cable placement. Avoid looping the wires outside the body, and check each wire once it is connected to ensure that there is no tension on the electrodes or leads.

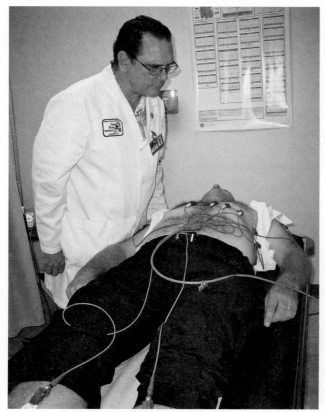

A. Correct Lead Wire Placement

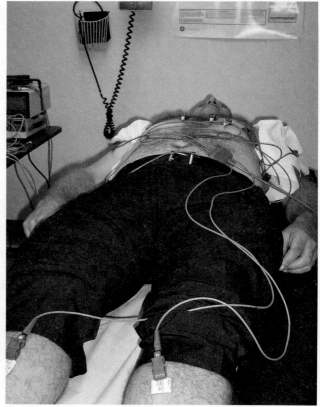

B. Incorrect Lead Wire Placement

Checkpoint Questions (LO 4.4)

1. How can you be certain you are attaching the lead wires to the electrodes properly?

   _____

   _____

2. Why should you place the limb electrodes before the chest electrodes?

   _____

   _____

4.5 Safety and Infection Control

When performing an ECG, you must always follow precautions. You must practice universal or standard precautions at all times. These precautions are followed in all situations in which job exposure to blood or body fluids is likely. Wash your hands carefully before and after the procedure to prevent transfer of microorganisms. Wear gloves if there is a risk of exposure to the patient's blood or other body fluids.

In the hospital, you will need to follow additional precautions for patients in isolation. Depending on the type of isolation, masks, eye protection, and gowns may also be necessary when entering the room. Follow the facility's policy and the guidelines provided in Table 4-3. You should know standard precautions related to all hospitalized patients and maintain them throughout the procedure. As a rule, it is better to wear gloves even if it is not necessary. Do not forget to wash your hands or perform hand hygiene before putting on the gloves and after removing them. See Appendix B for more information about Standard and Isolation Precautions including hand hygiene and personal protective equipment (PPE).

General safety guidelines and safety measures specific to the ECG procedure must also be practiced. Before beginning the procedure, you must identify, verify, and ensure that you are performing the procedure on the correct

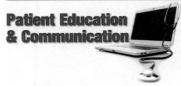

Patient Education & Communication

Relocating Electrodes

When moving the electrodes to a different location due to an amputation or bandages, you should document this on the 12-lead ECG recording.

Safety & Infection Control

Isolation Precautions

There are three types of isolation identified by the Centers for Disease Control and Prevention: airborne, droplet, and contact. Standard precautions include specific guidelines for caring for patients in isolation. See Appendix B for detail information about following these standards.

TABLE 4-3   Infection Control Guidelines for Isolation of Hospitalized Patients

In addition to standard precautions, follow these guidelines and the policy of your place of employment to prevent the spread of infections.

Airborne Precautions

For patients known or suspected to be infected with microorganisms transmitted by minute airborne droplets:

- Use a private room that has monitored negative air.
- Keep the room door closed and the patient in the room.
- Wear respiratory protection when entering the room of a patient with known or suspected infectious pulmonary tuberculosis.
- Wear special HEPA N-95, N-99, or N-100 masks when entering the room.
- Do not enter the room of a patient known or suspected to have rubeola or varicella if you are susceptible; if you must enter the room, wear respiratory protection.
- Limit the movement and transport of patients from the room to essential purposes only.
- Place a surgical mask on the patient if transport or movement is necessary.

Droplet Precautions

For patients known or suspected to be infected with microorganisms transmitted by droplets that can be generated by the patient during coughing, sneezing, talking, or the performance of procedures:

- Place patient in a private room (special air handling and ventilation are not necessary and the door may remain open).
- Wear a mask when working within 3 feet of the patient.
- Limit the movement and transport of the patient from the room to essential purposes only.
- Use a mask on the patient if transport or movement is necessary.

Contact Precautions

For patients known or suspected to be infected or colonized with microorganisms that can be transmitted by direct or indirect contact (*direct contact* includes hand or skin-to-skin contact that occurs when performing patient care that requires touching the patient's dry skin; *indirect contact* includes touching environmental surfaces or patient-care items in the patient's environment):

- Place patients in a private room.
- Wear gloves according to standard precautions.
- Wear gloves when entering the room and while providing patient care.
- Change gloves after having contact with infective material that may contain high concentrations of microorganisms, such as feces and wound drainage.
- Remove gloves before leaving the patient's room.
- Wash hands immediately.
- Do not touch potentially contaminated environmental surfaces or items in the patient's room after glove removal.
- All equipment must be disinfected after entering the patient's room. The 12-lead ECG machine needs to be wiped down immediately.

patient. Use two forms of identification, for example, the patient's name, birth date, and/or medical record number. Then you should raise the side rail on the unattended side of the patient's bed or exam table. If the patient is on an exam table, have him or her lie down and pull the extension out for his or her legs and feet. If the patient is on a gurney or hospital bed, remember to employ proper body mechanics by raising the bed to a comfortable working level and to raise the side rail on the opposite side of the bed for safety. Recall from Chapter 1, body mechanics is using movements that maintain proper posture and avoid muscle and bone injuries. Prior to performing the ECG, check to be sure that the grounding prong is securely attached to the plug. Plug the machine in securely. Ensure that the bed or exam table is not touching the wall or any electrical equipment. Be sure that the patient is not touching the

TABLE 4-4 Maintaining Safety During an ECG

- Check that the grounding prong is securely attached to the plug.
- Plug the machine in securely, making sure the cord is not separating from the receptacle.
- Ensure that the power cord insulation is intact.
- Remove the plug by pulling it out by the prong connection, not by pulling on the electrical cord.
- Raise the bed to a working height and return it to low position when completed.
- Keep the side rail up on the opposite side of the bed or exam table.
- Perform hand hygiene and wear gloves or other personal protective equipment as required.
- Use proper body mechanics at all times:
  - Feet apart and knees bent to lift and move
  - Have the patient assist or obtain assistance when necessary
  - Avoid twisting and reaching, and lift with your legs

bed or exam table frame or safety rail. Always check the insulation on the lead wires for cracks before each use. Ensure that all electronic devices the patient may have are turned off and removed from the patient (Table 4-4).

Prepare the patient for the procedure by first ensuring privacy and providing for the patient's safety and comfort during the ECG. The patient's door or curtain should be closed, and the patient's clothing appropriately removed and draped for privacy. Assist the patient to dress and undress as needed to provide for comfort and safety. Once the procedure is complete, you should clean the lead wires, leads, and machine. If you performed an ECG on a patient in isolation or with a contagious disease, you will need to clean the equipment properly to prevent the spread of infection. Observe the guidelines at your place of employment and the manufacturer's directions for the correct cleaning technique. Once you have completed the entire procedure, including cleanup, you should wash your hands. Remember to thank the patient and ask if he or she needs any further assistance.

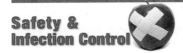

Safety & Infection Control

Practice proper body mechanics at all times to protect yourself from injuries when moving or lifting patients or other large or awkward items.

Checkpoint Questions (LO 4.5)

1. Name at least three things to do to ensure safety during an ECG.

   _____

   _____

2. Name at least three troubleshooting techniques during an ECG.

   _____

4.6 Operating the ECG Machine

Before operating the ECG machine, make sure you have done the following:

- Identified and communicated with the patient.
- Prepared the patient and the room.
- Provided for patient privacy.
- Provided for safety and infection control.
- Located and checked the equipment for functioning.
- Loaded the ECG graph paper, if necessary.
- Attached the electrodes and leads.

Now you should be ready to operate the ECG machine. For an automatic ECG, simply press the Run or Auto button. Check the LCD display for errors. If the ECG machine provides interpretation, it will print out along with the tracing. This process takes only about 15 to 20 seconds.

For a manual ECG machine, make sure the equipment is standardized and set to lead I. You may need to run a few complexes (complete ECG waveforms) and then insert a standardization mark. The mark should be set between the T wave of one complex and the P wave of the next. Follow specific directions provided in the operator's manual or according to your institution's policy and procedure.

Most ECG machines are automatic and mark the lead codes. If the equipment you are using does not, mark each code manually during the tracing. While the ECG is running, change the lead code dial, then mark each lead. You should run about 8 to 10 inches of complexes for leads I, II, and III. For the rest of the leads, 5 inches should be sufficient. Identify the recording with the patient's name, the date, and other required information. This is usually entered into the LCD display prior to the recording. With older machines you may need to mount the tracing upon completion of the ECG.

Checkpoint Questions (LO 4.6)

1. What must be done before you run the actual ECG tracing?

_____

_____

2. If you are running a manual ECG tracing, how long of a tracing do you need to run for leads I, II, and III?

_____

_____

4.7 Checking the ECG Tracing

Certain problems can occur when obtaining an ECG tracing. General troubleshooting guidelines should be followed to avoid these problems (Table 4-5). The most frequent problem is unwanted marks on the ECG. These marks are called artifact. The marks are not caused by the heart activity; they are caused by some other source of movement or electrical activity. When an ECG tracing has these unwanted marks, it is difficult or impossible to read. You are responsible for producing a correct tracing without artifact. In order to do this, you must first recognize artifact and then be able to eliminate it. The three most common causes of artifact are somatic tremor, wandering baseline, and alternating current interference (see Table 4-6 for ways to correct these causes of artifact).

TABLE 4-5 **Troubleshooting Techniques During an ECG**

- Perform and ensure good skin preparation.
- Use new (unused) electrodes and clean clips.
- Make sure personal electrical devices are turned off and removed from the patient.
- Ensure that the bed or examination table is not touching the wall or any electrical equipment.
- Ensure that the patient is not touching the frame, side rail, or any metal part of the bed or examination table.
- Always check the insulation on the lead wires for cracks before use.
- Ensure that there is no stress on the lead wires or electrodes.

TABLE 4-6 **Correcting Artifact**

Type of Artifact	Cause	Correction
Somatic tremor	Involuntary muscle movement: shivering, muscle tension, pain, fear	Reassure the patient, warm the patient, and encourage him or her to take slow, deep breaths.
	Voluntary movement: talking, chewing gum	Remind the patient not to make any movement during the procedure.
	Movement due to neuromuscular disorder such as Parkinson's disease	Have the patient put his or her hands, palms down, under the buttocks.
Wandering baseline	Improperly applied electrodes or poor skin preparation	Apply electrodes securely, make sure that the entire surface is in contact with the patient's skin.
	Pulling on electrodes from unsupported lead wires	Remove tension from lead wires.
	Oil, lotion, dirt, or hair on the skin under the electrodes	Clean the skin with alcohol and gauze or an alcohol prep pad.
	Old, corroded, or dirty electrodes or clips; Too little or dried out electrode gel	Use new disposable electrodes and store unused ones in a sealed plastic bag; if using gel, apply plenty of new solution to electrodes.
Alternating current (AC) interference	Improper grounding	Ensure that the plug has three prongs and is plugged into a grounded electrical outlet.
	Other electrical equipment	Unplug equipment and wait until any other procedure is done, if possible.
	Lead wires crossed and not pointed toward the hands and feet	Reposition the lead wires to ensure that they follow limbs and are pointed in the proper direction.
	Electrical wiring in the walls or ceiling	Move the patient's bed away from the wall (use a 45-degree angle if necessary).
	Corroded or dirty leads	Clean the leads after each use.

Somatic Tremor

Sometimes a patient's muscles will move, either voluntarily or involuntarily, which can produce **somatic tremor**, also known as body tremor. Movement of the muscles of the body is controlled by electrical voltages. These voltages are erratic, unlike the cardiac voltage, which is consistent. Somatic tremor appears as erratic spikes on the ECG tracing (Figure 4-6).

Troubleshooting

Multiple ECGs

If your hospitalized patient requires daily ECGs for comparison by the physician, the ECG tracing may look different if the electrodes are placed in different sites on the chest and limbs. Each time you record an ECG on the patient, place the leads on the same site or as close as possible to the placement from the previous ECG. Some facilities will permit placing small marks on the patient to ensure that electrode placement will be consistent for multiple (serial) ECGs.

You are doing your third ECG on a patient in three days. Where should the electrodes be placed?

_____

_____

Voluntary muscle movements are due to tension, fear, gum chewing, talking, uncomfortable position, or pain. They may also be due to shivering or tense muscles. You should identify the correct cause before proceeding with the ECG. Knowing the cause will help you eliminate the artifact. Warm or reassure the patient if he or she is cold or frightened. Encourage slow, deep breaths to help calm the patient. Remind the patient to refrain from moving or talking.

Sometimes involuntary muscle movements are due to Parkinson's disease or other neuromuscular disorders. These are more difficult to control. Have patients who suffer from neuromuscular disorders put their hands, palms down, under their buttocks. This will decrease the tremor and improve the tracing. If a patient has this type of tremor, it should be recorded on the ECG tracing.

Interrupted baseline (Flatline) - leads are not placed correctly

Figure 4-6 Somatic tremor appears as erratic spikes on the ECG tracing.

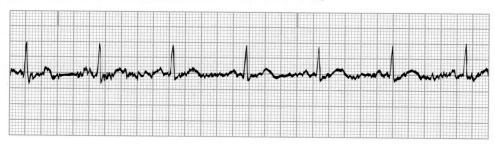

Figure 4-7 Wandering baseline occurs when the baseline of the ECG tracing drifts away from the center of the ECG graph paper.

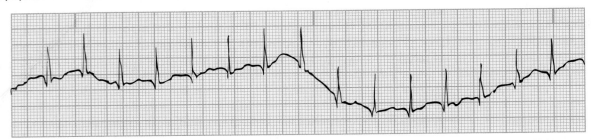

Wandering Baseline (Baseline Shift)

Wandering baseline, or baseline shift, occurs when the tracing drifts away from the center of the graph paper (Figure 4-7). Baseline shift can have many causes. Typically, it is due to improper electrode application such as the following:

- Too loose or incorrect electrode application
- Tension or pulling on electrode lead wires
- Too little electrode gel or solution
- Old or dried out electrode gel or solution
- Corroded or dirty electrodes
- Oil, lotion, dirt, or hair under the electrodes
- Poor or no skin preparation

To avoid problems with wandering baseline, apply the electrodes securely and make sure they are not too loose or tight. Be certain that the entire surface is in contact with the patient's skin. Check the lead wires and remove any tension from them. Use fresh electrode gel or new disposable electrodes. Make sure that previously opened electrodes have been stored in a plastic bag or container. Clean the reusable leads after each use. Clean the patient's skin carefully before applying electrodes.

Alternating Current (AC) Interference

Alternating current is normally present in all electrical equipment and wiring in the walls. Sometimes the wires can radiate or leak a small amount of energy into the immediate surrounding area. When a patient is present in this area, the patient's body may pick up some of the current. This current is then registered on the ECG and is called **AC (alternating current) interference**. AC interference will appear as uniform small spikes on the ECG tracing (Figure 4-8).

Many different things can cause AC interference artifact. These include improper grounding, other electrical equipment, lead wires crossed, and corroded or dirty electrodes. Eliminating the cause and using proper technique can prevent AC interference artifact. Eliminating sources of electrical current, ensuring proper grounding of the machine, and attaching the lead wires correctly can reduce AC interference.

The cause of AC interference is sometimes difficult to determine. You may still have AC interference even after you have checked that the machine is properly grounded, the lead wires are correct, and other equipment is turned off. In order to find the source, time permitting, you can try this technique. Run lead I, lead II, and lead III, and look for interference.

Figure 4-8 Alternating current (AC) interference appears as uniform small spikes on the ECG tracing.

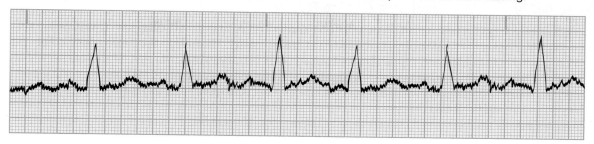

TABLE 4-7 Troubleshooting AC Interference

Leads with Most AC Interference Noted	Source of Interference or Direction
Leads I and II	Right arm
Leads I and III	Left arm
Leads II and III	Left leg

Evaluate each strip for interference to determine the direction or source of interference (Table 4-7). For example, if you have the most interference in leads II and III, the source is probably near or on the left leg. You may need to rotate the bed or exam table at a 45-degree angle away from the source. Also, do not forget the proper placement of the lead cables. They should follow the body contours and be lying flat against the skin. In addition, the power cord should not touch the bed or exam table frame. This is another possible source of electrical interference.

Artifact can also be caused by other sources. High-tension wires and transformers on a power pole and diathermy machines used to give high-frequency currents as heat treatments can cause AC interference. Electro-cautery, IV pumps, feeding tubes, and x-ray machines can also interfere if they are in the room or an adjacent room. Even the electrical wires in the walls, ceiling, and floor, although they are not visible, can cause artifact. Most ECG machines have a battery that allows you to unplug and still perform the ECG. Unplugging the machine eliminates any AC interference that may be produced from the electrical outlet.

There are some additional problems you may encounter when obtaining an ECG. One example is an interrupted baseline on one or more leads. This appears as a flat line on the tracing. This could occur when a wire is not plugged in correctly or is loose. If a flat line occurs on more than one lead, it may be that the wires have been switched. Check your machine cables and connections. Ensure that the machine is set to obtain a tracing. Do not forget to check for loose or broken lead wires, which may also cause a break in the complexes or an interrupted baseline.

After troubleshooting any problem, if you cannot correct it, report it to your supervisor. If it is an AC interference problem, the biomedical engineering department, if available, may need to track down the source of the interference. It could also be that the machine requires service. In this case, the manufacturer should be called for information and assistance.

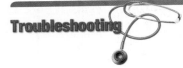

Troubleshooting

Handling a Flatline Tracing

If a flat line without deflections occurs during the tracing, it could be asystole (indicates no heart beat). Remain calm and check the patient first, since the patient is your number one concern. If the patient is able to respond, check the electrodes, lead wires, and cables.

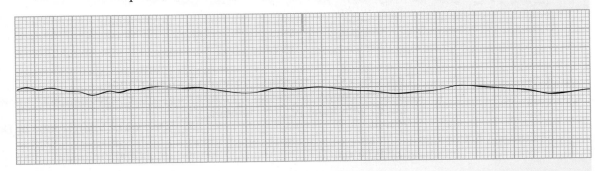

The patient's ECG tracing looks like the one pictured here. What should you do?

_____

Checkpoint Questions (LO 4.7)

1. What is the most likely cause of the following artifact?

_____

_____

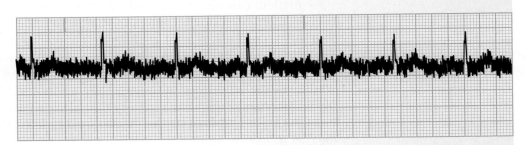

2. Name three causes of wandering baseline.

_____

_____

4.8 Reporting ECG Results

When you have completed an ECG, use the method your facility requires for reporting the results. Check your facility policy to be certain you are placing the completed ECG tracings in the appropriate place. In many situations, you will be required to make two copies, one to be placed on the patient's chart and the other to be read by the consulting physician. In the hospital, the second copy is often taken back to the ECG department or stored on the computer for evaluation in the ECG laboratory. The second copy may also be placed in a box at the nursing station where the patient is located. In an ambulatory care facility, it may be attached to the front of the chart and/or placed on the physician's desk.

Some facilities have a computer that can read the ECG electronically and/or store it electronically in a central database for future reference. In addition, sometimes ECG tracings are faxed or electronically sent to other locations. These procedures require special equipment. You may be asked to perform either of these procedures. If so, you must be trained using your facility's equipment. If the ECG was ordered stat (immediately), you will need to give the results directly and immediately to your superior or the physician. If your supervisor is not available, place the results on top of the chart, find your supervisor, and inform him or her that the ECG has been completed. Remember, in a stat situation, the patient may have a condition that needs immediate treatment, and no time should be wasted.

As previously discussed, billing is another issue to consider when reporting completion of an ECG. When you enter the data into the machine or on the designated form, it must be complete and accurate. If the patient is not charged for the procedure, this can have an adverse effect on the hospital's finances and subsequently on your job. Check the facility policy to be certain you have completed the necessary steps to ensure that the patient will be charged.

In many facilities, the information is entered into a computer to be sent to the billing department. You may need to enter the patient's diagnosis, which is provided by the physician and is found on the chart. Each diagnosis has a special diagnostic code, known as an *ICD-9 code.* In addition, as of 2011 ICD-10 codes will be in effect. In most cases, you will need to identify the correct code, either ICD-9 or ICD-10, when entering the information for the billing department. Using these codes helps ensure that the facility is reimbursed for the procedure.

Checkpoint Questions (LO 4.8)

1. How should you report a stat ECG?

   _____

   _____

2. Why is it critical to enter the correct and complete data into the computer when performing an ECG?

   _____

   _____

4.9 Equipment Maintenance

Care and maintenance of the ECG machine must be done and is your responsibility. Become familiar with the manufacturer's instructions for operation and maintenance of the ECG machine. The operator's manual for the machine you are using will include specific directions about routine care and maintenance. General day-to-day care and maintenance include

Figure 4-9 This alligator-type clip is frequently used for the ECG. Wipe such clips clean after use to prevent electrolyte gel or paste from getting stuck between the teeth of the clip.

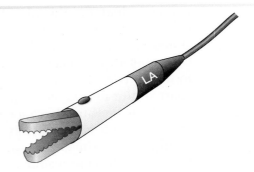

Safety & Infection Control

Maintaining the ECG Equipment

Cleaning the ECG machine and maintaining the supplies are necessary for safe and efficient ECG recording and accurate tracings.

cleaning the ECG machine and stocking the supplies, such as electrodes, skin preparation, paper, and cleaning supplies.

Keep the ECG machine clean to prevent transmission of infection and to create a positive image of yourself and the facility where you are employed. Use a small amount of nonabrasive cleaner on the equipment case, cover, and control panel. Wipe the machine dry with a soft cloth. Follow the specific directions in the operator's manual for the disinfection procedure.

The cables and reusable electrodes should be disinfected frequently. Use a soft cloth moistened with disinfectant and wipe the entire cable and reusable electrode. You can also use packaged disinfectant wipes if they are available. To determine the type of disinfectant you should use, check the policy at the facility where you are working. Keep these available on the ECG cart. Do not place the cables or ECG machine in fluid or use heat sterilization. Do not use acetone, ether, or other harsh chemicals or solvents. Always follow the manufacturer's directions for best results.

When using disposable electrodes, carefully maintain the alligator clips used for attachment. Check them to ensure that the pins fit snugly on the electrode. Check for small amounts of electrolyte paste or gel that may cling to the clips. These bits of paste may prevent good contact with the electrodes (Figure 4-9).

Wipe down the patient cables and lead wires with a damp cloth. Replace them neatly on the ECG machine for storage (Figure 4-10). Inspect them regularly for cracks or fraying. Replace any cables that are damaged. See Procedure Checklist 4-1 at the end of this chapter to practice recording an ECG.

Checkpoint Question (LO 4.9)

1. Why should you know how to troubleshoot and maintain the equipment for an ECG?

_____

_____

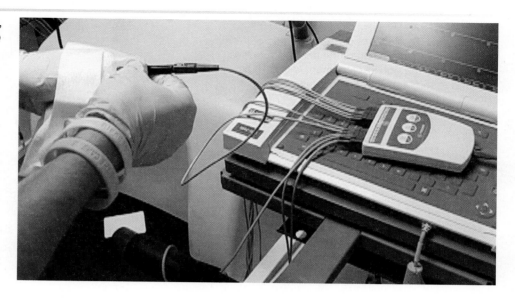

Figure 4-10 Before storing, clean each lead wire and clip with disinfectant. For safety, inspect each wire for cracks or fraying.

4.10 Pediatric ECG

When preparing a child for an ECG, it is important to give simple directions that he or she can understand. Identify yourself and explain what you are going to do. Allow the child to ask questions. Avoid technical words like *electrodes* and *electrocardiogram.* Use the word "stickers" to describe electrodes. If the child is fearful of the "stickers," allow him to place the stickers on a toy, doll, or parent. This will show the child that the procedure does not hurt. Explain that you are going to take a "picture" of the child's heart. Because children can usually identify with picture taking, this will help them understand that they need to be still during the "picture."

Always identify the child by name and check his or her identification wristband. If the parents are present, you may allow them to stay. For a small child or infant, the parent can assist by letting the child lie quietly in his or her arms. A fussy infant may be soothed by using a pacifier. If you are unable to soothe an irritable infant, you may need to wait until he or she falls asleep. For older children, you can allow them to apply their own arm and leg electrodes. Adolescents may prefer to be alone with you during the procedure. Ask them if they would like their parent(s) to stay or leave.

When the ECG tracing is completed, talk about the procedure. Give verbal praise and be supportive. Reward the child with an age-appropriate item or activity such as stickers or a special trip to the playroom.

Special smaller electrodes are available and should be used for pediatric patients. In addition, for infants or children with very fast heart rates, you may find it necessary to adjust the paper speed to 50 mm/sec. This will allow the physician to view each of the deflections on the ECG tracing. If you make this adjustment, don't forget to note on the ECG recording when completed.

An ECG for a child is performed with the same lead placement as for an adult. The chest lead V6 must be placed exactly on the midaxillary line. Because of the small size of the chest, correct placement becomes even

Figure 4-11 For infants and small children, you may need to place V3 on the right side of the chest to prevent crowding of the chest electrodes. This alternate method of placement is known as V3R and is sometimes used on adults.

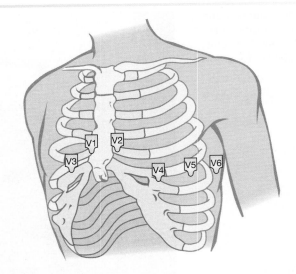

more important. Small differences in placement can make a difference in the ECG tracing. Because of crowding on the chest, it may be necessary to move the V3 lead to the right side of the chest. It should be placed on the right side in the same location as it normally would be on the left. This is known as a V3 right (V3R) (Figure 4-11).

Checkpoint Questions (LO 4.10)

1. Why do you frequently need to adjust the paper speed to 50 mm/sec for infants and small children?

_____

_____

2. When you change the paper speed to 50 mm/sec, what should you do?

_____

4.11 Cardiac Monitoring

Patients may require continuous cardiac monitoring at the scene of an emergency, in the hospital during or after surgery, or when they have cardiac, pulmonary, or electrolyte problems. In addition to the cables, monitor, and disposable supplies (electrodes), the monitoring systems used in a hospital may include devices that monitor the heart rate and rhythm, blood pressure, cardiac output, and arterial blood oxygen saturation.

During continuous cardiac monitoring, typically either lead II or a modified chest lead (MCL) is used because they provide the best ability to view the P wave. Exact placement of the electrodes affects the view of the heart and the resulting waveform. Three electrodes are placed, and the placement may vary depending upon the system used.

- White cable with electrode (labeled RA) at the right arm location
- Black cable with electrode (labeled LA) at the left arm location
- Red cable with electrode (labeled F or LL) at the left leg location

During continuous cardiac monitoring, a 12-lead ECG also can be performed. See Procedure Checklist 4.2 at the end of this chapter to review and practice this procedure.

Checkpoint Question (LO 4-11)

1. What is the difference between continuous cardiac monitoring and a routine ECG?

4.12 Special Patient Considerations

Occasionally you will need to record lead tracings other than the basic 12. You may need to record a heart rhythm strip, which is a single strip showing only one lead tracing. The heart rhythm is usually produced in lead II and is about 10 seconds of running time. Many ECG machines will print this strip on the bottom of the 12-lead tracing or following the completion of the 12-lead recording. A rhythm strip will be used to check for heart rhythm abnormalities. You may also be asked to provide a V4R on an adult for cases of right ventricular infarction.

You may encounter other circumstances that require you to make modifications to the basic 12-lead procedure. When changes in the placement of leads is necessary for any reason, a note should be included on the tracing. Consider the following when placing leads and recording tracings in a patient's chart:

- V1 and V2 may have to be placed higher due to recently placed breast implants.
- Do not place the electrode on a woman's breast. Move the breast with the back of your hand and place the electrode under it. If this is done, note on the ECG tracing that the electrodes (V3, V4, and V5) are placed lower than required.
- If a woman has had a mastectomy, be careful placing the electrodes, the skin may be fragile. Note that the patient had a mastectomy and which breast is affected on the ECG tracing.
- If the patient is an amputee, place the limb leads on the upper chest and lower abdomen instead of on the arms and legs. Make sure the leads are in the same place on each side of the body.
- Alternate locations may be necessary due to interference from burns, dressings, chest tubes, etc. Remember to document if electrodes are moved to a different location and why.
- A pregnant woman should have the lower limb leads placed on the thighs, not the abdomen. Place the patient on her left side slightly, by using a small rolled towel under the right hip to reduce pressure on

the inferior vena cava. Document on the ECG that the patient is pregnant and the number of months.

- Geriatric patients generally have thin skin, which is part of the normal aging process. Apply the electrodes carefully and remove gently to prevent damage to their skin. Geriatric patients may have some readings on the ECG tracing that are age-related and are considered normal.

- If the patient is unable to lie on his or her back, be sure to indicate on the tracing the position of the patient during the tracing.

- When someone is in a permanent fetal position with arms drawn tightly over his or her chest, you may need to place the electrodes on the back. They will need to be positioned over the heart on the left side of the back. Today's small, thin, disposable electrodes are easier to place under a patient's arms, so place on the back only if necessary.

- A condition known as **dextrocardia,** is when the heart is on the right side of the chest rather than on the left. In this case the physician would order a right-side 12-lead ECG. The leads are reversed (mirror image) from the usual lead placement. This is the only case where the aVR tracing will produce a positive deflection. On the ECG tracing report, you should indicate that you did a right-side ECG (Figure 4-12).

You may be asked to perform a right side or posterior ECG as ordered by the physician. These expanded data tracings enable the physician to detect problems with the right ventricle and posterior wall of the left ventricle.

The leads are commonly identified as right precordial leads V1R, V2R, V3R, V4R, V5R, V6R and posterior leads V7, V8, V9, V9R, V8R, and V7R. These additional leads are periodically requested by the physician after a standard 12-lead ECG has been obtained.

Some facilities will have specialized equipment, but it is not essential. You can obtain the ECG tracing by adding these leads with the standard 12-lead ECG machine. This procedure can be simple when you know where to place the electrodes. First, run a standard 12-lead ECG as described earlier. Second, using the precordial cables (V1-V6), place additional electrodes in the appropriate locations and run a second 12-lead ECG. It is important that you do not forget to write on the labels of the new leads.

NOTE: As with all 12-lead ECGs, it is important that the patient lie as still as possible to avoid artifact.

dextrocardia When the heart is on the opposite or right side of the chest.

Figure 4-12 Use these lead placements for patients with dextrocardia, a condition in which the left ventricle, left atrium, and aortic arch are located on the right side of the chest.

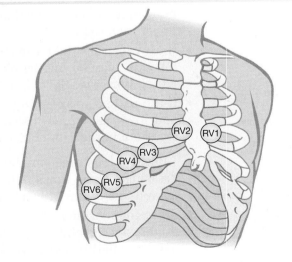

The *right side 12-lead ECG* will have the right side of the chest leads placed in a "mirror" image of the standard 12-lead ECG, meaning the same anatomic levels but on the opposite side of the chest. V1 is placed on the 4th intercostal space, left sternal margin, V2 is placed on the 4th intercostal space, right sternal margin, skip V3 (as always), and continue toward the patient's right (see Figure 4-13*A*).

The *posterior 12-lead ECG* (or leads on the patient's back) is focusing on the posterior aspect of the heart:

- **V7** is located at the left **posterior axillary line** (an imaginary line on the back of the chest that runs vertically from the shoulder down on the outer edge of the rib cage) in a straight line from V6. You will reposition the V1 lead to this location.
- **Skip V8** is located at the left **midscapular line** (an imaginary line on the back of the chest that runs vertically through the center of the scapula) in a straight line from V7; it will be placed half-way between V7 and V9. You will reposition the V2 lead to this location.
- **V9** is located at the left **paraspinous line** (an imaginary line next to the spine that runs vertically along the side of the spine) in a straight line from the V7 lead. You will move the V3 lead to this location. (Go back and place V8 half-way between V7 and V9 in a straight line.)
- **V9R** is placed at the right paraspinous line in a straight line from the V9 lead. You will reposition the V4 lead to this location.
- **V8R** is located at the right midscapular line (an imaginary line on the back of the chest that runs vertically through the center of the scapula) in a straight line from V7; it will be placed half-way between V7R and V9R. You will reposition the V5 lead to this location.
- **V7R** is located at the right posterior axillary line (an imaginary line on the back of the chest that runs vertically from the shoulder down on the outer edge of the rib cage). You will reposition the V6 lead to this location (see Figure 4-13*B*)

When you record any ECG tracing, it is critical that you indicate any modification in electrode placement as it will effect the ECG tracing because the electrodes are focused on a different aspect of the heart and could potentially provide the wrong information if not noted.

NOTE: Limb lead cables and electrode locations do not change. The only electrode and cable changes are on the patient's chest.

posterior axillary line Imaginary line on the back that runs vertically from the shoulder down on the outer edge of the rib cage.

midscapular line Imaginary line on the back that runs vertically through the center of the scapula.

paraspinous line Imaginary line on the spine that runs vertically through the side of the spine.

Checkpoint Questions (LO 4.12)

1. What should you remember when asked to record a 15-lead or 18-lead ECG?

_____

_____

2. What additional ECG procedure may the doctor order for a patient with dextrocardia? Why?

_____

_____

Figure 4-13 (A.) Right Side Precordial leads, showing mirror image of standard chest lead placement. (B.) Posterior 12-Lead locations. Cables V1 through V6 are placed going from the patient's posterior left in order to the patients posterior right.

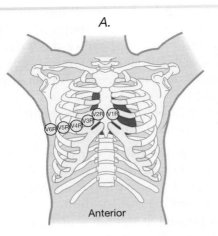

A.

Anterior

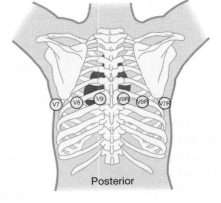

B.

Posterior

V1R	Fourth intercostal space left sternal margin
V2R	Fourth intercostal space right sternal margin
V3R	Midway between locations V1 and V4R, right chest
V4R	Midclavicular line in the fifth intercostal space, right chest
V5R	Anterior axillary line on the same horizontal level as V4R. right chest
V6R	Midaxillary line on the same horizontal level as V4R and V5R, right chest

V7	Left posterior axillary line, V6 level
V8	V8 (skip) place at midpoint on a horizontal line between V7 and V9
V9	Left paraspinal border, V6 level
V9R	Right paraspinous border
V8R	V8R (Skip) place at midpoint on a horizontal line between V7R and V9R
V7R	Right posterior axillary line

4.13 Handling Emergencies

Cardiac or Respiratory Arrest

During a cardiac or respiratory arrest, frequently called a Code Blue emergency, be ready to perform the tracing as quickly and efficiently as possible. An ECG is usually ordered "stat" in these situations. If possible, enter the patient's information into the ECG machine. Remain available but out of the way until the ECG is needed. You may need to take just the machine into the room and not the cart, if space is limited.

Because the patient's condition changes frequently during a Code Blue emergency, you may need to perform two ECGs in a row. Perform the first ECG and leave the electrodes in place in order to perform the second ECG quickly. Indicate on the tracing "repeat ECG—same lead placement." This will make the physician aware that the electrodes were not removed in between tracings.

Seizure

seizure An interruption of the electrical activity in the brain that causes involuntary muscle movement and sometimes unconsciousness.

If a patient has a **seizure** during the ECG, stay with him or her. Protect the patient from injury. Do not try to restrain the patient. Call for help, and report the seizure. Once the seizure is over, perform the ECG again and write on the ECG strip "postseizure."

1. What should you do if your patient has a seizure while you are starting to record an ECG?

_____

_____

Chapter Summary

Learning Outcomes	Summary	Pages
4.1 Prepare the patient, room, and equipment for an ECG.	The patient, the room, and the equipment must be properly prepared prior to performing an ECG.	83–84
4.2 Describe the communication needed during the ECG procedure, including the actions to take if a patient refuses.	When a patient refuses an ECG, you should identify the cause, alleviate any fears, notify your supervisor, and document the refusal on the medical record.	85–86
4.3 Identify the anatomical landmarks needed to apply the ECG chest electrodes.	In order to place the electrodes properly for an ECG, you must be able to locate anatomical landmarks, including the midclavicular line, anterior axillary line, intercostal spaces, suprasternal notch, and the angle of Louis.	87
4.4 Demonstrate the procedure for applying the electrodes and lead wires for a 12-lead ECG and cardiac monitoring.	An ECG is performed using the ECG machine, lead wires, and electrodes. The patient must be identified correctly, the tracing must be correct, and safety must be maintained during the procedure.	88–90
4.5 Identify at least three ways to prevent infection and provide for safety during the ECG procedure.	To ensure safety and prevent infection during an ECG: • follow standard precautions, most importantly hand hygiene; • follow isolation precautions and use personal protective equipment when necessary; • check the plug and power cord; • raise the bed and keep the side rail up; and • use two patient identifiers before the procedure.	92–94
4.6 Describe the procedure for recording and reporting a 12-lead ECG.	The ECG procedure includes identifying, communicating, and preparing the patient, maintaining safety, privacy, and infection control, checking and preparing the room and equipment, attaching the electrodes and leads, and then operating the ECG machine and reporting the results.	95
4.7 Identify types of artifact and how to prevent or correct them.	Three types of artifact include: • somatic tremor caused by muscle movement, • wandering baseline, usually caused by improperly applied electrodes, or poor skin prep, • AC interference, caused by some type of electrical interference.	95–100

(Continued)

Learning Outcomes	Summary	Pages
4.8 Describe how to report the ECG results.	ECGs are recorded electronically and in paper fashion. Although they may be "read" by the machine, they must be provided promptly in a proper format to the practitioner who will be interpreting them.	100–101
4.9 Identify the steps for cleaning and caring for the ECG equipment.	Upon completion of an ECG, the equipment must be cleaned and stored properly according to your facility guidelines and the manufacturer's recommendations.	101–103
4.10 Explain variations used for pediatric ECG procedures.	During a pediatric ECG, the chest lead V3 may need to be placed on the right side of the chest due to the small size of the chest.	103–104
4.11 Distinguish between a routine ECG and cardiac monitoring.	Cardiac monitoring uses three leads with different placements.	104–105
4.12 Summarize special patient circumstances when performing an ECG.	Many special patient considerations can occur during an ECG, such as for female patients, pregnant patients, amputees, and geriatric patients.	105–108
4.13 Recall the steps for handling an emergency during the ECG.	During a cardiac or respiratory arrest; perform the ECG stat; in some cases, just take the machine into the room and be prepared to run two ECGs in a row. During a seizure; remain calm, do not restrain the patient, and call for help.	108

Chapter Review

Matching I

Match the landmark with its location. Place the letter on the corresponding line. (LO 4.3)

_____ **1.** suprasternal notch

_____ **2.** fifth intercostal space

_____ **3.** manubrium

_____ **4.** right clavicle

a. extends from the sternum to the scapula

b. the space between the fifth and sixth ribs

c. the top of the sternum

d. the dip at the base of the neck just above where the clavicle attaches to the sternum

Match the lead to its correct placement. Place the letter on the corresponding line. (LO 4.4)

_____ **5.** V1

_____ **6.** V2

_____ **7.** V3

_____ **8.** V4

_____ **9.** V5

_____ **10.** V6

a. fifth intercostal space, at the anterior axillary line

b. fourth intercostal space, left sternal border

c. fifth intercostal space, at the midaxillary line

d. fifth intercostal space at the midclavicular line

e. fourth intercostal space, right sternal border

f. halfway between V2 and V4

Match the imaginary line with its location. Place the letter on the corresponding line. (LO 4.3)

_____ **11.** midclavicular line

_____ **12.** midaxillary line

_____ **13.** anterior axillary line

a. front of the axilla

b. middle of the axilla

c. usually passes through the nipple line

Multiple Choice

Circle the correct answer.

14. For placement of the electrodes, how is the ICS located? (LO 4.3)

    a. Locating the sternum and feeling for a dip at the edge

    b. Finding the ribs near the nipple line

    c. Locating the clavicle and feeling for a dent directly below it

    d. Locating the space between the clavicle and V4

15. What would be the first and most appropriate thing to say if a patient refuses an ECG? (LO 4.2)
    a. "Will you tell me why you don't wish to have an ECG done?"
    b. "Don't worry; it only takes a few seconds."
    c. "Your doctor has ordered this test, and it must be done."
    d. "I will have to report you to my supervisor immediately."

16. When applying chest leads, V4 is placed (LO 4.4)
    a. midway between V3 and V5.
    b. at the fourth ICS, right sternal border.
    c. at the fifth ICS, left midclavicular line.
    d. at the fourth ICS, left sternal border.

17. When applying chest leads, V2 is placed (LO 4.4)
    a. midway between V3 and V5.
    b. at the fourth ICS, right sternal border.
    c. at the fifth ICS, left midclavicular line.
    d. at the fourth ICS, left sternal border.

18. To prevent disease transmission during an ECG, you should (LO 4.5)
    a. check the ground prong.
    b. wash your hands.
    c. raise the side rail.
    d. lower the bed.

19. Safety procedures specific to the ECG include the following: (LO 4.5)
    a. Wash hands, clean up all spills immediately.
    b. Lower bed, raise the side rail.
    c. Check the ground prong, give the call signal.
    d. Check the lead wires, insulation, and ground prong.

20. Which of the following would *not* be done prior to performing an ECG? (LO 4.1)
    a. Receive and validate the order.
    b. Clean the leads, and write ECG variations on tracing.
    c. Check and change paper if necessary.
    d. Enter patient data into machine.

21. When applying chest leads, V1 is placed (LO 4.4)
    a. midway between V3 and V5.
    b. at the fourth ICS, right sternal border.
    c. at the fifth ICS, left midclavicular line.
    d. at the fourth ICS, left sternal border.

22. Marks on the ECG tracing caused by another source of activity are (LO 4.7)
    a. asystole.
    b. conduction marks.
    c. artifacts.
    d. wandering baseline.

23. Somatic tremors are caused by (LO 4.7)
    a. electrical current leak.
    b. tracing drifts away from center.
    c. muscle movement.
    d. contact with another electrical device.

24. You noticed a wandering baseline on the ECG tracing. What measure(s) should you do to correct the problem? (LO 4.7)
   a. Apply new electrodes.
   b. Reposition the electrodes.
   c. Ensure that the wires are not crossed.
   d. All of the above.

25. You notice that leads I and II have a lot of artifact while recording a 12-lead ECG. Which electrode is probably not placed appropriately? (LO 4.6)
   a. Right arm
   b. Left arm
   c. Left leg
   d. None of the above

26. Which of the following is *not* a specific type of isolation precaution implemented for hospitalized patients? (LO 4.5)
   a. AIDS precautions
   b. Droplet precautions
   c. Airborne precautions
   d. Contact precautions

27. Which of the following are ways to correct AC interference? (LO 4.7)
   a. Unplug electrical equipment, move bed away from wall.
   b. Apply electrodes securely, remove tension from lead wires.
   c. Have patient place hands under his or her buttocks, remind patient not to move.
   d. Replace loose electrodes and have the patient turn slightly to the side.

28. Which of the following are ways to correct somatic tremor? (LO 4.7)
   a. Unplug electrical equipment, move bed away from wall.
   b. Apply electrodes securely, remove tension from lead wires.
   c. Have patient place hands under his or her buttocks, remind patient not to move.
   d. Replace loose electrodes, have the patient turn slightly to the side.

29. Which of the following are ways to correct wandering baseline? (LO 4.7)
   a. Unplug electrical equipment, move bed away from wall.
   b. Apply electrodes securely, remove tension from lead wires.
   c. Have patient place hands under his or her buttocks, remind patient not to move.
   d. Replace loose electrodes, have the patient turn slightly to the side.

30. When applying chest leads, V6 is placed (LO 4.3)
   a. in line with V4 on the midaxillary line.
   b. at the fourth ICS, right sternal border.
   c. at the fifth ICS, left midclavicular line.
   d. at the fourth ICS, left sternal border.

31. If your patient has an amputated left lower leg, you should place the electrodes as follows: (LO 4.11)
   a. LL on left upper leg, RL on right lower leg
   b. LL on left lower abdomen, RL on right lower abdomen
   c. LL on left lower leg, RL on right upper leg
   d. LL on left lower abdomen, RL on right lower leg

32. When performing a 12-lead ECG on an infant or small child, do all of the following *except* (LO 4.10)

   a. speak in children's terms.
   b. use smaller ECG electrodes.
   c. perform a V3R tracing.
   d. use a special ECG machine.

33. Approach the patient from the _____ when performing an ECG. (LO 4.6)

   a. left side
   b. right side
   c. top
   d. bottom

True/False

Read each statement, and determine if it is true or false. Circle the T or F. For false (F) statements, correct them to "make them true" on the lines provided.

T   F   34. Natural skin oils, moisturizers, and perspiration can contribute to artifact on an ECG tracing. (LO 4.7)

_____

T   F   35. The letter *R* is placed after any tracing when the electrode is not in its usual position and has been placed on the right side of the patient's chest. (LO 4.11)

_____

T   F   36. Because an ECG is *not* an invasive procedure, it is not necessary to wear personal protective equipment (PPE) when performing this procedure under any circumstances. (LO 4.5)

_____

Matching II

_____ 37. intercostal space (ICS) (LO 4.3)

_____ 38. midaxillary line (LO 4.3)

_____ 39. stat (LO 4.12)

_____ 40. anterior axillary line (LO 4.3)

_____ 41. artifact (LO 4.7)

_____ 42. seizure (LO 4.12)

_____ 43. midclavicular line (LO 4.3)

a. an interruption of the electrical activity of the brain that causes involuntary muscle movement and sometimes unconsciousness

b. a boney prominence located approximately 1 inch below the suprasternal notch, where the manubrium and the body of the sternum are joined

c. outer edge of the sternum

d. the space between two ribs

e. an imaginary line on the chest that runs vertically through the center of the clavicle

f. when the tracing of an ECG drifts away from the center of the paper; also called baseline shift (It has many causes, all of which can be corrected.)

_____ **44.** somatic tremor
(LO 4.7)

_____ **45.** angle of Louis
(LO 4.3)

_____ **46.** AC interference
(LO 4.7)

_____ **47.** wandering baseline
(LO 4.7)

_____ **48.** sternal border
(LO 4.3)

_____ **49.** dextrocardia
(LO 4.11)

_____ **50.** midscapular line
(LO 4.3)

g. an imaginary vertical line that starts in the middle of the axillary region (armpit)

h. unwanted marks on the ECG caused by electrical activity from sources other than the heart

i. unwanted markings on the ECG tracing caused by other electrical sources

j. an imaginary vertical line on the back that starts in the middle of the scapula

k. immediately

l. voluntary or involuntary muscle movement; also known as body tremor

m. an imaginary vertical line starting at the edge of the chest where the axillary region begins

n. when the heart is on the reverse side of the chest

51. (1.–9.) Identify the landmarks on the chest drawing. Label each line. (LO 4.3)

1. _____
2. _____
3. _____
4. _____
5. _____
6. _____
7. _____
8. _____
9. _____

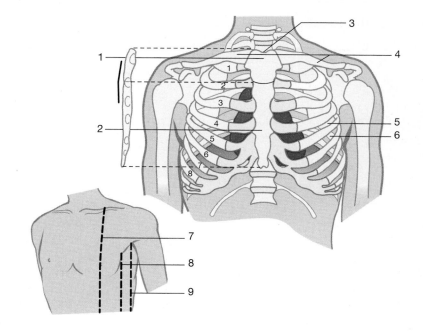

52. Identify each lead and describe its location for a 12-lead ECG. (LO 4.4)

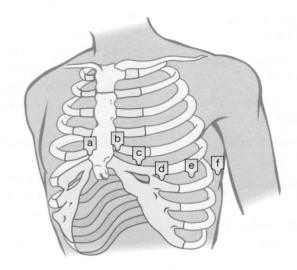

a. _____

b. _____

c. _____

d. _____

e. _____

f. _____

Critical Thinking Application *What Should You Do?*

Read the following situations, and use your critical thinking skills to determine how you would handle each. Write your answer in detail in the space provided.

53. You are working in a local hospital and are called to perform an ECG on a patient who is in a coma and was admitted to the hospital because of a myocardial infarction. You set up the machine and begin to run the ECG, and the tracing is a flat line. You know that a flat line is serious. What would be the first thing you do? (LO 4.11)

_____

_____

54. Your patient has Parkinson's disease. During the procedure, you notice a lot of artifact. What kind of artifact would you expect it to be? How could you reduce the artifact? (LO 4.7)

_____

_____

55. You are performing an ECG on a patient, and he or she begins to complain of chest pain. What should you do? (LO 4.12)

_____

_____

56. When you finish performing an ECG, the patient asks you for a copy. What do you do? (LO 4.8)

_____

_____

Get Connected *Internet Activity*

Visit the McGraw-Hill Higher Education Online Learning Center *Electrocardiography for Healthcare Professionals* Web site at **www.mhhe.com/boothecg3e** to complete the following activity.

1. 15- and 18-lead ECG. The American Association of Critical Care Nurses describes the steps and lead placement for obtaining more than the normal 12-lead ECG. Search their Web site or use a search engine to find information that will help you understand the rationale and placement of the electrodes. (LO 4.11)

Using the Student CD

Now that you have completed the material in the chapter text, return to the student CD and complete any chapter activities you have not yet done. Practice your terminology with the "Key Term Concentration" game. Review the chapter material with the "Challenge" and "Spin the Wheel" games. Take the final chapter test, and complete the troubleshooting question; email or print your results to document your proficiency for this chapter.

Procedures

Use the following Procedure Checklists 4-1 and 4-2 to practice and perform the skills presented in this chapter. (LO 4.4 and 4.13)

PROCEDURE CHECKLIST 4-1
Recording an Electrocardiogram

Procedure Steps (*Rationale*)	Practice Yes	No	Practice Yes	No	Test Yes	No	Mastered Date	Initials
Preprocedure								
1. Receive and validate order.								
2. Check machine for proper functioning, including electrical cord, lead wires, and paper.								
3. Obtain necessary supplies.								
4. Read specific information from manufacturer's instructions.								
5. Ensure adequate paper is available.								
6. Change or add paper if necessary.								
7. Enter data into ECG machine if available.								
Procedure								
1. Identify patient using two forms of identification. (Ensures HIPAA standards)								
2. Explain procedure.								
3. Wash hands.								
4. Position and prepare patient. Turn off and remove electronics. (Prevents artifact)								
5. Provide for privacy and prevent exposure. (Provides comfort, alleviates stress)								
6. Ensure bed or exam table is not touching wall. (Prevents artifact)								
7. Move the bed or exam table away from electrical equipment. (Prevents artifact)								
8. Ensure patient is not touching headboard, footboard, or side rails. (Prevents artifact)								
9. Cleanse and prepare skin as necessary.								
10. Apply electrodes to limbs and chest.								

(Continued)

Procedure Steps (*Rationale*)	Practice Yes	No	Practice Yes	No	Test Yes	No	Mastered Date	Initials
Procedure (*continued*)								
11. Attach lead wire, assuming that no tension is on wires. Make a stress loop. (Prevents discomfort to patient and artifact)								
12. Enter additional patient data in the LCD panel if necessary.								
13. Press Run button.								
14. Check tracing for quality. Observe for artifact.								
15. Run additional ECG if necessary.								
16. Observe LCD display for errors.								
17. Turn off machine and unplug when completed.								
18. Remove electrodes and clean skin, if necessary.								
19. Assist the patient to a safe and comfortable position.								
Postprocedure								
1. Write on ECG any variations in lead placement, reason for poor quality tracing, or change in tracing speed. (Ensures accurate evaluation)								
2. Provide the results to the licensed practitioner.								
3. Place completed ECG tracing in the appropriate area.								
4. Clean the leads.								
5. Drape the lead wires of the machine in an orderly fashion.								
6. Return the machine to the designated storage location.								

Comments: _____

_____

_____

_____

_____

Signed

Evaluator: _____

Student: _____

PROCEDURE CHECKLIST 4-2

Continuous Cardiac Monitoring

Procedure Steps (*Rationale*)	Practice Yes	No	Practice Yes	No	Test Yes	No	Mastered Date	Initials
Preprocedure								
Gather supplies and equipment: • Cardiac monitor (check monitor before applying to the patient) • Cable and lead wires • Electrodes • Skin prep supplies, i.e., alcohol, gauze pads, razor as necessary • Gloves								
Procedure								
Identify the patient.								
Introduce yourself.								
Explain what you are going to do to the patient, and ask if patient has any questions.								
Ask the patient to undress from the waist up (assist as necessary). Provide patient with a gown or drape to use for privacy.								
Wash your hands, and don medical exam gloves.								
Expose only the areas necessary to perform the procedure (maintain patient privacy).								
Select appropriate locations, and prep the skin (brisk circular rub with dry gauze, rasp, or alcohol. (Let alcohol dry.) *** Note: avoid bony prominences • Right arm — just under the clavicle and medial to the right shoulder • Left arm — just under the clavicle and medial to the left shoulder • Left leg — upper abdomen at the margin where the abdomen and lowest rib meet.								
Shave or clip hair if necessary (follow facility policy).								
Attach electrodes to the ends of the cables.								
Place white cable with electrode (labeled RA) on the right arm location.								
Place black cable with electrode (labeled LA) on the left arm location.								

(Continued)

Procedure Steps (*Rationale*)	Practice Yes	No	Practice Yes	No	Test Yes	No	Mastered Date	Initials
Procedure (*continued*)								
Place the red cable with electrode (labeled F or LL) on the left leg location.								
***Remember to press around the outer edge of the electrode to ensure good adhesive contact with the skin.								
*** Remember to press around the center of the electrode to ensure good gel-to-skin contact with conductive media (reduces artifact).								
***It may be necessary to make stress loops and tape them directly to the patient.								
Attach cable clip to the sheet or patient gown to reduce tugging on electrodes (reduces artifact).								
Turn cardiac monitor on and select lead II.								
Select heart rate limits according to local policy.								
Observe heart rate and rhythm — troubleshoot if artifact is noted.								
Print a rhythm strip for further analysis and reporting to licensed healthcare practitioner.								
Postprocedure								
Remove gloves, and wash hands.								
Document procedure.								

Comments: _____

_____

_____

_____

_____

Signed

Evaluator: _____

Student: _____

5 Rhythm Strip Interpretation and Sinus Rhythms

Chapter Outline

- Rhythm Interpretation (p. 123)
- Identifying the Components of the Rhythm (p. 123)
- Normal Sinus Rhythm (p. 130)
- Sinus Bradycardia (p. 133)
- Sinus Tachycardia (p. 135)
- Sinus Dysrhythmia (p. 136)
- Sinus Arrest (p. 138)

Learning Outcomes

5.1 Explain the process of evaluating ECG tracings and determining the presence of dysrhythmias.

5.2 Describe the criteria used for classification of the dysrhythmias, including rhythm, rate, P wave configuration, PR interval measurement, and QRS duration measurement.

5.3 Identify normal sinus rhythm using the criteria for classification, and explain how the rhythm may affect the patient, including basic patient care and treatment.

5.4 Identify sinus bradycardia using the criteria for classification, and explain how the rhythm may affect the patient, including basic patient care and treatment.

5.5 Identify sinus tachycardia using the criteria for classification, and explain how the rhythm may affect the patient, including basic patient care and treatment.

5.6 Identify sinus dysrhythmia using the criteria for classification, and explain how the rhythm may affect the patient, including basic patient care and treatment.

5.7 Identify sinus arrest using the criteria for classification, and explain how the rhythm may affect the patient, including basic patient care and treatment.

Key Terms

asystole
bradycardia
cardiac output
hypotension
ischemia

J point
palpitations
syncope
tachycardia
vagal tone

5.1 Rhythm Interpretation

As discussed in Chapter 1, the ECG is an important tool used for the diagnosis and treatment of various cardiac and other related diseases. The recorded tracing of the ECG waveforms produced by the heart can tell you basic information about a patient's condition. The ability to evaluate various ECG waveforms is an important skill for many healthcare professionals, including nurses, doctors, and medical assistants. In addition, as a multiskilled healthcare employee you may be required to determine if an ECG is normal or abnormal and be able to respond to a cardiac emergency, if necessary. You will follow your scope of practice and the policy at your place of employment when evaluating and reporting dysrhythmias.

As you have already learned, the ECG waveform has various components—such as waves, segments, and intervals—that are evaluated and classified based on their size, length of time, and location on the tracing. All of these different components determine the type of cardiac rhythm. In order to evaluate a rhythm, you must first understand each component and its normal appearance. When these components differ from the expected norm, a dysrhythmia (or arrhythmia) is indicated. Remember, an abnormal ECG tracing may only be the result of artifact. The tracing must be evaluated for artifact prior to the evaluation of the heart rhythm.

The process of determining or labeling the type of cardiac dysrhythmia can be challenging. The best approach in determining the actual rhythm is to take on the role of a detective. Detectives will gather all the information they can before determining who is the suspect or how something has happened. The process of ECG analysis is similar. We first gather all the data regarding the different waveforms and their patterns. The next step is to match all the information to the specific ECG rhythm criteria in order to classify the various cardiac dysrhythmias.

In this chapter, you are introduced to the rhythm criteria used to identify the various cardiac dysrhythmias. You will continue to apply this process as you learn about the categories of dysrhythmias taught in Chapters 5 through 10. You will learn the process of evaluating dysrhythmia, which will lay a strong foundation for your beginning practice or continued education in electrocardiography. Most importantly, after completing this chapter you should be able to recognize abnormalities in the cardiac rhythm and respond appropriately.

Checkpoint Question (LO 5.1)

1. What is evaluated and classified when determining dysrhythmias?

_____

_____

5.2 Identifying the Components of the Rhythm

Although the following process is introduced in this chapter, it is the same process that will be utilized when analyzing all dysrhythmias, regardless of the category or complexity of the tracing.

ECG analysis consists of a five-step process of gathering data about each rhythm strip. These steps include evaluating the following components of the ECG rhythm strips:

- Rhythm (regularity)
- Rate
- P wave configuration
- PR interval
- QRS duration and configuration

Once the information is gathered, the data are compared to the specific criteria for each dysrhythmia. Cardiac dysrhythmia interpretation is an art. Frequently, you will find practitioners discussing how to classify a dysrhythmia because patients may experience a variety of different cardiac dysrhythmias at the same time. This makes it difficult to determine the origin of the dysrhythmia or to classify it. The more interpretations you perform, the more efficient you become in classifying the rhythm.

Before you begin the steps, you should know that lead II is the most common monitoring lead. Unless otherwise specified, it is lead II that is being used in this chapter.

Step 1: Determining the ECG Rhythm or Regularity

Determining the rhythm involves evaluating the pattern of how the atria and ventricles contract. The rhythm can occur in regular or irregular intervals. Each chamber of the heart is assessed for its type of pattern. In Chapter 3, you learned that the P wave represents atrial depolarization and the QRS complex represents ventricular depolarization. The rhythm of atrial contraction is evaluated by assessing the regularity or irregularity of the occurrence of the P waves. The QRS complexes are assessed to evaluate ventricular contraction. Calipers are used for this portion of the analysis to measure the distance between the P waves and the width of the QRS complex (Figure 5-1).

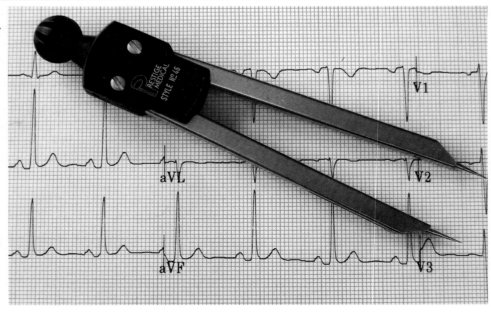

Figure 5-1 Calipers are used to measure ECG tracings.

Figure 5-2 Measuring the P-P wave interval.

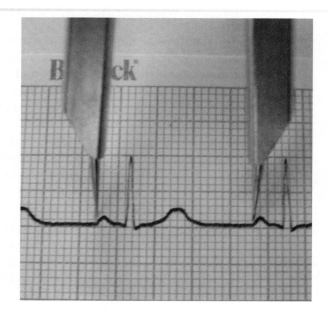

The P-P wave interval should be evaluated first. The caliper interval is established when the first point of the caliper is placed on the beginning of one P wave and the second point on the beginning of the next P wave. Measuring several of these intervals determines if the P waves are occurring in a regular sequence. At least 10 seconds of the ECG tracing of P waves are measured to determine if the P waves occur in a regular or irregular rhythm throughout the rhythm strip (Figure 5-2).

Next, determine the rhythm of the QRS complex. Since the QRS complex is a configuration of three possible waveforms, it is important to analyze this interval from the same waveform in each of the QRS complexes. For example, it is often easier to see the R wave of the QRS complex. Measuring the R-R wave interval is easy due to its upward deflection (Figure 5-3). Occasionally, the QRS complex does not exhibit an R wave, in which case you can use the point of the Q and S wave junction as an easy point of evaluation. Most importantly, you must measure the same part of the waveform for each QRS complex to determine the regularity of the ventricular depolarization. The first point of the caliper should be placed on the first QRS complex and the other point placed on the next QRS complex. The interval should be evaluated throughout at least a 6-second strip to determine the rhythm of the QRS complexes.

Figure 5-3 Waves, Intervals, and Segments.

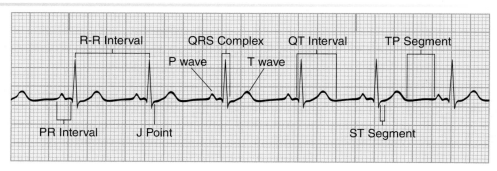

Step 2: Determining the Atrial and Ventricular Rate

The method used to calculate the heart rate is based on whether the rhythm is regular or irregular. The heart rate must be determined for both atria and ventricles. The atrial rate is determined by the P-P wave interval measurements, and the ventricular rate is determined by the R-R wave measurement. Most frequently, the atrial and ventricular rates will be the same; sometimes, however, the rates may be different due to conditions occurring in the myocardium. It is important to note if the atrial rate is different from the ventricular rate since this will help narrow the selection of dysrhythmias. The methods used to differentiate the rates are described in the following sections.

Regular Rhythm

Once you have determined that the rhythm is regular, you can use this method to calculate the atrial and ventricular rate. The caliper interval of the P-P or R-R measurement is placed on the ECG paper to determine the number of small boxes or duration of time. (Remember from Chapter 3 that each small box is equal to 0.04 seconds.) Move the caliper interval to the top or the bottom of the page so that the number of boxes can be determined without interference from the ECG tracing. Once you have counted the small boxes, divide the number into 1500 to calculate the heart rate. The ventricular rate is determined in the same manner except you will need to count the number of boxes *between* the QRS complexes. Table 5-1 provides the heart rates based on the number of small boxes between the two P or two R waves. Unlike the method described in Chapter 3 (which provides only an estimate), this method of calculation provides an accurate heart rate similar to measuring a person's pulse. The actual rate is extremely important when the heart rate is either **tachycardia** (more than 100 beats per minute [bpm]) or **bradycardia** (less than 60 beats per minute).

tachycardia A fast heart rate, usually greater than 100 beats per minute.

bradycardia A slow heart rate, usually less than 60 beats per minute.

Irregular Rhythm

When the rhythm is irregular, as determined in Step 1, the interval between the P waves or the QRS complexes is not constant. To determine the heart rate for an irregular rhythm, use the 6-second method as described in Chapter 3. Simply multiply the number of P waves and QRS complexes in a 6-second strip by 10. This method is often used in emergencies to determine an estimated heart rate (pulse rate) for the patient.

Interpret-TIP

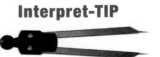

Many variables affect QT interval, i.e., heart rate, coronary heart disease, electrolyte imbalance, antidysrhythmic medications, to name a few. A shorter or longer than normal QTi may indicate that the patient is at an increased risk for certain dysrhythmias and sudden death.

Step 3: Identifying the P Wave Configuration (Shape)

Analyzing P waves and their relationship with the QRS complex is necessary to determine the type of dysrhythmia. The P wave reflects the atrial contraction and how the electrical current is moving through the atria. The relationship between the P wave and QRS complex provides information regarding the coordination between atrial and ventricular contractions. Several questions need to be answered when analyzing the P wave.

TABLE 5-1 Calculating Heart Rates with a Regular Rhythm

Small Boxes in P-P or R-R Interval	Heart Rate	Small Boxes in P-P or R-R Interval	Heart Rate	Small Boxes in P-P or R-R Interval	Heart Rate
4	375	20	75	36	42
5	300	21	71	37	40
6	250	22	68	38	39
7	214	23	65	39	38
8	188	24	62	40	38
9	167	25	60	41	37
10	150	26	58	42	36
11	136	27	55	43	35
12	125	28	54	44	34
13	115	29	52	45	33
14	107	30	50	46	33
15	100	31	48	47	32
16	94	32	47	48	31
17	88	33	45	49	31
18	83	34	44	50	30
19	79	35	43		

A rate calculator can also be used for regular rhythms. The start mark is placed at the first P wave or R wave, whichever you are using. Where the next consecutive P or R wave lines up is the approximate heart rate. See the following figure.

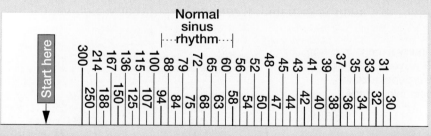

- *Are the shapes and waveforms all the same?* If they appear to be different, the route in which the current is moving through the atria is not on the same pathway. Sometimes the P wave may not exist.
- *Does each P wave have a QRS complex following it?* In normal conduction pathways, the QRS complex always follows the P wave. If there are additional P waves or QRS complexes present without a P wave in front, the normal conduction pathway may not have been used, and the atria and ventricles are not contracting together.

Step 4: Measuring the PR Interval

The PR interval measures the length of time it takes the electrical current to be initiated at the sinoatrial node and travel through the electrical current pathway to cause a ventricular contraction. The PR interval is determined by measuring from the beginning of the P wave, or its up slope, to the beginning of the QRS complex. This is the first indication of ventricular depolarization. Not all tracings will show a Q wave. In the absence of a Q wave, the second caliper tip is placed at the beginning of the R wave. (Please review Figure 2-11 if necessary.) The normal range of the PR interval is 0.12 to 0.20 second (Figure 5-4).

When determining the measurements, the time interval should always be in multiples of 0.02 second, which represents one-half of the smallest box. To effectively determine measurements to 0.01 second, the small box on the ECG paper would need to be divided into four smaller divisions. *This can be done effectively only with a computer, not a practitioner's eyes.*

PR intervals are also evaluated to ensure that the measurements are the same from one PR interval to the next. If the intervals have different measurements, either the electrical current is being delayed for some reason or it may be initiating from locations other than the sinoatrial node.

Step 5: Measuring the QRS Duration and Analyzing the Configuration (Shape)

Measuring the QRS complex is essential in determining the duration of time it takes for the ventricles to depolarize or contract. This information is helpful in discriminating between different dysrhythmias. If the QRS complex is narrow, or within the normal limits of 0.06 to 0.10 second, current has traveled through the normal ventricular conduction pathways to activate the ventricles to contract. When the QRS complex is wide, 0.12 second or greater, the current is taking longer than normal to contract the ventricles.

J point A point on the QRS complex where the depolarization is completed and repolarization starts.

To measure the QRS duration and configuration, place the first caliper point where the QRS complex starts and the second point at the **J point** (Figure 5-5). The J point is located where the S wave stops and the ST segment is initiated. It marks the point at which ventricular depolarization is

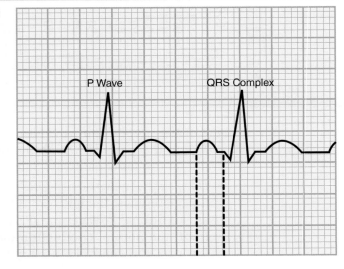

Figure 5-4 The PR interval measured from the beginning of the P wave to the first indication of ventricular depolarization, which is usually the beginning of the QRS complex.

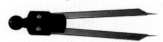

QRS Measurement

Although a QRS measurement of 0.11 secon~~d~~
the normal range, it would only be a mea~~s~~
ECG machine. The human eye cannot ~~d~~
measurements.

completed and repolarization begins. It is i~~n~~
this ending point of the QRS complex, sinc~~e~~
may not be at the isoelectric line.

Several questions need to be answered when determining the QRS
measurement and configuration (Figure 5-6).

- Are all the QRS complexes of equal length?
- What is the actual measurement, and is it within the normal limits?
- Do all QRS complexes look alike, and are the unusual QRS complexes associated with an ectopic beat?

Figure 5-5 The J point is where the S wave stops and the ST segment is initiated.

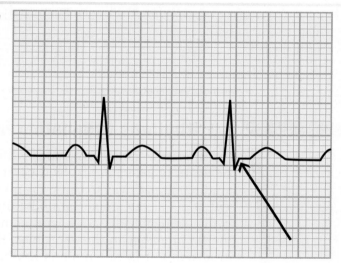

Figure 5-6 Measure the QRS duration from the beginning of the QRS complex to the J point.

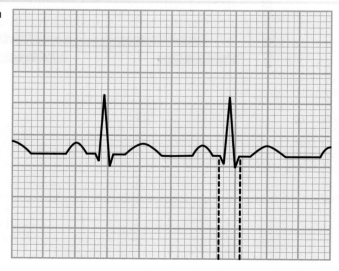

After you have completed these five steps of identifying the components of the rhythm, you will then compare the information to the specific criteria for classifying each of the dysrhythmias. The rest of this chapter explains the specific criteria for classification related to common rhythms and dysrhythmias that will help you identify the various ECG rhythms.

Checkpoint Questions (LO 5.2)

1. Name the five components that must be evaluated on a rhythm strip.

_____

_____

2. A regular rhythm has 19 small boxes between the P-P interval. What is the heart rate?

_____

_____

3. After you measure the QRS duration and configuration, what other questions need to be answered?

_____

_____

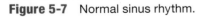

5.3 Rhythms Originating from the Sinus Node

The sinoatrial node (SA node) is the normal or "primary" pacemaker of the heart. It generates an electrical impulse that travels through the normal conduction pathway to cause the myocardium to depolarize. Electrical current starts at the sinoatrial node, travels the normal conduction pathway to the atrioventrical node, and continues through the bundle of His and bundle branches to the ventricles. Because the rhythm starts at the sinoatrial node, it is called sinus rhythm. The electrical current is produced at the sinus node at a rate of 60 to 100 beats per minute. The rates of the rhythm will vary, and the types of sinus beats may include sinus rhythm, sinus bradycardia, sinus tachycardia, and sinus dysrhythmia.

Normal sinus rhythm is reflective of a normally functioning conduction system (Figure 5-7). The electrical current is following the normal

Figure 5-7 Normal sinus rhythm.

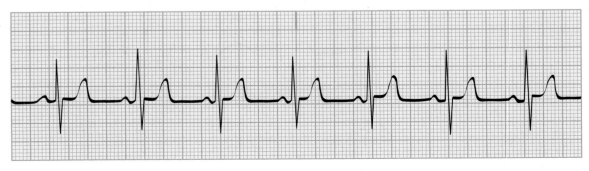

conduction pathway without interference from other bodily systems or disease processes.

Criteria for Classification

- *Rhythm:* The intervals between the two P and two R waves will occur in a consistent pattern.
- *Rate:* Both the atrial and ventricular rate will be between 60 and 100 beats per minute.
- *P wave configuration:* The P waves will have the same shape and are usually upright in deflection on the rhythm strip. A P wave will appear in front of every QRS complex.
- *PR interval:* The PR interval measurement will be between 0.12 and 0.20 second, which is within normal limits. Each PR interval will be the same, without any variations.
- *QRS duration and configuration:* The QRS duration and configuration measurement will be between 0.06 and 0.10 second, which is within normal limits. Each QRS duration and configuration will be without any variations from PQRST complex to complex.

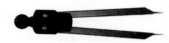

Interpret-TIP

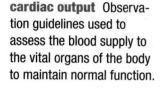

Normal Sinus Rhythm

Sinus rhythm is the only rhythm for which all five steps are within normal limits.

How the Patient Is Affected and What You Should Know

cardiac output Observation guidelines used to assess the blood supply to the vital organs of the body to maintain normal function.

Sinus rhythm is the desired rhythm. Patients with this rhythm should have normal **cardiac output.** Normal cardiac output means that the heart is beating adequately, pumping blood to the body's organs to maintain normal function. Signs and symptoms of adequate cardiac output include an alert and oriented patient with no difficulty breathing, no chest pain or pressure, and a stable blood pressure.

Because this is a normal rhythm, no intervention is necessary. If the patient's rhythm returns to sinus rhythm from another dysrhythmia, it is always important to make sure that the patient is not experiencing problems with low cardiac output, which indicates that the heart is not pumping adequately (Table 5-2). Any time a patient displays symptoms of low cardiac output, a licensed practitioner needs to be informed for further assessment.

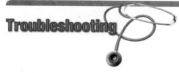

Troubleshooting

Report the Patient Condition, Not the Tracing

The patient you are monitoring is very pale and appears to be breathing very fast. His monitor indicates a sinus rhythm. What should you do?

_____

_____

TABLE 5-2 Signs and Symptoms of Decreased Cardiac Output

Observe for any of these signs and symptoms associated with decreased cardiac output during ECG monitoring.

Neurological	Cardiac	Respiratory	Urinary	Peripheral
• Change in mental status • Light-headedness • Dizziness • Confusion • Loss of consciousness	• Chest pain • Palpitation • Chest discomfort • Enlarged cardiac size • Congestive heart failure	• Difficulty breathing • Shortness of breath • Frothy sputum • Fluid present in lungs • Lung congestion	• Decreased urinary output of less than 30 mL in one hour	• Hypotension • Pale skin • Skin cool and clammy to the touch

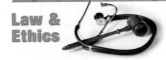

Law & Ethics

Documenting the ECG Rhythm and Tracing

The ECG rhythm, which is considered a legal document, needs to be included in the patient's medical record. The patient's name, date, and time plus the initials of the person performing the ECG must be identified on each rhythm strip. Documentation of the ECG rhythm and the patient's response help support the reason for the medical treatment.

Check Point Question (LO 5.3)

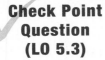

1. Using the criteria for classification, select the rhythm that most closely resembles normal sinus rhythm.

A.

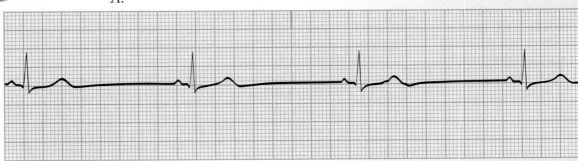

B.

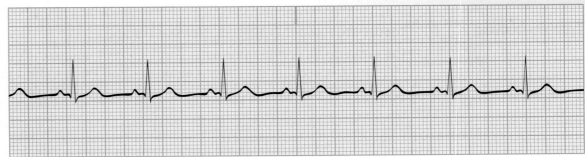

(Continued)

Which unique feature(s) led you to make the selection?

_____

_____

_____

5.4 Sinus Bradycardia

Sinus bradycardia is a rhythm of less than 60 beats per minute (Figure 5-8). Sinus bradycardia originates from the SA node and travels the normal conduction pathway. The only difference between this rhythm and sinus rhythm is that the rate is less than the normal inherent rate of the SA node.

Figure 5-8   Sinus bradycardia.

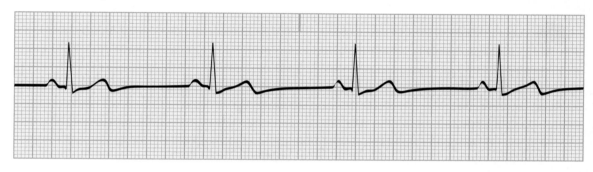

Criteria for Classification

- **Rhythm:** The R-R interval and P-P interval will occur on a regular and constant basis.
- **Rate:** The atrial and ventricular rates will be equal and less than 60 beats per minute.
- **P wave configuration:** The shapes of each of the P waves are upright and uniform. There is a P wave in front of each of the QRS complexes. No additional P waves or QRS complexes are noted.
- **PR interval:** The PR interval measurement will be between 0.12 and 0.20 second, which is within normal limits. Each PR interval will be the same.
- **QRS duration and configuration:** The QRS duration and configuration measurement will be between 0.06 and 0.10 second, which is within normal limits. Each QRS duration and configuration will be the same, without any variations from QRS complex to complex.

Interpret-TIP

Sinus Bradycardia

For sinus bradycardia, the heart rate is less than 60 beats per minute, and all other measurements are within normal limits.

How the Patient Is Affected and What You Should Know

The patient who exhibits sinus bradycardia may or may not experience signs and symptoms of low cardiac output. When administering an ECG to a patient with a slow heart rate, it is important to observe for the symptoms of low cardiac output (see Table 5-2). Remember, although the patient may look all right, he or she can quickly experience difficulties with low cardiac output. When you observe symptoms of low cardiac output, report any findings to a licensed practitioner immediately. This rhythm may require drug administration or application of a pacemaker.

Check Point Question (LO 5.4)

1. Using the criteria for classification, select the rhythm that most closely resembles sinus bradycardia rhythm.

A.

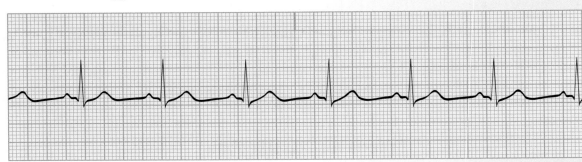

B.

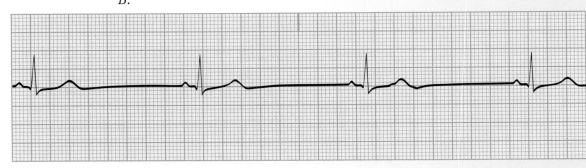

Which unique feature(s) led you to make the selection?

_____

_____

_____

5.5 Sinus Tachycardia

Sinus tachycardia is a condition in which the SA node fires and the electrical impulse travels through the normal conduction pathway but the rate of impulse firing is faster than 100 beats per minute (Figure 5-9).

Figure 5-9 Sinus tachycardia.

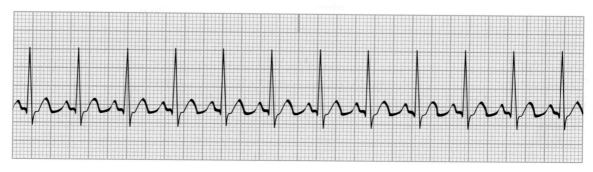

Criteria for Classification

- *Rhythm:* The R-R interval and P-P interval will be equal and constant.
- *Rate:* Both the atrial and ventricular rates will be the same, between 100 and 150 beats per minute.
- *P wave configuration:* The P waves will have the same shape and usually are upright in deflection on the rhythm strip. There will be a P wave in front of every QRS complex.
- *PR interval:* The PR interval measurement will be between 0.12 and 0.20 second. This is within normal limits. Each PR interval will be the same, without any variations.
- *QRS duration and configuration:* The QRS duration and configuration measurement will be between 0.06 and 0.10 second, which is within normal limits. Each QRS duration and configuration will be the same, without any variations from QRS complex to complex.

Interpret-TIP

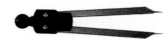

Sinus Tachycardia

For sinus tachycardia, the heart rate is greater than 100 beats per minute, and all other measurements are within normal limits.

How the Patient Is Affected and What You Should Know

The effect of this rhythm on the patient depends on the rate of tachycardia above the patient's normal resting heart rate. For example, if the patient's normal resting heart rate is 90 and now the patient is exhibiting a rate of 108 beats per minute after walking the hallway, the tachycardia would be expected and is viewed as the patient's normal response to exercise. However, if the patient's normal heart rate is 60 and it is now 140, the patient is probably experiencing symptoms of low cardiac output. Often the patient

palpitations Fast, irregular heartbeat sensation felt by the patient, which may or may not be associated with complaints of chest pain.

will complain of **palpitations** or "heart fluttering" with faster rates. If the patient has had a recent myocardial infarction, sinus tachycardia is considered to be more serious or even life threatening.

When caring for a patient who is experiencing sinus tachycardia, first observe for signs and symptoms of low cardiac output. If evidence of low cardiac output is observed, a licensed practitioner should be notified immediately. Medication may need to be administered by a licensed practitioner.

Check Point Question (LO 5.5)

1. Using the criteria for classification, select the rhythm that most closely resembles sinus tachycardia rhythm.

A.

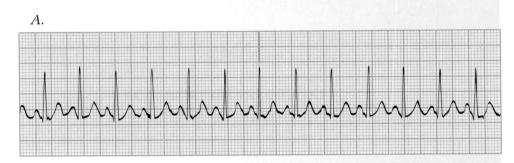

B.

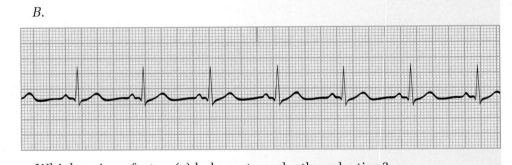

Which unique feature(s) led you to make the selection?

_____

_____

_____

5.6 Sinus Dysrhythmia

vagal tone Condition in which impulses over the vagus nerve exert a continuous inhibitory effect upon the heart and cause a decrease in heart rate.

Sinus dysrhythmia (sinus arrhythmia) is a condition in which the heart rate remains within normal limits but is influenced by the respiratory cycle and variations of **vagal tone** (a condition in which impulses over the vagus nerve cause a decrease in heart rate), causing the rhythm to be irregular. For instance, when a patient inhales air, the pressure inside the chest cavity increases, causing pressure on the heart. The heart rate will increase as the

Figure 5-10   Sinus dysrhythmia.

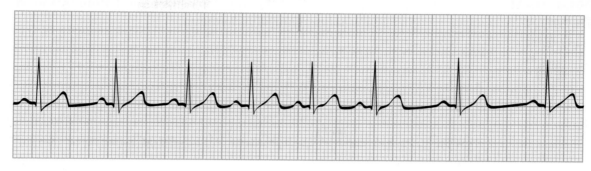

patient inhales. As the patient exhales, the chest cavity pressure decreases, along with the heart rate (Figure 5-10).

Criteria for Classification

- *Rhythm:* The interval between the P-P and R-R waves will occur at irregular periods.
- *Rate:* Both the atrial and ventricular rates will be the same, between 60 and 100 beats per minute.
- *P wave configuration:* The P waves will have the same shape and usually are upright in deflection on the rhythm strip. There will be a P wave in front of every QRS complex.
- *PR interval:* The PR interval measurement will be between 0.12 and 0.20 second. Each PR interval will be the same, without any variations.
- *QRS duration and configuration:* The QRS duration and configuration measurement will be between 0.06 and 0.10 second. Each QRS duration and configuration will be the same, without any variations from QRS complex to complex.

Interpret-TIP

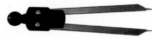

Sinus Dysrhythmia

For sinus dysrhythmia, the P-P and R-R intervals will progressively widen then narrow, following the patient's breathing pattern.

How the Patient Is Affected and What You Should Know

Patients usually show no clinical signs or symptoms with sinus dysrhythmia. If the irregularity is severe enough to decrease the heart rate to 40 to 50 beats per minutes, the patient may complain of palpitations or dizziness. This depends on how slowly the heart beats when the SA node is suppressed from the respiratory or vagal influences. You should notify the physician or other licensed practitioner when the heart rate slows below 50 or the patient complains of dizziness or palpitations. A copy of the rhythm strip should be mounted on the patient's medical record for documentation.

**Check Point
Question
(LO 5.6)**

1. Using the criteria for classification, select the rhythm that most closely resembles sinus dysrhythmia.

A.

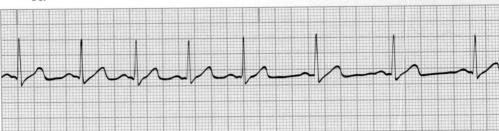

B.

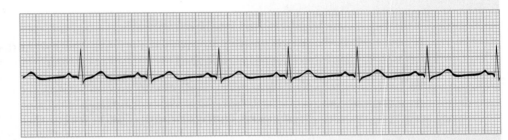

Which unique feature(s) led you to make the selection?

_____

_____

_____

5.7 Sinus Arrest

Sinus arrest, sometimes referred to as sinus pause, occurs when the SA node stops firing, causing a pause in electrical activity. During the pause, no electrical impulse is initiated or sent through the normal conduction system to cause either an atrial or a ventricular contraction (Figure 5-11).

Figure 5-11 Sinus arrest.

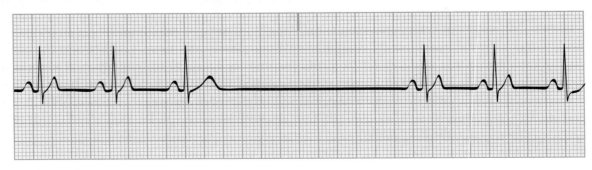

Criteria for Classification

- **Rhythm:** The cardiac complexes are regular before and after the sinus arrest period, but this rhythm is considered irregular due to the absence of electrical activity during the pause.
- **Rate:** Both the atrial and ventricular rates will be the same. The rate will vary, depending on the amount of electrical activity occurring from the sinoatrial node.
- **P wave configuration:** The P waves will have the same shape and are upright in deflection on the rhythm strip. There will be a P wave in front of every QRS complex.
- **PR interval:** The PR interval measurement will be between 0.12 and 0.20 second, which is within normal limits. Each PR interval will be the same, without any variations.
- **QRS duration and configuration:** The QRS duration and configuration measurement will be between 0.06 and 0.10 second, which is within normal limits. Each QRS duration and configuration will be the same, without any variations from QRS complex to complex.
- **Length of pause:** The length of pause needs to be measured to determine how long the heart had no rhythm. To measure, place the calipers on the R-R interval around the pause. Once the time frame is determined, calculate the length of time for the pause by multiplying the number of boxes by 0.04 second. The frequency of pauses is also noted because the more frequent the pauses, the more urgent the situation.

It should be noted that the arrest period may be terminated by an escaped beat from one of the subsidiary pacemakers when the heart rate is less than 60 beats per minute. In this instance, there would be a junctional or ventricular escape beat then resumption of the usual electrical activity.

Alert! When sinus arrest reaches or exceeds 6 seconds, it is considered a medical emergency. Code Blue procedures must be initiated.

Interpret-TIP

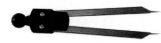

Sinus Arrest

You will observe regularly occuring PQRSTs both before and after the arrest period. No electrical activity occurs during the arrest period.

How the Patient Is Affected and What You Should Know

The seriousness of sinus arrest depends on the length of the pause. The patient will experience signs and symptoms of decreased cardiac output if the pause is 2 seconds long and occurs on a frequent basis. The pauses may also cause periods of ischemia (when cells are deprived of oxygen), hypotension, dizziness, and syncope (loss of consciousness).

The patient may initially appear to be asymptomatic (without symptoms) and then develop signs and symptoms of low cardiac output. Therefore, it is important to observe the patient frequently for signs of low cardiac output. Notify a licensed practitioner of these symptoms, and provide information about the frequency and length of pauses. The patient will require immediate treatment. If sinus arrest reaches 6 seconds, this is considered a Code Blue medical emergency.

ischemia Lack of blood supply to an area of tissue due to a blockage in the circulation to that area.

hypotension low blood pressure

syncope Condition when the patient loses consciousness (fainting).

Sinus Arrest

A patient is in sinus arrest that lasts longer than 6 seconds. This indicates that no electrical current is traveling through the cardiac conduction system and is known as **asystole**. What should you do?

asystole When no rhythm or electrical current is traveling through the cardiac conduction system.

_____

_____

Check Point Question (LO 5.7)

1. Using the criteria for classification, select the rhythm that most closely resembles sinus arrest.

A.

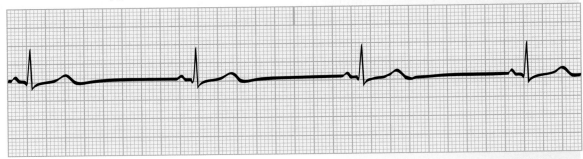

B.

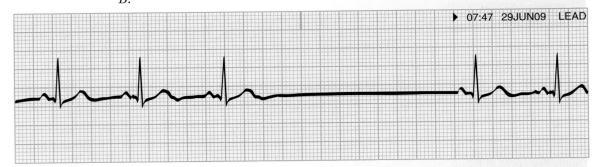

▶ 07:47 29JUN09 LEAD

Which unique feature(s) led you to make the selection?

_____

_____

_____

Chapter Summary

Learning Outcomes	Summary	Pages
5.1 Explain the process of evaluating ECG tracings and determining the presence of dysrhythmias.	Evaluating an ECG requires basic knowledge of the waves, segments, and intervals of the tracing and the rate, rhythm, and regularity of the heartbeat.	123
5.2 Describe the criteria used for classification of the dysrhythmias, including rhythm, rate, P wave configuration, PR interval measurement, and QRS duration measurement.	The process of evaluating an ECG tracing includes determining the ECG rhythm or regularity, determining the atrial and ventricular rate, identifying the P wave configuration, measuring the PR interval, measuring the QRS duration, and analyzing the configuration.	123–130
5.3 Identify normal sinus rhythm using the criteria for classification, and explain how the rhythm may affect the patient, including basic patient care and treatment.	Normal sinus rhythm is effectively a normal-functioning electrical conduction system and requires no specialized patient care or treatment.	130–132
5.4 Identify sinus bradycardia using the criteria for classification, and explain how the rhythm may affect the patient, including basic patient care and treatment.	Sinus bradycardia is a rhythm of less than 60 beats per minute, with electrical activity originating in the SA node. The other four criteria are within "normal" limits.	133–134
5.5 Identify sinus tachycardia using the criteria for classification, and explain how the rhythm may affect the patient, including basic patient care and treatment.	Sinus tachycardia is a rhythm of greater than 100 beats per minute, with electrical activity originating in the SA node. The other four criteria are within "normal" limits.	135–136
5.6 Identify sinus dysrhythmia using the criteria for classification, and explain how the rhythm may affect the patient, including basic patient care and treatment.	Sinus dysrhythmia is a condition in which the heart rate remains within normal limits but is influenced by the respiratory cycle and variations of vagal tone, causing the rhythm to be irregular. The other four criteria are within "normal" limits.	136–137
5.7 Identify sinus arrest using the criteria for classification, and explain how the rhythm may affect the patient, including basic patient care and treatment.	Sinus arrest occurs when the SA node stops firing; this creates a pause in electrical activity, causing the rhythm to be irregular. The length of the pause may cause the heart rate to be less than 60 beats per minute. Otherwise, the other criteria are within "normal" limits.	138–141

Chapter Review

Matching

Match the terms related to rhythm strip interpretation to the best definition.

_____ 1. heart rate less than 60 bpm (LO 5.2)

_____ 2. the amount of blood being pumped by the heart (LO 5.3)

_____ 3. low blood pressure (LO 5.6)

_____ 4. lack of blood supply (LO 5.6)

_____ 5. depolarization is completed and repolarization starts (LO 5.2)

_____ 6. fast, irregular heartbeats felt by the patient (LO 5.4)

_____ 7. loss of consciousness (fainting) (LO 5.6)

_____ 8. heart rate greater than 100 bpm (LO 5.2)

_____ 9. continuous inhibitory effect on the heart (LO 5.6)

a. vagal tone
b. bradycardia
c. tachycardia
d. cardiac output
e. hypotension
f. palpitations
g. J point
h. syncope
i. ischemia

Multiple Choice

Circle the correct answer.

10. What is the rate of a normal sinus rhythm? (LO 5.3)
    a. 60 to 100 beats per minute
    b. 50 to 90 beats per minute
    c. 100 to 150 beats per minute
    d. 60 to 80 beats per minute

11. What sinus rhythm has a rate of less than 60 beats per minute? (LO 5.4)
    a. Sinus tachycardia
    b. Sinus bradycardia
    c. Sinus dysrythmia
    d. Sinus rhythms

12. Which question does *not* need to be answered when determining the QRS measurement? (LO 5.2)
    a. Are all the QRS complexes of equal length?
    b. What is the actual QRS measurement, and is it within the normal limits?
    c. Do all QRS complexes look alike, and are the unusual QRS complexes associated with an ectopic beat?
    d. Is the R-R pattern regular?

13. What sinus rhythm has a rate of more than 100 beats per minute? (LO 5.5)
    a. Sinus tachycardia
    b. Sinus bradycardia
    c. Sinus dysrhythmia
    d. Sinus rhythms

14. What rhythm shows an irregularity during inspiration and expiration? (LO 5.6)
    a. Sinus tachycardia
    b. Sinus bradycardia
    c. Sinus dysrhythmia
    d. Sinus rhythms

15. The normal PR interval is (LO 5.2)
    a. 0.04 to 0.10 second.
    b. 0.12 to 0.20 second.
    c. 0.22 to 0.26 second.
    d. 0.28 to 0.32 second.

16. If a QRS complex measures 0.12 second or wider, it most likely indicates (LO 5.2)
    a. normal ventricular conduction.
    b. delayed ventricular conduction.
    c. increased delay at the AV node.
    d. myocardial infarction.

17. What is a common sign of low cardiac output? (LO 5.3)
    a. High blood pressure
    b. Alert and oriented
    c. Increased perfusion of vital organs
    d. Low blood pressure

Fill in the Blank

18. Sinus tachycardia may be a normal finding in persons as a result of _____. (LO 5.5)

19. When sinus arrest continues for 6 seconds or more it is considered _____. (LO 5.7)

20. The rhythm originating in the sinoatrial node that is considered normal is _____. (LO 5.3)

21. Two rhythms originating in the sinoatrial nodes that only affect the heart rate are _____ and _____. (LO 5.4, 5.5)

22. The rhythm originating in the node that affects the breathing pattern is _____. (LO 5.6)

Short answer

23. What rhythm originating in the sinus node is considered "normal"? _____
(LO 5.3)

24. Name the two sinus rhythms whose only difference from Normal Sinus Rhythm is the
rate. _____ (LO 5.4, 5.5)

25. What rhythm originating in the sinus node is affected by the breathing
pattern? _____ (LO 5.6)

Critical Thinking Application *Rhythm Identification*

Review the dysrhythmias pictured here and, using the criteria for classification provided in the
chapter as clues, identify each rhythm and provide what information you used to make your
decision. (LO 5.3 to 5.7)

26.

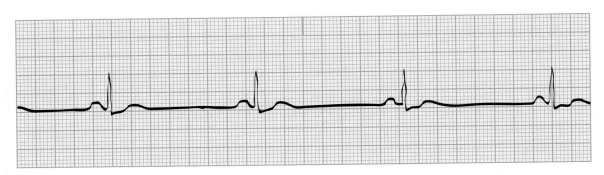

Rhythm (Regular or Irregular): _____   PR interval: _____

Rate: _____   QRS: _____

P wave: _____   Interpretation: _____

27.

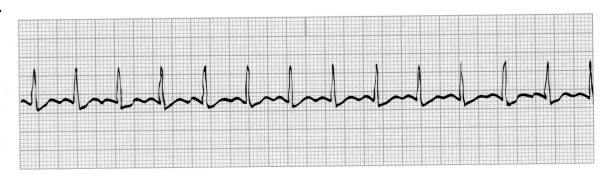

Rhythm (Regular or Irregular): _____   PR interval: _____

Rate: _____   QRS: _____

P wave: _____   Interpretation: _____

28.

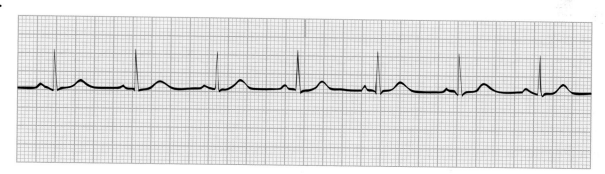

Rhythm (Regular or Irregular): _____   PR interval: _____

Rate: _____   QRS: _____

P wave: _____   Interpretation: _____

29.

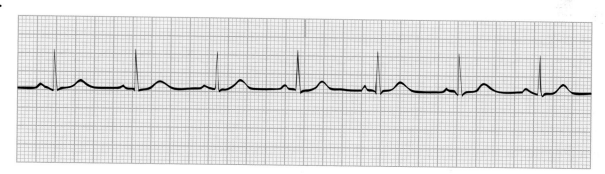

Rhythm (Regular or Irregular): _____   PR interval: _____

Rate: _____   QRS: _____

P wave: _____   Interpretation: _____

30.

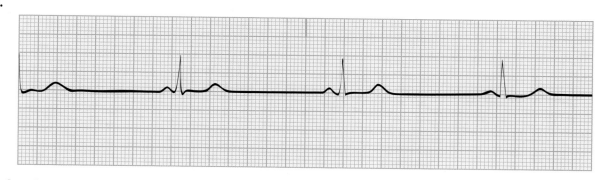

Rhythm (Regular or Irregular): _____   PR interval: _____

Rate: _____   QRS: _____

P wave: _____   Interpretation: _____

31.

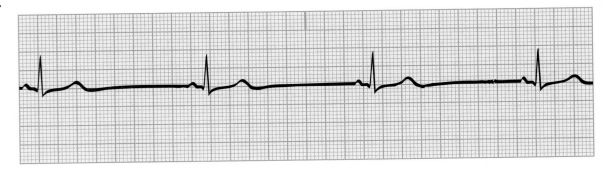

Rhythm (Regular or Irregular): _____   PR interval: _____

Rate: _____   QRS: _____

P wave: _____   Interpretation: _____

32.

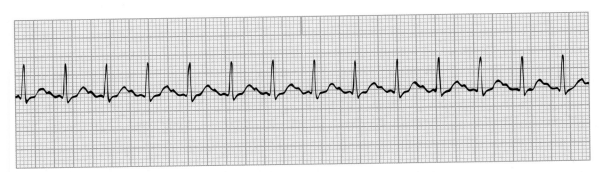

Rhythm (Regular or Irregular): _____   PR interval: _____

Rate: _____   QRS: _____

P wave: _____   Interpretation: _____

33.

Rhythm (Regular or Irregular): _____   PR interval: _____

Rate: _____   QRS: _____

P wave: _____   Interpretation: _____

34.

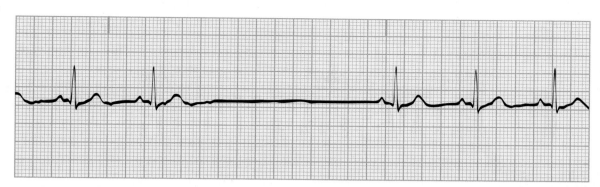

Rhythm (Regular or Irregular): _____   PR interval: _____

Rate: _____   QRS: _____

P wave: _____   Interpretation: _____

35.

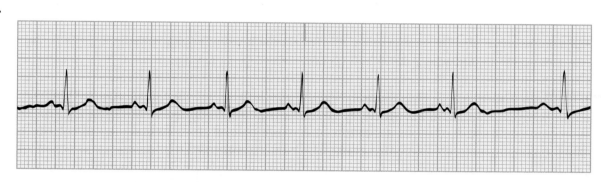

Rhythm (Regular or Irregular): _____   PR interval: _____

Rate: _____   QRS: _____

P wave: _____   Interpretation: _____

Get Connected *Internet Activity*

Visit the McGraw-Hill Higher Education Online Learning Center *Electrocardiography for Healthcare Professionals* Web site at **www.mhhe.com/boothecg3e** to complete the following activity.

1. For practice and review of common cardiac rhythms and dysrhythmias try the dynamic rhythm simulator, The Six Second ECG, at the Web site: http://skillstat.com/Flash/ECG_Sim_2004.html.

 ## Using the Student CD

Now that you have completed the material in the chapter text, return to the student CD and complete any chapter activities you have not yet done. Practice your terminology with the "Key Term Concentration" game. Review the chapter material with the "Spin the Wheel" and "ECG Challenge" games. Take the final chapter test, and complete the troubleshooting question; email or print your results to document your proficiency for this chapter.

6 Atrial Dysrhythmias

Chapter Outline

- Introduction to Atrial Dysrhythmias (p. 149)
- Premature Atrial Complexes (PACs) (p. 149)
- Wandering Atrial Pacemaker (WAP) (p. 151)
- Multifocal Atrial Tachycardia (MAT) (p. 153)
- Atrial Flutter (p. 155)
- Atrial Fibrillation (p. 157)

Learning Outcomes

6.1 Summarize the similarities between atrial dysrhythmias.

6.2 Identify premature atrial complexes using the criteria for classification and explain how the rhythm may affect the patient, including basic patient care and treatment.

6.3 Identify wandering atrial pacemaker using the criteria for classification and explain how the rhythm may affect the patient, including basic patient care and treatment.

6.4 Identify multifocal atrial tachycardia using the criteria for classification and explain how the rhythm may affect the patient, including basic patient care and treatment.

6.5 Identify atrial flutter using the criteria for classification and explain how the rhythm may affect the patient, including basic patient care and treatment.

6.6 Identify atrial fibrillation using the criteria for classification and explain how the rhythm may affect the patient, including basic patient care and treatment.

Key Terms

atrial kick
automaticity
biphasic
cerebrovascular accident (CVA)
ectopic impulse
focus or foci

myocardial infarction (MI)
neurological
pulmonary embolism
renal infarction
thrombus
trigeminy

6.1 Introduction to Atrial Dysrhythmias

ectopic impulse Ectopic impulse refers to an electrical impulse that comes from outside of the normal pacemaker site or electrical conduction pathway.

Atrial dysrhythmias, also known as arrythmias, are caused by an **ectopic impulse** in either the right or the left atria. However, the atrial origin is outside the SA node, which interrupts the inherent rate of the SA node. The heart works on the principle that the fastest impulse will control the heart rate. Since the atrial ectopic beat is generating electrical impulses faster than the sinoatrial node, the ectopic beat will override the sinoatrial node impulse and cause the atria and ventricles to depolarize. Dysrhythmias that are caused by the atrial ectopic site include premature atrial complexes, atrial tachycardia, atrial flutter, and atrial fibrillation. The P wave is affected by rhythms in this category.

neurological Pertaining to the nervous system, its diseases, and its functions.

Atrial dysrhythmias occur from conditions that cause pressure on the atria such as damage to the atria from myocardial infarction, valvular problems, or **neurological** influences (pertaining to the nervous system). When the area is stressed or damaged, the cells become unstable and the electrical state may cause depolarization to occur more easily.

CheckPoint Question (LO 6.1)

1. Which wave form is affected by the change in electrical activity within the atria?

_____

_____

6.2 Premature Atrial Complexes

Premature atrial complexes (PACs) are electrical impulses that originate in the atria and initiate an early impulse that interrupts the inherent regular rhythm (Figure 6-1).

Criteria for Classification

- ***Rhythm:*** The regularity between the P-P interval and R-R interval is constant with the exception of the early complexes. There will be a section of the rhythm that is regular and occasionally an early complex.
- ***Rate:*** The rates of the atria and ventricles will usually be within normal limits of 60 to 100, depending on the frequency of the PACs.
- ***P wave configuration:*** The P waves will have the same configuration and shape. The early beat usually will have a different shape than the rest of the P waves on the strip. This P wave may be flattened, notched, biphasic or equiphasic (have two phases), or otherwise unusual. It may even be hidden within the T wave of the preceding complex. Evidence that the P wave is hidden within the T wave includes a notch in the T wave, a pointed shape, or being taller than the other T waves.

biphasic The waveform that has an equally positive (upward) and negative (downward) deflection on the ECG tracing.

- ***PR interval:*** The PR interval will measure within normal limits of 0.12 to 0.20 second. The early beat will probably have a different PR measurement than the normal complexes but will be within normal limits.
- ***QRS duration and configuration:*** The QRS duration and configuration will be within normal limits of 0.06 to 0.10 second.

Figure 6-1 Premature atrial complex (PAC).

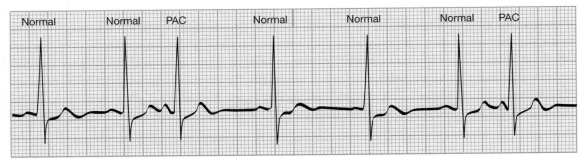

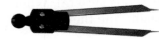

Interpret-TIP

Premature Atrial Complexes

A PAC is a cardiac complex that occurs too soon. It has a positively deflected P wave. Other than being "early," this complex does not possess any abnormal features.

Determine the underlying rhythm of sinus rhythm, sinus bradycardia, sinus tachycardia, or sinus dysrhythmia when identifying PACs. The rhythm strip must be labeled with this underlying rhythm and the type of PAC. An example of this terminology is "sinus rhythm with trigeminal PACs" (**trigeminy** refers to a pattern in which every third complex is a premature beat).

trigeminy Pattern in which every third complex is a premature beat.

How the Patient Is Affected and What You Should Know

With each PAC, the atria do not achieve the maximum blood capacity prior to contraction. This lack of blood causes a decrease in cardiac output and less volume in the ventricles prior to ventricular contraction. Therefore, in the patient who has prior cardiac disease, frequent PACs can cause the patient to experience symptoms of low cardiac output.

When caring for a patient with PACs, observe the patient for signs and symptoms of low cardiac output. Monitoring the amount or frequency of PACs is essential. The patient may complain of palpitations from the early beats. The severity of the patient's complaints is related to the frequency of the PACs. In addition, frequent PACs may indicate that a more serious atrial dysrhythmia may follow. The more frequent occurrence indicates that the ectopic **focus** (cardiac cell that functions as an ectopic beat) may continue and take control of the heart rate. Any observation of low cardiac output should be communicated to a licensed practitioner for appropriate treatment.

focus or foci A cardiac cell or group of cells that function as an ectopic beat.

CheckPoint Question (LO 6.2)

Using the criteria for classification, select the rhythm that most closely resembles premature atrial complex (PAC).

(Continued)

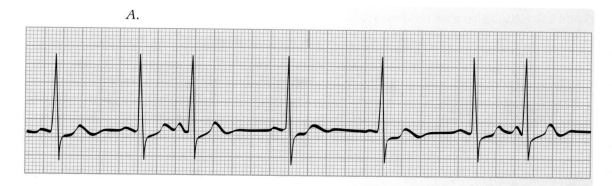

A.

B.

1. Which unique feature(s) led you to make the selection?

_____

_____

_____

6.3 Wandering Atrial Pacemaker

Wandering atrial pacemaker (WAP) is a rhythm in which the pacemaker site shifts between the SA node, atria, and/or the AV junction. The P wave configuration changes in appearance during the pacemaker shift. At least three different P wave configurations in the same lead indicate a wandering atrial pacemaker (Figure 6-2).

Criteria for Classification

- *Rhythm:* Slightly irregular
- *Rate:* Should be within normal limits of 60 to 100 beats per minute
- *P wave configuration (shape):* Continuous change in appearance
- *PR interval:* Varies
- *QRS duration and configuration:* Usually within normal limits

Figure 6-2 Wandering atrial pacemaker.

Wandering atrial pacemaker arises from different sites in the atria.

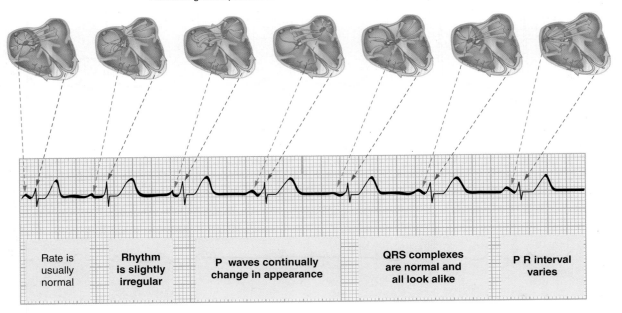

| Rate is usually normal | Rhythm is slightly irregular | P waves continually change in appearance | QRS complexes are normal and all look alike | P R interval varies |

How the Patient Is Affected and What You Should Know

WAP is a normal finding in children, older adults, and well-conditioned athletes and does not usually cause clinical signs and symptoms. However, it may also be related to some types of organic heart disease and drug toxicity.

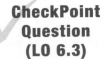

Interpret-TIP

Wandering Atrial Pacemaker Rhythm

WAP has a changing P wave configuration with at least three variations in one lead. The rhythm may be irregular.

CheckPoint Question (LO 6.3)

Using the criteria for classification, select the rhythm that most closely resembles the wandering atrial pacemaker (WAP) rhythm.

A.

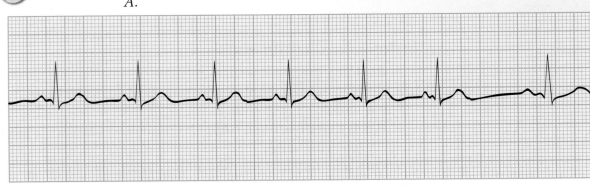

(Continued)

B.

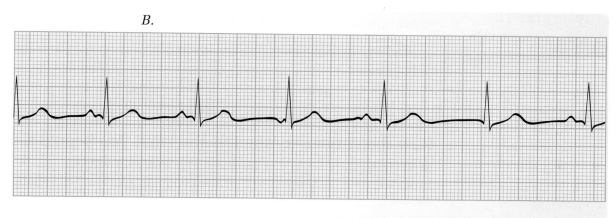

1. Which unique feature(s) led you to make the selection?

_____

_____

_____

6.4 Multifocal Atrial Tachycardia

Multifocal atrial tachycardia (MAT) has a P wave that changes from beat to beat and a heart rate of 101 to 150 (Figure 6-3). It has the same characteristics as wandering atrial pacemaker (WAP), with the only difference being that the rate is in excess of 100. It can be distinguished by looking closely for visible changing P waves.

Figure 6-3   Multifocal atrial tachycardia.

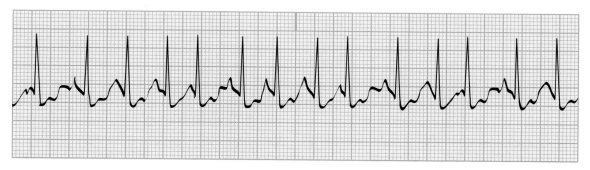

Criteria for Classification

- **Rhythm:** Irregular
- **Rate:** Between 101 and 150 beats per minute
- **P wave configuration:** P waves change in appearance from beat to beat. They may be upright, rounded, notched, inverted, biphasic, or buried in the QRS complex.
- **PR interval:** Varies due to the changing origin of the electrical activity
- **QRS duration and configuration:** Normal in duration and all complexes look alike

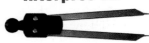
Multifocal Atrial Tachycardia

MAT has a clearly changing P wave and a heart rate of 101 to 150 beats per minute.

How the Patient Is Affected and What You Should Know

MAT is usually triggered by an acute attack of emphysema, congestive heart failure (CHF), or acute mitral valve regurgitation. This rhythm should be reported to the licensed practitioner, and the patient's vital signs and condition should be monitored.

CheckPoint Question (LO 6.4)

Using the criteria for classification, select the rhythm which most closely resembles wandering atrial pacemaker (WAP) Rhythm.

A.

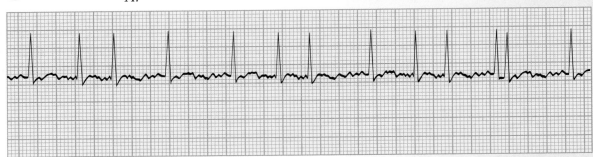

B.

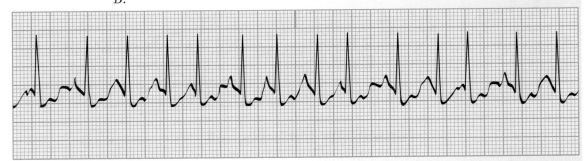

1. Which unique feature(s) led you to make the selection?

_____

_____

_____

6.5 Flutter

Sawtooth-
Appereance

Rythym usually
regular

Atrial flutter (A flutter) occurs when a rapid impulse originates in the atrial tissue. The ectopic focus may be originating from ischemic areas of the heart with enhanced **automaticity** (ability to initiate an electrical current) or from a reentry pathway. A reentry pathway is an extra pathway that has developed where a group of cells will generate an impulse faster than the SA node. This impulse then follows a route that allows the impulse to reach the AV node quicker than the normal conduction pathway. The reentry pathway is similar to finding a shortcut to work or school to bypass the normal traffic route to get you to your destination faster. The electrical current or rhythm is recorded in a characteristic sawtooth pattern (Figure 6-4). This atrial activity is called flutter (F) waves. As shown in Figure 6-4, F waves are often seen in a ratio of 2, 3, 4, and even 5 F waves to each QRS complex. This means that the atria (represented by the F waves) are depolarizing and contracting at a rate equal to the ratio of F waves to QRS complexes. When interpreting this rhythm, it is often described to include the ratio of F waves to QRS complexes; that is, atrial flutter 3:1. Most often this is a transient dysrhythmia that will lead to more serious atrial dysrhythmia if not treated.

Figure 6-4   Atrial flutter.

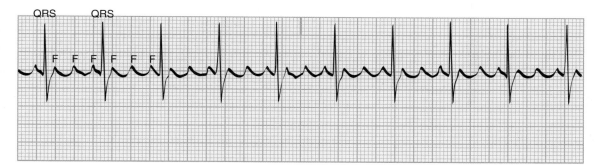

Criteria for Classification

- **Rhythm:** The P-P interval or flutter-to-flutter waves will be regular. The interval set with the calipers will stay constant throughout the rhythm. The R-R interval is usually irregular, but occasionally it may be regular in pattern. The regularity of the R-R interval will depend on the ability of the AV node to limit impulses to ventricles.
- **Rate:** The atrial rate will be between 250 and 350 beats per minute.
- **P wave configuration:** P waves are not seen, and only flutter (or F) waves are present. These flutter waves resemble a "sawtooth" or "picket fence." They will be seen best in leads II, III, and aVF. The correlation between P waves and QRS complexes no longer exists. There will be more flutter waves than QRS complexes.
- **PR interval:** No identifiable P wave exists, so the PR interval cannot be measured.
- **QRS duration and configuration:** The QRS duration will be within normal limits of 0.06 to 0.10 second.

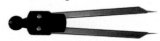
Atrial Flutter

Atrial flutter has a "sawtooth" atrial pattern between the QRS complexes.

How the Patient Is Affected and What You Should Know

atrial kick When blood is ejected into the ventricles by the atria immediately prior to ventricular systole.

The atrial kick, which occurs when blood is ejected into the ventricles by the atria immediately prior to ventricular systole, is no longer present since the atria do not contract completely, followed by a delay in the ventricular contraction. This loss in atrial kick contributes to a 10% to 30% decrease in cardiac output. Some patients may tolerate this if the heart rate is within normal limits of 60 to 100 beats per minute. But once the heart rate increases significantly and loss of the atrial kick occurs, the patient will demonstrate signs and symptoms of low cardiac output.

When atrial flutter occurs, notify the licensed practitioner to implement a treatment plan, which usually includes oxygen therapy to ensure adequate supply to the vital organs. The patient is monitored continuously to determine if the rhythm converts to a sinus rhythm or progresses to atrial fibrillation. A continuous rhythm strip is needed to document if any changes occurred as a result of the medical intervention. Always indicate on the rhythm strip the type of intervention that is being implemented. The ECG strips are then mounted and saved in the patient's medical record or chart.

CheckPoint Question (LO 6.5)

Using the criteria for classification, select the rhythm that most closely resembles atrial flutter rhythm.

A.

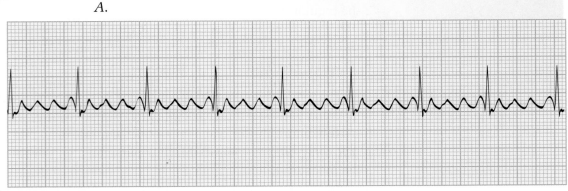

(Continued)

B.

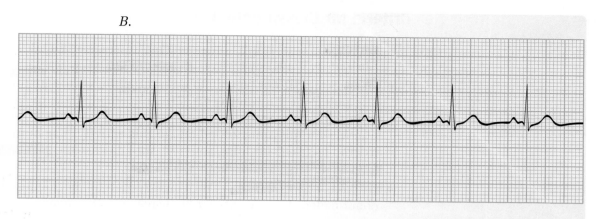

Which unique feature(s) led you to make the selection?

_____

_____

_____

6.6 Atrial Fibrillation

Atrial fibrillation (A fib) occurs when electrical impulses come from areas of reentry pathways or multiple ectopic foci. Each electrical impulse results in depolarization of only a small group of atrial cells rather than the whole atria. This results in the atria not contracting as a whole, causing it to quiver, similar to a bowl of Jell-O™ when shaken. The result of this disorganized electrical activity is that the atria are not really pumping blood as they normally do. This ineffective electrical activity can cause a cardiac output of up to 30%. Multiple atrial activity is recorded as a chaotic wave, often with the appearance of fine scribbles (Figure 6-5). No P wave can be identified. The waveform of the chaotic "scribbles" is referred to as fibrillatory waves or f waves.

Figure 6-5 Atrial fibrillation.

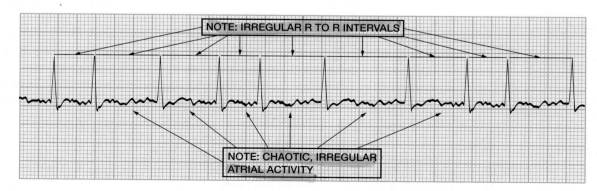

Criteria for Classification

- **Rhythm:** The P-P interval is unable to be determined because of the fibrillatory waves or f waves. The R-R interval is irregular.
- **Rate:** You will *not* be able to determine the atrial rate due to the chaotic nature of the waveforms. This electrical chaos makes it virtually impossible to identify or measure the atrial rate. The atria are not contracting and pumping blood due to this activity. The numbers referred to are electrical impulse activity, not contraction. Electrical impulse activity often is in the range of 375–700.
- **P wave configuration:** The P waves cannot be identified. There is chaotic electrical activity, or "f" waves may be seen.
- **PR interval:** The PR interval cannot be measured, since the P wave is not identifiable.
- **QRS duration and configuration:** The QRS duration and configuration will be within normal limits of 0.06 to 0.10 second and irregular.

Interpret-TIP

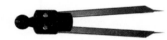

Atrial Fibrillation

Atrial fibrillation shows chaotic atrial electrical activity with irregular R-R intervals.

How the Patient Is Affected and What You Should Know

The patient will exhibit signs and symptoms of decreased cardiac output. The patient usually has limited cardiac function because of preexisting cardiac conditions, so with the loss of atrial kick, the patient's cardiac output will decrease significantly. When patients first present with atrial fibrillation the ventricular response is often over 100 beats per minute. This is referred to as "uncontrolled" A-fib. Patients with "new onset" A-fib will often complain of dizziness, nausea, etc. These are signs of low cardiac output. The initial goal in the treatment of uncontrolled A-fib is to stabilize the patient by slowing the ventricular response via the use of medications first, then cardioversion if necessary. Once the heart rate is controlled within the range of 60 to 100 beats per minute, the patient may be able to tolerate the loss of the atrial kick.

Blood will begin to collect in the atria because they are not contracting completely, allowing the opportunity for a clot or **thrombus** to form. Therefore, the patient has an increased risk of developing and sending an embolism (traveling blood clot) out into the body's systemic circulation, which can then migrate to other vital organs, such as the lungs or brain. The patient may develop a **cerebral vascular accident (CVA), myocardial infarction (MI), pulmonary embolism, renal infarction,** or an embolism in any place that the arterial blood is transported. Essentially, the heart is playing Russian roulette with us because there is no way to predict where the embolism will travel in the body to cause serious damage or even sudden death.

thrombus A blood clot that forms on the inside of an injured blood vessel wall.

cerebrovascular accident A stroke caused by a hemorrhage in the brain or more often by a clot lodged in cerebral artery.

myocardial infarction A blockage of one or more of the coronary arteries causing lack of oxygen to the heart and damage to the muscle tissue.

pulmonary embolism A blocked artery in the lungs, usually caused by a blood clot.

renal infarction A lack of oxygen to lung tissue due to a blocked blood vessel.

Patients who exhibit atrial fibrillation must be observed for low cardiac output. The rhythm needs to be monitored closely as the medication or electrical cardioversion is attempted. Report any complications or vital sign changes to the licensed practitioner immediately.

CheckPoint Question (LO 6.6)

Using the criteria for classification, select the rhythm that most closely resembles atrial fibrillation rhythm.

A.

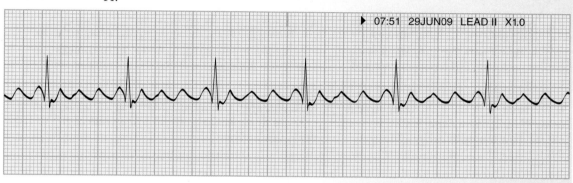

▶ 07:51 29JUN09 LEAD II X1.0

B.

1. Which unique feature(s) led you to make the selection?

_____

_____

_____

Chapter Summary

Learning Outcomes	Summary	Pages
6.1 Summarize the similarities between atrial dysrhythmias.	Atrial dysrhythmias also known as arrhythmias are caused by an ectopic impulse in either of the atria.	149
6.2 Identify premature atrial complexes using the criteria for classification and explain how the rhythm may affect the patient, including basic patient care and treatment.	Premature atrial complexes (PACs) are electrical impulses that originate in the atria and initiate an early impulse that interrupts the inherent regular rhythm.	149–151
6.3 Identify wandering atrial pacemaker using the criteria for classification and explain how the rhythm may affect the patient, including basic patient care and treatment.	A wandering atrial pacemaker (WAP) is a rhythm in which the pacemakersite shifts between the SA node, atria, and/or the AV junction. The P wave configuration changes in appearance during the pacemaker shift.	151–153
6.4 Identify multifocal atrial tachycardia using the criteria for classification and explain how the rhythm may affect the patient, including basic patient care and treatment.	Multifocal atrial tachycardia (MAT) has a P wave that changes from beat to beat and a heart rate of 101 to 150 beats per minute.	153–154
6.5 Identify atrial flutter using the criteria for classification and explain how the rhythm may affect the patient, including basic patient care and treatment.	Atrial flutter (A flutter) occurs when a rapid impulse originates in the atrial tissue. This dysrhythmia presents with a classic sawtooth or picket fence appearance known as flutter or F waves.	155–157
6.6 Identify atrial fibrillation using the criteria for classification and explain how the rhythm may affect the patient, including basic patient care and treatment.	Atrial fibrillation (A fib) occurs when electrical impulses come from areas of reentry pathways or multiple ectopic foci. Each electrical impulse results in depolarization of only a small group of atrial cells rather than the whole atria. This dysrhythmia presents with classic chaotic ("f" or fibrillatory) waves between the irregular R- R intervals	157–159

Chapter Review

Matching

_____ 1. ectopic (L O 6.1)

_____ 2. trigeminy (L O 6.2)

_____ 3. focus (L O 6.2)

_____ 4. neurological (L O 6.1)

_____ 5. automaticity (L O 6.5)

_____ 6. atrial kick (L O 6.5)

_____ 7. thrombus (L O 6.6)

_____ 8. biphasic (L O 6.2)

_____ 9. cerebrovascular accident (L O 6.6)

_____ 10. renal (L O 6.6)

_____ 11. pulmonary embolism (L O 6.6)

_____ 12. myocardial (L O 6.6)

a. pertaining to the heart

b. pertaining to the kidneys

c. outside the normal pacemaker site

d. blood is ejected completely by the atria prior to ventricular systole

e. cell functions as an ectopic impulse formation

f. every third complex is premature

g. pertaining to the nervous system

h. cardiac cell initiates an electrical impulse

i. stroke

j. traveling blood clot in the lungs

k. blood clot

l. lack of oxygen due to a blocked blood vessel

Multiple Choice

Circle the correct answer.

13. What is the rate of wandering atrial pacemaker rhythm? (LO 6.3)
    a. 60 to 100 beats per minute
    b. 50 to 90 beats per minute
    c. 100 to 150 beats per minute
    d. 60 to 80 beats per minute

14. What dysrhythmia is similar to wandering atrial pacemaker, but the rate exceeds 100 beats per minute? (LO 6.4)
    a. Sinus tachycardia
    b. Multfocal atrial tachycardia
    c. Atrial flutter
    d. Atrial fibrillation

15. What is the major health risk for patients who have atrial fibrillation? (LO 6.6)
    a. Hypertension?
    b. Thrombus formation and embolization?
    c. Bundle branch block
    d. Bleeding problems

16. What atrial dysrhythmia has capital "F" waves and a classic sawtooth or picket fence appearance? (LO 6.5)
    a. PACs
    b. Multifocal atrial tachycardia
    c. Atrial fibrillation
    d. Atrial flutter

17. What atrial dysrhythmia has lowercase "f" waves, chaotic atrial electrical activity and irregular R to R intervals? (LO 6.6)
    a. PACs
    b. Multifocal atrial tachycardia
    c. Atrial fibrillation
    d. Atrial flutter

18. Wandering atrial pacemaker rhythm must have _____ or more different shaped "P" waves. (LO 6.3)
    a. Two
    b. Three
    c. Four
    d. None of the above

19. When premature complexes occur in a rhythm, they interrupt the underlying rhythm, causing it to be _____ when analyzing it. (LO 6.2)
    a. Regular
    b. Irregular
    c. A wider QRS complex
    d. Bradycardic

20. What is a common sign of low cardiac output? (LO 6.1)
    a. High blood pressure
    b. Alert and oriented
    c. Increased perfusion of vital organs
    d. Low blood pressure

Fill in the Blank

21. Multifocal atrial tachycardia may occasionally be confused with _____ . (LO 6.4)

22. When analyzing atrial flutter, you note that there are four "F" waves for each QRS complex. How will you represent this pattern in your interpretation? _____ . (LO 6.5)

Short Answer

23. The patient has coronary artery disease. How would you expect PACs to affect this patient? (LO 6.1)

_____

_____

24. What treatment is usually indicated for patients with atrial flutter? (LO 6.5)

_____

_____

25. What is the best way to describe the rhythm pattern for atrial fibrillation? (LO 6.6)

_____

_____

26. Which rhythm is considered more serious, MAT or WAP, and why? (LO 6.3, 6.4)

_____

_____

Critical Thinking Applications _Rhythm Identification_

Review the dysrhythmias pictured here and, using the criteria for classification provided in the chapter as clues, identify each rhythm and provide what information you used to make your decision. (LO 6.2–6.6)

27.

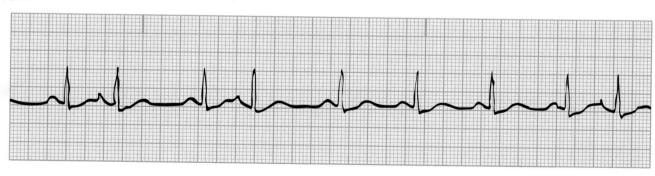

Rhythm (Regular or Irregular): _____ PR interval: _____

Rate: _____ QRS: _____

P wave: _____ Interpretation: _____

28.

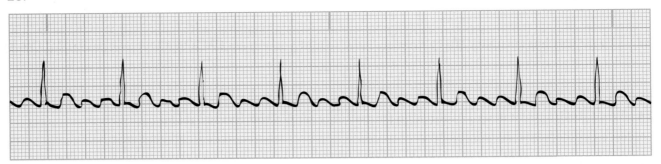

Rhythm (Regular or Irregular): _____ PR interval: _____

Rate: _____ QRS: _____

P wave: _____ Interpretation: _____

29.

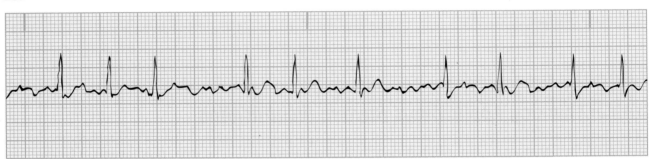

Rhythm (Regular or Irregular): _____ PR interval: _____

Rate: _____ QRS: _____

P wave: _____ Interpretation: _____

30.

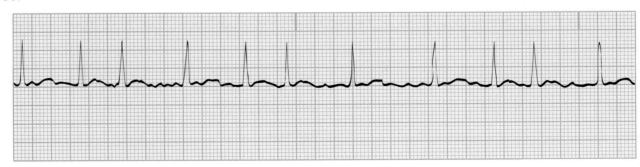

Rhythm (Regular or Irregular): _____ PR interval: _____

Rate: _____ QRS: _____

P wave: _____ Interpretation: _____

31.

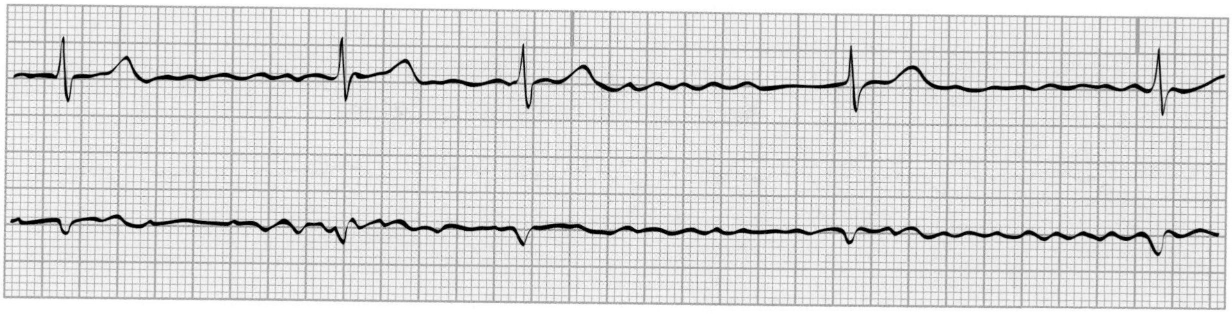

Rhythm (Regular or Irregular): _____ PR interval: _____

Rate: _____ QRS: _____

P wave: _____ Interpretation: _____

32.

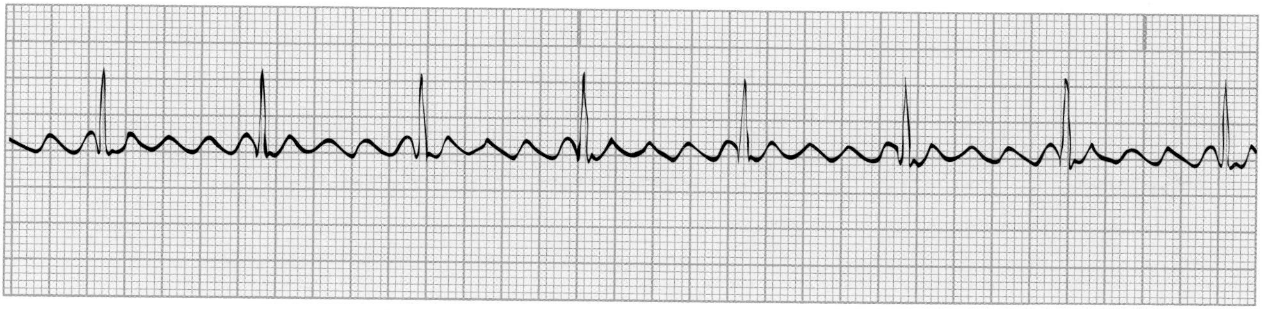

Rhythm (Regular or Irregular): _____ PR interval: _____

Rate: _____ QRS: _____

P wave: _____ Interpretation: _____

33.

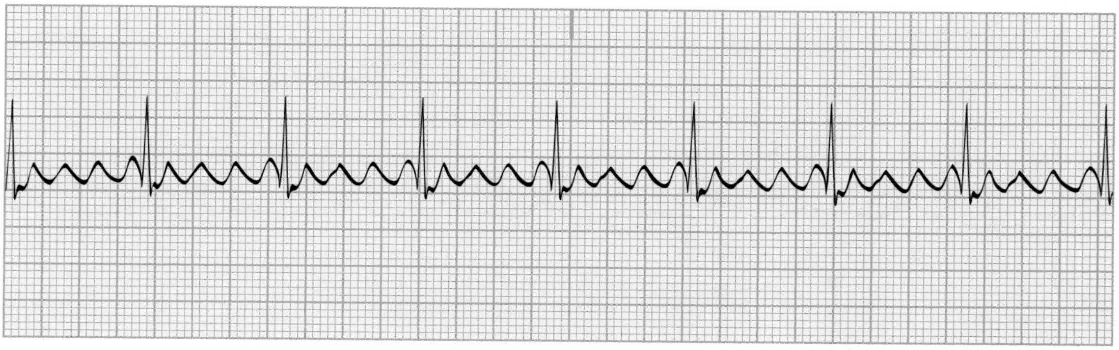

Rhythm (Regular or Irregular): _____ PR interval: _____

Rate: _____ QRS: _____

P wave: _____ Interpretation: _____

34.

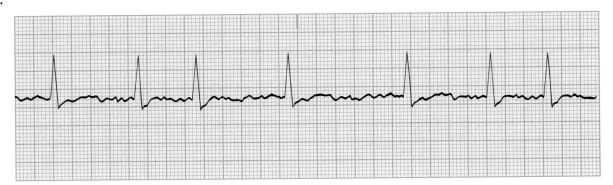

Rhythm (Regular or Irregular): _____ PR interval: _____

Rate: _____ QRS: _____

P wave: _____ Interpretation: _____

35.

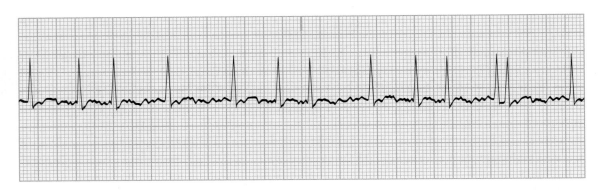

Rhythm (Regular or Irregular): _____ PR interval: _____

Rate: _____ QRS: _____

P wave: _____ Interpretation: _____

36.

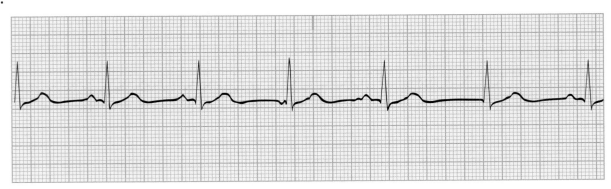

Rhythm (Regular or Irregular): _____ PR interval: _____

Rate: _____ QRS: _____

P wave: _____ Interpretation: _____

37.

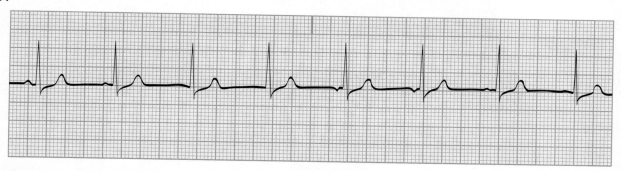

Rhythm (Regular or Irregular): _____ PR interval: _____

Rate: _____ QRS: _____

P wave: _____ Interpretation: _____

Internet Activity

Visit the McGraw-Hill Higher Education Online Learning Center *Electrocardiography for Healthcare Professionals* Web site at **www.mhhe.com/boothecg3e** to complete the following activity.

1. Go to the National Heart, Lung, and Blood Institute Diseases and Conditions Index and review Atrial Fibrillation http://www.nhlbi.nih.gov/health/dci/Browse/Heart.html. Create a list of things that can be done to prevent and treat this condition.

 ## Using the Student CD

Now that you have completed the material in the chapter text, return to the student CD and complete any chapter activities you have not yet done. Practice your terminology with the "Key Term Concentration" game. Review the chapter material with the "Spin the Wheel" and "ECG Challenge" game. Take the final chapter test and complete the troubleshooting question and email or print your results to document your proficiency for this chapter.

7 Junctional Dysrhythmias

Chapter Outline

- Introduction to Junctional Dysrhythmias (p. 169)
- Premature Junctional Complex (PJC) (p. 169)
- Junctional Escape Rhythm (p. 171)
- Accelerated Junctional Rhythm (p. 173)
- Junctional Tachycardia (p. 175)
- Supraventricular Tachycardia (SVT) (p. 177)

Learning Outcomes

7.1 Describe the various junctional dysrhythmias.

7.2 Identify premature junctional complexes using the criteria for classification, and explain how the rhythm may affect the patient, including basic patient care and treatment.

7.3 Identify junctional escape rhythm using the criteria for classification, and explain how the rhythm may affect the patient, including basic patient care and treatment.

7.4 Identify accelerated junctional rhythm using the criteria for classification, and explain how the rhythm may affect the patient, including basic patient care and treatment.

7.5 Identify junctional tachycardia rhythm using the criteria for classification, and explain how the rhythm may affect the patient, including basic patient care and treatment.

7.6 Identify supraventricular tachycardia rhythm using the criteria for classification, and explain how the rhythm may affect the patient, including basic patient care and treatment.

Key Terms

escape rhythm
hypotension
palpitations

retrograde
supraventricular
underlying rhythm

7.1 Introduction to Junctional Dysrhythmias

The atrioventricular node is sometimes referred to as the AV junction or AV tissue. Though abnormal, these AV node cells, which possess the property of automaticity, can function as a pacemaker. The inherent rate of the AV node is between 40 and 60 beats per minute. Junctional rhythms are a result of electrical impulses coming from the AV node rather than from the SA node. With junctional rhythms, it is important to understand that the electrical current is initiated *from* the AV junction. As a result of the electrical activity coming from the AV node or junction, the electrical impulses causing depolarization of the atria are flowing retrograde, or backward. This reverse flow of electrical activity causes the unique inverted P wave morphology seen in junctional dysrhythmias. Junctional rhythms are suggestive of more serious conditions with the electrical conduction system in the heart. The AV node is the backup pacemaker for the heart after the SA node. Junctional rhythm, accelerated junctional rhythm, and junctional tachycardia are all conditions in which the SA node has been injured and the AV node functions as the pacemaker of the heart.

Checkpoint Question (LO 7.1)

1. Explain what causes the inverted P wave morphology found with junctional rhythms?

_____

_____

7.2 Premature Junctional Complex (PJC)

underlying rhythm Occurs before the next expected sinus impulse, causing an irregularity.

A premature junctional complex (PJC) is a single early electrical impulse that originates in the atrioventricular junction. It occurs before the next expected sinus impulse, causing an irregularity in the underlying rhythm (Figure 7-1).

Criteria for Classification

- *Rhythm:* May be occasionally irregular or frequently irregular, depending upon the number of PJCs present
- *Rate:* Will depend upon the underlying rhythm
- *P wave configuration:* The P wave is inverted and may immediately precede or follow the QRS complex, or it may be buried within the QRS complex.
- *PR interval:* May be shorter than normal if the P wave precedes the QRS complex, absent if the P wave is buried in the QRS, and not measurable if it occurs after the QRS complex.
- *QRS duration and configuration:* The QRS duration and configuration will be between 0.06 and 0.10 second, which is within normal limits.

    NOTE: Remember that the PR interval can only be measured if the P wave (regardless of shape) occurs prior to the QRS complex.

Figure 7-1   Premature junctional contraction at 6th beat of sinus rhythm.

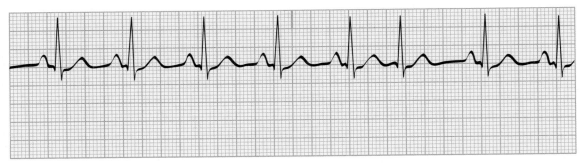

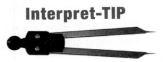

Interpret-TIP

Premature Junctional Complexes?

PJCs will cause the rhythm to be irregular, and the P wave may appear before, during, or after the QRS complex. Regardless of location, if the P wave is seen, it will be inverted.

hypotension Condition in which the patient's blood pressure is not adequate to maintain good blood supply to the vital organs.

How the Patient Is Affected and What You Should Know

When the patient has a healthy heart, isolated PJCs cause no signs or symptoms. If PJCs occur more than four to six per minute, this warns of a more serious condition. An irregular pulse would be noted, and the patient may experience **hypotension** due to low cardiac output.

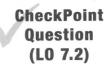

CheckPoint Question (LO 7.2)

Using the criteria for classification, select the rhythm that most closely resembles premature junctional complex.

A.

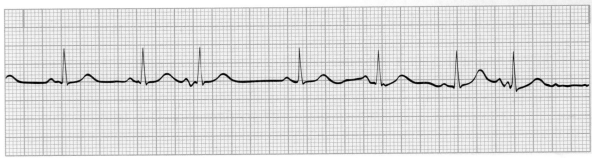

(Continued)

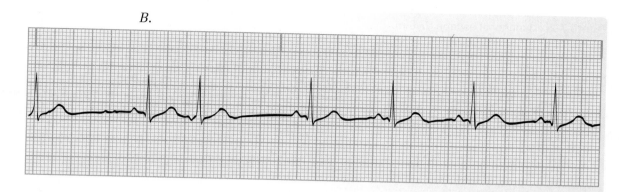

B.

1. Which unique feature(s) led you to make the selection?

_____

_____

_____

7.3 Junctional Escape Rhythm

escape rhythm A rhythm that occurs when the SA node fails to initiate the electrical activity and one of the backup pacemaker sites takes over.

Junctional rhythm, also known as junctional **escape rhythm,** originates at atrioventricular junctional tissue, producing retrograde (backward) depolarization of atrial tissue, and, at the same time, stimulates the depolarization of ventricles (Figure 7-2).

Note: escape rhythms occur when the SA node fails to initiate the electrical activity. When this happens one of the backup pacemaker sites takes over.

Criteria for Classification

- **Rhythm:** The P-P and R-R intervals are regular and at similar intervals. The P-P interval may be difficult to measure due to the location of the P wave.
- **Rate:** If the P wave is identifiable, the rate will be 40 to 60 beats per minute. The ventricular rate will be 40 to 60 beats per minute.
- **P wave configuration:** The P wave is usually inverted and may precede, follow, or fall within the QRS complex. It may not be visible at all on the rhythm strip.
- **PR interval:** If the P wave is before the QRS complex, the PR interval will measure less than 0.12 second and will be constant. If the P wave is not before the QRS complex, the PR interval cannot be determined. This is because this P wave is not associated with the next QRS complex.
- **QRS duration and configuration:** The QRS duration and configuration will be within normal limits of 0.06 to 0.10 second.

Figure 7-2 Junctional escape rhythm.

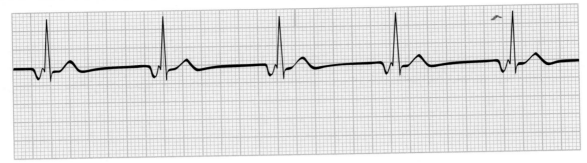

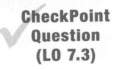

Interpret-TIP

Junctional Escape Rhythm

The P wave may occur before, during (buried), or after the QRS. If the P wave is seen, it will be inverted. The heart rate is between 40 to 60 beats per minute.

How the Patient Is Affected and What You Should Know

The patient with junctional escape rhythm has a slower heart rate than normal and loses the atrial kick due to the shortening of the interval between the atrial depolarization and ventricular depolarization. These conditions often cause the patient to exhibit symptoms of low cardiac output. Common signs and symptoms of low cardiac output displayed include hypotension (low blood pressure) and altered mental status, such as confusion or disorientation. Observe for symptoms and monitor the ECG tracing in case a more serious dysrhythmia occurs. Report the presence of junctional rhythm and your observations of the patient to a licensed practitioner for appropriate medical treatment.

CheckPoint Question (LO 7.3)

Using the criteria for classification, select the rhythm that most closely resembles junctional escape rhythm.

A.

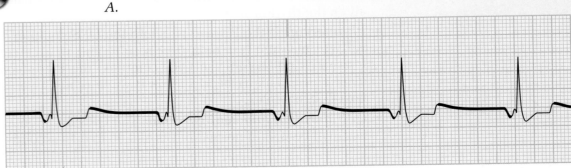

(Continued)

B.

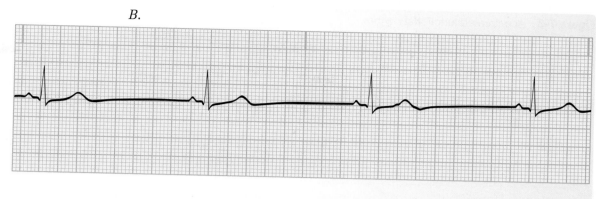

1. Which unique feature(s) led you to make the selection?

   _____

   _____

2. What are differences between a PJC rhythm and a junctional rhythm?

   _____

   _____

   _____

7.4 Accelerated Junctional Rhythm

Accelerated junctional rhythm shares the same unique morphology as junctional escape rhythm, with the distinguishing difference being the heart rate. This rhythm originates at atrioventricular (AV) junctional tissue, producing **retrograde** (backward) depolarization of atrial tissue, and, at the same time, stimulates the depolarization of ventricles (Figure 7-3).

retrograde moving backward

Criteria for Classification

- *Rhythm:* The P-P and R-R intervals are regular and at similar intervals. The P-P interval may be difficult to measure due to the location of the P wave.
- *Rate:* If the P wave is identifiable, the rate will be 60 to 100 beats per minute. The ventricular rate will be at the same rate of 60 to 100 beats per minute.
- *P wave configuration:* The P wave is usually inverted and may precede, follow, or fall within the QRS complex. *It may not be visible at all on the rhythm strip.*
- *PR interval:* If the P wave is before the QRS complex, the PR interval will measure less than 0.12 second and will be constant. *If the P wave is not before the QRS complex, the PR interval cannot be determined.* This is because this P wave is not associated with the next QRS complex.
- *QRS duration and configuration:* The QRS duration and configuration will be within normal limits of 0.06 to 0.10 second.

Figure 7-3 Accelerated junctional rhythm.

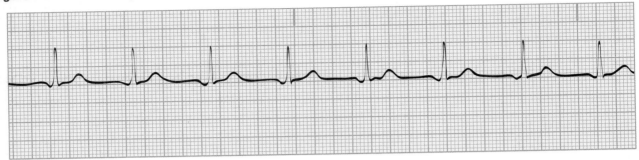

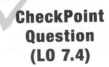

Interpret-TIP

Accelerated Junctional Rhythm

A junctional rhythm may have an inverted or absent P wave or a P wave that follows the QRS complex. Heart rate is between 60 and 100 beats per minute.

How the Patient Is Affected and What You Should Know

It is unlikely that the patient will show signs and symptoms of low cardiac output because the rate is the same as normal sinus rhythm. It is still very important to observe your patient for symptoms and to monitor the ECG tracing in case a more serious dysrhythmia occurs. Report the presence of accelerated junctional rhythm and your observations of the patient to a licensed practitioner for appropriate medical treatment.

CheckPoint Question (LO 7.4)

Using the criteria for classification, select the rhythm that most closely resembles accelerated junctional rhythm.

A.

(Continued)

B.

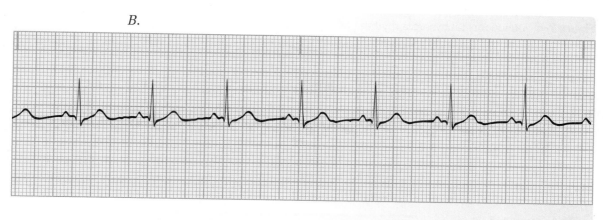

1. Which unique feature(s) led you to make the selection?

_____

_____

_____

7.5 Junctional Tachycardia Rhythm

Junctional tachycardia rhythm shares the same unique morphology as junctional escape rhythm and accelerated junctional rhythm, the only difference again being the heart rate is faster in junctional tachycardia. The electrical activity originates at the atrioventricular (AV) junctional tissue, producing retrograde (backward) depolarization of atrial tissue, and at the same time stimulates the depolarization of ventricles (Figure 7-4).

Criteria for Classification

- **Rhythm:** The P-P and R-R intervals are regular and at similar intervals. The P-P interval may be even more difficult to measure because of the combination of location of the P wave couple and the increased rate of automaticity.

- **Rate:** If the P wave is identifiable, the rate will be between 100 and 150 beats per minute. The ventricular rate will be at the same rate (between 100 and 150 beats per minute).

- **P wave configuration:** The P wave is usually inverted and may precede, follow, or fall within the QRS complex. It may not be visible at all on the rhythm strip. *At the upper limit of this range, it may be very difficult to determine the origin of the atrial electrical activity without increasing the paper speed of your cardiac monitor.*

- **PR interval:** If the P wave is before the QRS complex, the PR interval will measure less than 0.12 second and will be constant. If the P wave is not before the QRS complex, the PR interval cannot be determined because this P wave is not associated with the next QRS complex.

- **QRS duration and configuration:** The QRS duration and configuration will be within the normal limits of 0.06 to 0.10 second.

Figure 7-4   Junctional tachycardia rhythm.

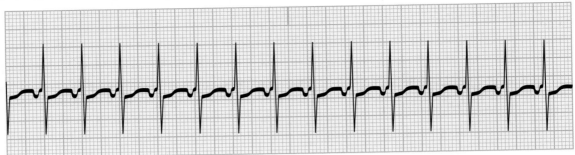

Interpret-TIP

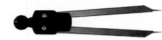

Junctional Tachycardia Rhythm

A junctional tachycardia rhythm may have an inverted or absent P wave or a P wave that follows the QRS complex. Heart rate is between 100 and 150 beats per minute.

How the Patient Is Affected and What You Should Know

The effect of this rhythm on the patient depends on the rate of junctional tachycardia. For example, if the patient's normal resting heart rate is 90 and now the patient is exhibiting a rate of 108 beats per minute after walking the hallway, tachycardia would be expected and is viewed as the patient's normal response to exercise. However, if the patient's normal heart rate is 60 and it is now 140, the patient is probably experiencing symptoms of low cardiac output. Often the patient will complain of **palpitations** or "heart fluttering" with faster rates. If the patient has had a recent myocardial infarction, junctional tachycardia or tachycardia of any type is considered to be more serious or even life threatening.

Observe the patient for symptoms, and monitor the ECG tracing in case a more serious dysrhythmia occurs. Report the presence of junctional tachycardia rhythm and your observations of the patient to a licensed practitioner for appropriate medical treatment. Medication may need to be administered to terminate this dysrhythmia.

palpitations Fast, irregular heartbeat sensation felt by the patient, which may or may not be associated with complaints of chest pain.

CheckPoint Question (LO 7.5)

Using the criteria for classification, select the rhythm that most closely resembles junctional tachycardia rhythm.

A.

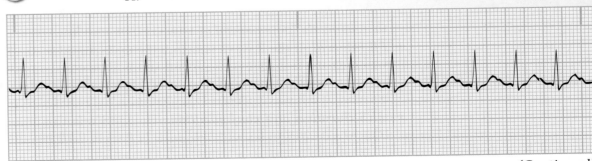

(Continued)

B.

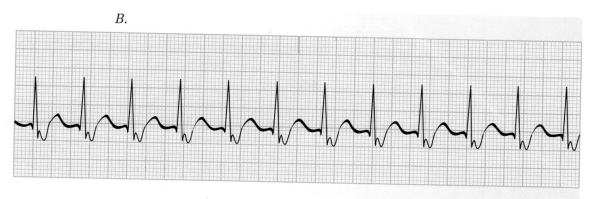

1. Which unique feature(s) led you to make the selection?

_____

_____

_____

7.6 Supraventricular Tachycardia (SVT)

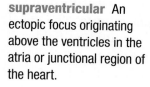

supraventricular An ectopic focus originating above the ventricles in the atria or junctional region of the heart.

A supraventricular tachycardia (SVT) is a classification of rapid heartbeats occurring at a rate greater than 150 beats per minute (Figure 7-5). Although supraventricular tachycardia (SVT) is not specifically a junctional dysrhythmia, the origin causing this rapid heart rhythm may come from any location "above the ventricles." As its name implies, supra means "above". Impulse activity may come from anywhere within the atria, SA node, AV node or other locations within the atria. Supraventricular refers to an ectopic focus originating above the ventricles, in the atria, or in the junctional region of the heart. The heart is beating so fast that it is difficult to determine if the source of origin is from the sinus node, atria, or the AV junction. Because the heart rate is so rapid, the atria are contracting as soon as the ventricles are relaxing. This causes the P waves (atrial contraction) to become difficult to identify because they may occur at the same time as the QRS or T waves (ventricle relaxation). Rhythms that fall into this category are identified in Table 7-1.

SVTs, as well as the rhythms in the table below, are often referred to as re-entry dysrhythmias. Re-entry dysrhythmias occur when there is essentially a blockage or short-circuit in the normal electrical conduction pathway. This forces the electrical impulse to follow an aberrant pathway, which often leads

Figure 7-5 Supraventricular tachycardia.

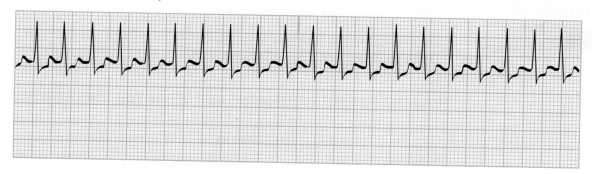

TABLE 7-1 Dysrhythmias Associated with Supraventricular Tachycardia

Sinus Node	Atrium	Junctional
Sinus tachycardia	Atrial flutter Atrial fibrillation	Junctional tachycardia

to a series of rapid depolarizations that in turn lead to tachydysrhythmias such as atrial fibrillation, atrial flutter, or junctional tachycardia, to name a few.

The primary difficulty in classifying the actual rhythm is identifying where the tachycardia originates. The P wave may appear before, after, or during the QRS complex, depending on the origin. The PR interval measurement is difficult to assess because you cannot often see the initial upswing of the P wave. Frequently, the licensed practitioner will request the paper speed be increased to pull the cardiac complexes apart in an attempt to expose the P wave and determine the origin or source of the electrical activity. However, be sure to mark the tracing if this is done.

Criteria for Classification

- *Rhythm:* The ventricular (R-R) rhythm is usually regular or with minimal irregularity from R-R interval. The atrial rhythm may or may not be seen. This is because other electrical activity is occurring at the same time. Remember, the ECG will record only the activity it "sees" in each lead. The atrial activity is small compared to ventricular activity; therefore, the ventricular activity is the largest amount of energy seen when the ECG tracing is recorded. Depending on whether the P waves are seen, you may not be able to determine regular P waves. If identifiable, they are usually regular.
- *Rate:* The ventricular rate is 150 to 250 beats per minute. The atrial rate will be difficult to determine when P waves are unidentifiable.
- *P wave configuration:* The P waves are usually not identified when the heart rate is this rapid. Remember that when the heart rate increases, the time interval between atrial contraction and ventricular relaxation decreases. Therefore, if there is a P wave present, it may occur simultaneously with the T wave and may be buried within it. The P wave may occur before, during, or after the QRS complex.
- *PR interval:* Usually the PR interval is unable to be determined because the beginning of the P wave cannot be clearly identified.
- *QRS duration and configuration:* The QRS measurement is considered within normal limits when measured at 0.06 to 0.10 second.

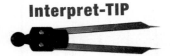

Interpret-TIP

Supraventricular Dysrhythmias

Supraventricular tachycardia presents with a normal–narrow-appearing QRS complex and a rate of greater than 150 beats per minute.

How the Patient Is Affected and What You Should Know

There are various supraventricular dysrhythmias, all of which may cause the patient to exhibit the same signs and symptoms. The patient may be in either a stable or an unstable condition. The stable patient (one

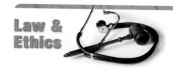

Law & Ethics

Scope of Practice

Your role regarding evaluation of the rhythm strip and assessment of the patient will depend on your training and place of employment. Working outside of your scope of practice is illegal, and you could be held liable for performing tasks that are not part of your role as a healthcare professional.

without signs and symptoms of decreased cardiac output) may only complain of palpitations and state, "I'm just not feeling right" or "My heart is fluttering." When the patient's condition is *unstable,* he or she may experience any symptom of low cardiac output, which is reflective of the heart not pumping effectively to other body systems. Many patients may present initially with a stable condition and then a few minutes later experience unstable symptoms such as those presented in Table 5-2.

Observe the patient for signs and symptoms of low cardiac output. Signs, symptoms, and rhythm changes need to be communicated quickly to a licensed practitioner for appropriate medical treatment. Because tachycardia significantly increases myocardial oxygen demand, treatment should begin as early as possible. It is difficult to predict how long a patient's heart can beat at a rapid rate before it begins to affect the other body systems.

Check Point Questions (LO 7.6)

1. What are the rate and the origination point of a supraventricular tachycardia?

   _____

   _____

2. What might you be asked to do when a patient has a supraventricular dysrhythmia?

   _____

   _____

3. List common sensations described by patients experiencing SVT.

   _____

   _____

4. Using the criteria for classification, select the rhythm that most closely resembles supraventricular tachycardia (SVT) rhythm.

   A.

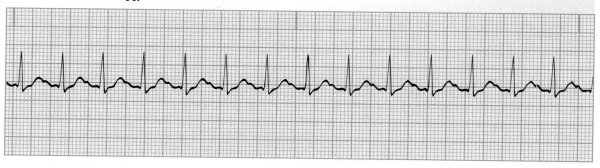

(Continued)

B.

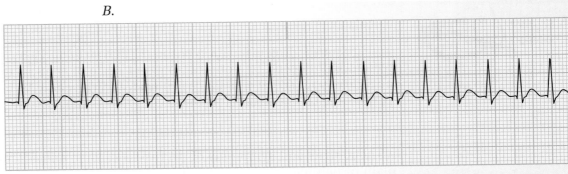

Which unique feature(s) led you to make the selection?

_____

_____

Chapter Summary

Learning Outcomes	Summary	Pages
7.1 Describe the various junctional dysrhythmias.	Junctional rhythms occur as a result of electrical impulses coming from the AV node or junction rather than the SA node. As a result of this change in origination site for the electrical activity, the electrical impulses causing depolarization of the atria are flowing retrograde (backward). This reverse flow of electrical activity causes the unique inverted P wave morphology seen in junctional dysrhythmias.	169
7.2 Identify premature junctional complex using the criteria for classification, and explain how the rhythm may affect the patient, including basic patient care and treatment.	A premature junctional complex (PJC) is a single early electrical impulse that originates in the AV junction. It occurs before the next expected sinus impulse, causing an irregularity in the rhythm.	169–170
7.3 Identify junctional escape rhythm using the criteria for classification, and explain how the rhythm may affect the patient, including basic patient care and treatment.	Junctional rhythm, also known as junctional escape rhythm, originates at AV junctional tissue, producing retrograde (backward) depolarization of atrial tissue, and, at the same time, stimulates the depolarization of ventricles.	171–173
7.4 Identify accelerated junctional rhythm using the criteria for classification, and explain how the rhythm may affect the patient, including basic patient care and treatment.	Accelerated junctional rhythm shares the same unique morphology as junctional escape rhythm, with the distinguishing difference being the heart rate, which is between 60 and 100 beats per minute for accelerated junctional rhythm.	173–175
7.5 Identify junctional tachycardia rhythm using the criteria for classification, and explain how the rhythm may affect the patient, including basic patient care and treatment.	Junctional tachycardia rhythm shares the same unique morphology as junctional escape rhythm and accelerated junctional rhythm, the only difference again being the heart rate exceeds 100 beats per minute.	175–177
7.6 Identify supraventricular tachycardia rhythm using the criteria for classification, and explain how the rhythm may affect the patient, including basic patient care and treatment.	Although supraventricular tachycardia is not specifically a junctional dysrhythmia, the origin causing this rapid heart rhythm may come from any location "above the ventricles." Supraventricular tachycardia presents with a normal–narrow-appearing QRS complex and a rate of greater than 150 beats per minute.	177–180

Chapter Review

Multiple Choice

Circle the correct answer.

1. What is the normal, inherent rate for the AV junction? (LO 7.1)
   a. 60–100 beats per minute
   b. 40–60 beats per minute (bpm)
   c. 100–160 beats per minute
   d. 20–40 beats per minute

2. Which of the following dysrhythmias is not considered part of the supraventricular tachycardia classification? (LO 7.6)
   a. Atrial fibrillation
   b. Sinus tachycardia
   c. Ventricular tachycardia
   d. Junctional tachycardia

3. What sign or symptom might a patient complain about when experiencing a supraventricular tachycardia in an unstable condition? (LO 7.6)
   a. Back pain
   b. Palpitations
   c. Hypothyroidism
   d. Chest pain and discomfort

4. The criterion needed to classify the dysrhythmia as a supraventricular tachycardia is (LO 7.6)
   a. heart rate between 150 and 350 beats per minute.
   b. a wide QRS complex.
   c. a clear, easily identifiable P wave with the entire wave visualized.
   d. atrial and ventricular rates that are not the same.

5. What is the primary difficulty in determining a supraventricular rhythm? (LO 7.6)
   a. Determining the ventricular rate
   b. Determining the regularity
   c. Measuring the QRS interval
   d. Determining the origin of the tachycardia

6. When is the identification of the specific dysrhythmia important in terms of treatment of the patient? (LO 7.6)
   a. When the patient first complains of any signs or symptoms.
   b. When the patient's heart rate has decreased to a rate of 100 to 150 beats per minute.
   c. During the treatment of a fast tachycardia situation.
   d. After the rhythm has been converted to a normal rhythm and/or the heart rate is between 60 and 100 beats per minute.

7. What is the heart rate range for junctional escape rhythm? (LO 7.2)
   a. 20–40 beats per minute
   b. 100–150 beats per minute
   c. 40–60 beats per minute
   d. 60–100 beats per minute

8. What is the heart rate range for accelerated junctional rhythm? (LO 7.3)
   a. 20–40 beats per minute
   b. 100–150 beats per minute
   c. 40–60 beats per minute
   d. 60–100 beats per minute

9. What is the heart rate range for junctional tachycardia rhythm? (LO 7.4)
   a. 20–40 beats per minute
   b. 100–150 beats per minute
   c. 40–60 beats per minute
   d. 60–100 beats per minute

Short Answer

10. Describe why P waves are inverted or buried within the QRS complex with junctional dysrhythmias (LO 7.1)

   _____

   _____

Critical Thinking Application *Rhythm Identification*

Review the dysrhythmias pictured here and, using the criteria for classification provided in the chapter as clues, identify each rhythm and provide what information you used to make your decision. (LO 7.2–7.6)

11.

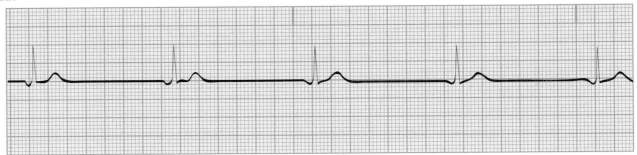

Rhythm (Regular or Irregular): _____   PR interval: _____

Rate: _____   QRS: _____

P wave: _____   Interpretation: _____

12.

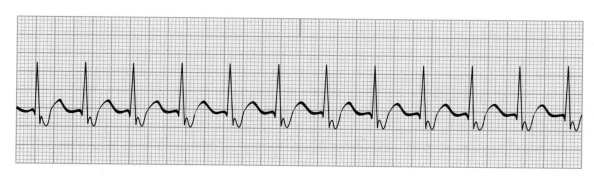

Rhythm (Regular or Irregular): _____ PR interval: _____

Rate: _____ QRS: _____

P wave: _____ Interpretation: _____

13.

Rhythm (Regular or Irregular): _____ PR interval: _____

Rate: _____ QRS: _____

P wave: _____ Interpretation: _____

14.

Rhythm (Regular or Irregular): _____ PR interval: _____

Rate: _____ QRS: _____

P wave: _____ Interpretation: _____

15.

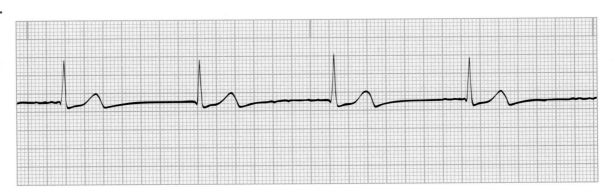

Rhythm (Regular or Irregular): _____ PR interval: _____

Rate: _____ QRS: _____

P wave: _____ Interpretation: _____

16.

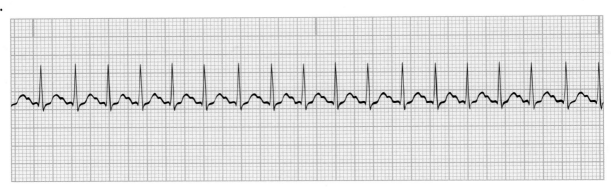

Rhythm (Regular or Irregular): _____ PR interval: _____

Rate: _____ QRS: _____

P wave: _____ Interpretation: _____

17.

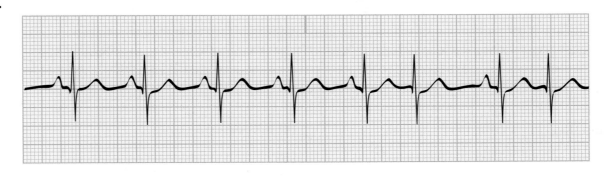

Rhythm (Regular or Irregular): _____ PR interval: _____

Rate: _____ QRS: _____

P wave: _____ Interpretation: _____

18.

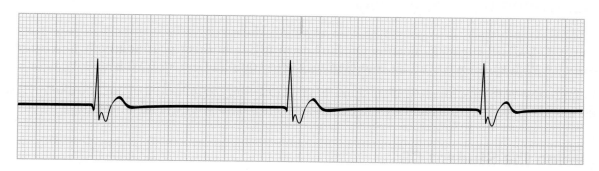

Rhythm (Regular or Irregular): _____ PR interval: _____

Rate: _____ QRS: _____

P wave: _____ Interpretation: _____

19.

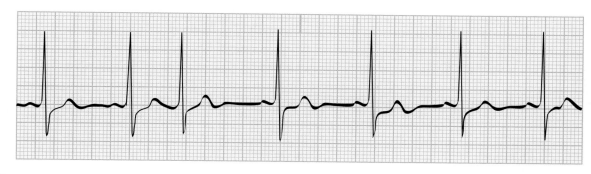

Rhythm (Regular or Irregular): _____ PR interval: _____

Rate: _____ QRS: _____

P wave: _____ Interpretation: _____

20.

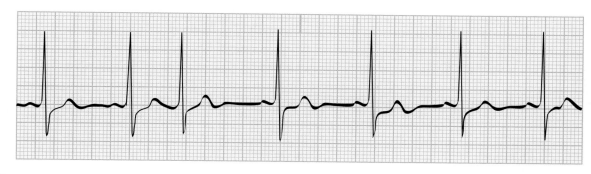

Rhythm (Regular or Irregular): _____ PR interval: _____

Rate: _____ QRS: _____

P wave: _____ Interpretation: _____

21.

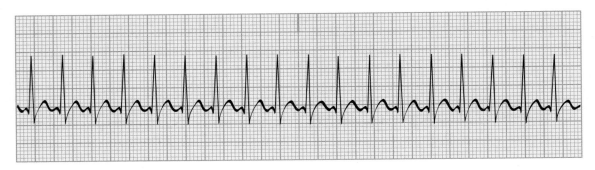

Rhythm (Regular or Irregular): _____ PR interval: _____

Rate: _____ QRS: _____

P wave: _____ Interpretation: _____

Get Connected *Internet Activity*

Visit the McGraw-Hill Higher Education Online Learning Center *Electrocardiography for Healthcare Professionals* Web site at **www.mhhe.com/boothecg3e** to complete the following activity.

1. Refer to the Web link http://skillstat.com/Flash/ECG_Sim_2004.html for practice and review of common cardiac rhythms and dysrhythmias. This is a dynamic rhythm simulator.

Using the Student CD

Now that you have completed the material in the chapter text, return to the student CD and complete any chapter activities you have not yet done. Practice your terminology with the "Key Term Concentration" game. Review the chapter material with the "Spin the Wheel" and "ECG Challenge" game. Take the final chapter test, and complete the troubleshooting question; email or print your results to document your proficiency for this chapter.

Heart Block Dysrhythmias

8

Chapter Outline

- Introduction to Heart Block Dysrhythmias (p. 187)
- First Degree Atrioventricular (AV) Block (p. 188)
- Second Degree Atrioventricular (AV) Block, Mobitz I (Type I or Wenckebach) (p. 189)
- Second Degree Atrioventricular (AV) Block, Type II (Mobitz II) (p. 192)
- Third Degree Atrioventricular (AV) Block (Complete) (p. 194)

Learning Outcomes

8.1 Describe the various heart block dysrhythmias.

8.2 Identify first degree heart block using the criteria for classification, and explain how the rhythm may affect the patient, including basic patient care and treatment.

8.3 Identify second degree atrioventricular (AV) block, Mobitz I, using the criteria for classification, and explain how the rhythm may affect the patient, including basic patient care and treatment.

8.4 Identify second degree atrioventricular (AV) block, Mobitz II, using the criteria for classification, and explain how the rhythm may affect the patient, including basic patient care and treatment.

8.5 Identify third degree atrioventricular (AV) block using the criteria for classification, and explain how the rhythm may affect the patient, including basic patient care and treatment.

Key Terms

blocked or nonconducted impulse
cardiac output parameters
dissociative

8.1 Introduction to Heart Block Dysrhythmias

In heart block rhythms, the electrical current has difficulty traveling along the normal conduction pathway, causing a delay in or absence of ventricular depolarization. The degree of blockage is dependent on the area affected and the cause of the delay or blockage. There are three levels of heart blocks. The P-P interval is regular with all heart blocks.

1. What is the cause of a heart block dysrhythmia?

_____

_____

8.2 First Degree Atrioventricular (AV) Block

First degree AV block is a *delay* in electrical conduction from the SA node to the AV node, usually around the AV node, which prevents an electrical impulse from traveling to the ventricular conduction system (Figure 8-1). The condition is similar to being in a traffic jam. You still arrive at your destination, but it takes you longer to get there. Electrical current from the SA node will still stimulate ventricular depolarization, but the time it takes to arrive in the ventricles is longer than normal.

Figure 8-1 First degree AV block.

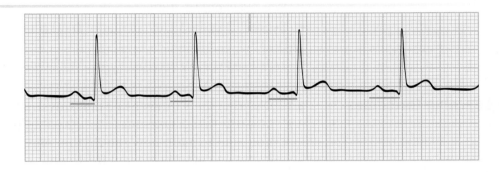

Criteria for Classification

- *Rhythm:* The regularity between the P-P interval and the R-R interval is constant.
- *Rate:* The rate of the atria and ventricles will usually be within normal limits of 60 to 100 beats per minute.
- *P wave configuration:* The P waves will have the same configuration and shape. Each QRS complex will have a P wave before it. There will be the same number of P waves as QRS complexes.
- *PR interval:* The PR interval will be greater than 0.20 second.
- *QRS duration and configuration:* The QRS duration and configuration will be within normal limits of 0.06 to 0.10 second.

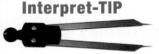

Interpret-TIP

First Degree AV Block

With first degree atrioventricular block, the PR interval is constant and measures greater than 0.20 second.

How the Patient Is Affected and What You Should Know

The patient will be able to maintain normal cardiac output. No change in the patient should occur with this rhythm. Monitor and observe for further degeneration and development of other heart blocks and report if they

cardiac output parameters
Observation guidelines used to assess the blood supply to the vital organs of the body to maintain normal function.

occur. It is important to observe the **cardiac output parameters**—to assess the blood supply to the vital organs—and to determine how well the patient is tolerating the dysrhythmia.

CheckPoint Question (LO 8.2)

Using the criteria for classification, select the rhythm that most closely resembles first degree AV block.

A.

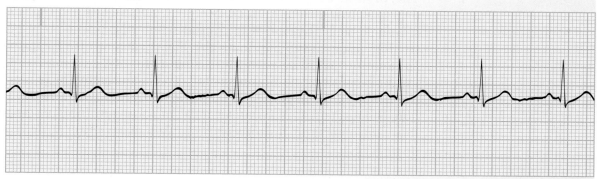

B.

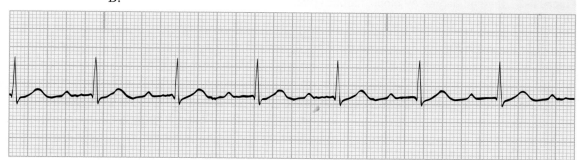

1. Which unique feature(s) led you to make the selection?

_____

_____

_____

blocked or nonconducted impulse Impulse occurs too soon after the preceding impulse, causing a period when no other impulses can occur in the ventricles.

8.3 Second Degree Atrioventricular (AV) Block, Mobitz I (Type I or Wenckebach)

There are two types of second degree heart blocks, second degree type I and second degree type II. This category of heart block has some **blocked or nonconducted** electrical impulses from the SA node to the ventricles at the atrioventricular junction region. As a result, there are missing QRS complexes. The impulses from the atria are regular but depending upon which second degree type of block, the conduction through the AV node may be delayed and at some point blocked in a pattern or the impulse is blocked entirely, resulting in missing QRS complexes.

Note: Second degree heart blocks are the only blocks with an irregular ventricular response.

There are currently two different types of second degree heart blocks, which were first discovered by Dr. Woldemar Mobitz, a German internist, in the early 20th century. Dr. Karel Frederik Wenckebach further investigated the rhythm and was able to identify a similar blockage pattern, but it was different from the one Dr. Mobitz observed. The rhythm Dr. Wenckebach observed was specifically labeled second degree atrioventricular block, Mobitz I, although it is often referred to as a Wenckebach rhythm. It is caused when diseased or injured atrioventricular node tissue conducts the electrical impulse to the ventricular conduction pathway with increasing difficulty, causing a delay in time until one of the atrial impulses fails to be conducted or is blocked. *After the dropped atrial impulse, the atrioventricular node resets itself to be able to handle future impulses more quickly and then progressively gets more difficult until it drops or is blocked again.* This pattern will repeat itself (Figure 8-2).

Figure 8-2   Second degree AV block, Mobitz I (Wenckebach).

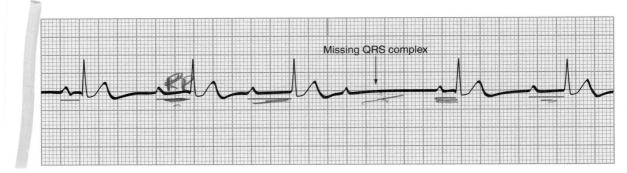

Missing QRS complex

Criteria for Classification

- **Rhythm:** The P-P interval will be regular. The R-R interval will be irregular due to the blocked impulse(s).
- **Rate:** Atrial rate will be within normal limits. The ventricular rate will be slower than the atrial rate.
- **P wave configuration:** The P wave configuration will be normal size with an upright P wave. There will be a P wave for every QRS complex, but there will be extra P waves.
- **PR interval:** The PR interval will vary from one measurement to the next. The PR interval will be progressively longer with each subsequent conducted P wave until the QRS wave is dropped. The PR interval will be short, and then the cycle will begin again.
- **QRS duration and configuration:** The QRS duration and configuration should be within normal limits of 0.06 to 0.10 second.

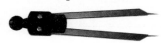

Second Degree AV Block, Mobitz I (Wenckebach)

A Mobitz I rhythm has a cyclical prolonging PR interval until the QRS is dropped. Then the cycle "resets" and begins again (irregular ventricular response).

How the Patient Is Affected and What You Should Know

The patient may or may not exhibit symptoms of decreased cardiac output, depending on the rate of ventricle contraction. As this rate decreases and reaches levels of 40 beats per minute or lower, the patient will show signs and symptoms of low cardiac output. This rhythm is usually due to inflammation around the atrioventricular node, and it is often a temporary condition that will resolve itself and return to a normal heart rhythm.

Since treatment is based on how the patient is tolerating the rhythm, the patient is observed for signs and symptoms of low cardiac output. If the patient is experiencing difficulties, a licensed practitioner administers medication; if not, the patient is monitored for further progression to third degree heart block.

CheckPoint Question (LO 8.3)

Using the criteria for classification, select the rhythm that most closely resembles second degree AV block, type I.

A.

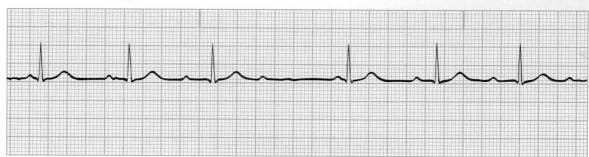

B.

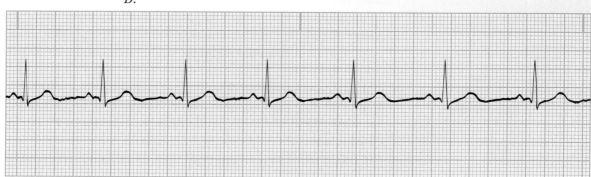

(Continued)

1. Which unique feature(s) led you to make the selection?

_____

_____

_____

8.4 Second Degree Atrioventricular (AV) Block, Type II (Mobitz II)

Second degree atrioventricular block, Mobitz II, is often referred to as the classical heart block because it was the first rhythm observed to have an occasional dropped complex (Figure 8-3). The atrioventricular node selects which electrical impulses it will block. Occasionally, the blocked QRS complexes will occur in a pattern. It might be seen as 2, 3, or 4 P waves between each QRS complex. When second degree type II occurs in this fashion, it is often referred to by the ratio of P waves to each QRS (e.g., second degree type II 3:1). When in doubt, refer to the Interpret-TIP for this dysrhythmia. There is usually no pattern or reason for the dropping of the QRS complex. **Frequently this dysrhythmia will progress to third degree atrioventricular block.**

Figure 8-3 Mobitz second degree type II.

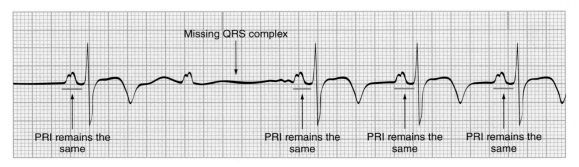

Criteria for Classification

- **Rhythm:** The P-P interval will be regular. The R-R interval may or may not be irregular due to the unpredictable nature of the blocked impulse(s). (R-R intervals are occasionally in a pattern.)
- **Rate:** Atrial rate will be within normal limits. The ventricular rate will be slower than the atrial rate. The atrial and ventricular rates will not be the same.
- **P wave configuration:** The P wave configuration will be normal, with a normal size and upright wave. There will be at least one P wave for every QRS complex, and there will be more P waves than QRS complexes.
- **PR interval:** The PR interval is constant and will remain constant even after the QRS drop occurs.
- **QRS duration and configuration:** The QRS duration and configuration should be within normal limits of 0.06 to 0.10 second.

TABLE 8-1 Differences Between Second Degree Heart Blocks

Type of Heart Block	PR Interval	Etiology	Treatment
Second degree AV block, Mobitz I (Type I, or Wenckebach)	Varies from one complex to another; will reset itself after the dropped complex	Temporary	May resolve itself; observe cardiac output and wait until the PR intervals vary and the dropped QRS complexes occur
Second degree AV block, Mobitz II (Type II, or classical block)	Constant PR interval throughout the rhythm strip	Chronic situation	Quickly leads to a complete heart block, a life-threatening situation that needs immediate attention: call 911 or Code Blue. Transcutaneous pacing may be placed on stand by. The use of this device may be directly related to the speed of ventricular depolarization or the frequency of dropped QRS complexes. Either of these circumstances may dramatically affect cardiac output.

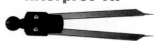

Interpret-TIP

Second Degree (AV) Block, Mobitz Type II

QRS complexes are missing, but, wherever a P is with the QRS complex, the PR interval will always measure the same.

How the Patient Is Affected and What You Should Know

Observe the patient for signs and symptoms of low cardiac output since this rhythm frequently will progress very quickly to a third degree atrioventricular block, or complete heart block (CHB), usually within seconds. Recognition of the classical block pattern versus the Wenckebach pattern is essential. See Table 8-1 for differences between second degree heart blocks. *The classical block is more critical and can quickly lead to a complete heart block and a Code Blue situation.* When your patient is experiencing

Troubleshooting

Mobitz I vs. Mobitz II

To quickly determine the difference between a second degree, Mobitz I (type I, or Wenckebach) and a second degree, Mobitz II (classical) AV block, first look for missing QRS complexes. Once this is determined, analyze the PR interval of the rhythm. If the PR interval is in a progressively pronging pattern, followed by a missing QRS, then you have second degree type I (Wenckebach). If the PR interval remains the same, then you have second degree type II.

Remember the mnemonic "Lengthen, Lengthen, drop equals Wenckebach."

Both rhythms should be reported; however, second degree type II is a highly unstable dysrhythmia and is a critical condition. Second degree type I is typically a much more stable rhythm; it is usually transient with a low degree for conversion to complete heart block.

What does the mnemonic "Lengthen, Lengthen, drop equals Wenckeback" mean?

second degree heart block, Mobitz II, you should immediately report it to a licensed practitioner; and, if trained, you should prepare for a Code Blue and application of a temporary external pacemaker.

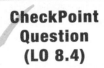
Using the criteria for classification, select the rhythm that most closely resembles second degree AV block type II.

A.

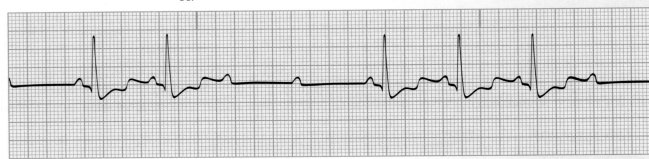

B.

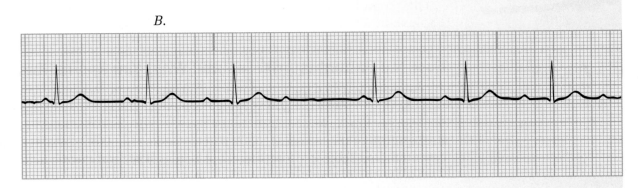

1. Which unique feature(s) led you to make the selection?

_____

_____

_____

8.5 Third Degree Atrioventricular (AV) Block (Complete)

dissociative To remove from association as with atrioventricular (AV) dissociation or a condition in which the atria and ventricles do not activate in a synchronous fashion but beat independent of each other.

Third degree atrioventricular block is also known as *third degree heart block* or *complete heart block* (CHB). All electrical impulses originating above the ventricles are blocked and prevented from reaching the ventricles. There is no correlation between atrial and ventricular depolarization. As a result, there will be noticeable and suspicious **dissociative** properties; namely the P-P and R-R intervals. Although the intervals are regular when measured, the atria and ventricles will be firing at completely different rates, resulting in a variable PR interval. This is due to the "block," and as a result the ventricular rate will be slower than the atrial rate (Figure 8-4).

The rate of the ventricular response and the configuration of the QRS complex will be dependent upon the level of the block. If the block is low in the bundle of His, the pacemaker would come from the slow (20 to 40 beats per minute) Purkinje network. The QRS complex in this instance would measure 0.12 second or greater.

If the block is higher and the impulse causing ventricular depolarization is coming from the area of the AV tissue, then the rate is likely to be 40 to 60 beats per minute and the QRS complex will present with a "normal to narrow" appearance measuring 0.06 to 0.10 second. The ventricular rate and QRS configurations are keys indicating the level of the heart block.

Figure 8-4   Third degree AV block (complete heart block).

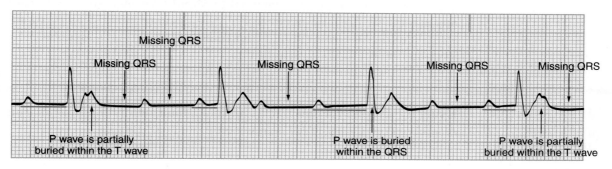

Criteria for Classification

- **Rhythm:** The P-P is regular. The R-R interval is also regular, but the P-P and R-R intervals will be different.
- **Rate:** The atrial rate will be within normal limits of 60 to 100 beats per minute. The ventricular rate is slow, between 20 and 40 or 40 to 60 beats per minute, depending upon the pacemaker site. (Either way, the ventricular rate will be less than the atrial rate.)
- **P wave configuration:** P waves will be of normal size and configuration, but the location may be buried within the QRS, either before or after the QRS complex. There will be no correlation seen between the P waves and the QRS complex. More P waves will be noted than QRS complexes, and not every P wave will have a QRS complex following it.
- **PR interval:** PR intervals will be variable due to the atrial and ventricular tissue depolarizing at different rates.
- **QRS duration and configuration:** The QRS duration and configuration will be the same but the measurements may be either within normal limits or wide, depending on the area of the blockage.

Interpret-TIP

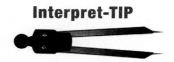

Third Degree (Complete) Heart Block

In third degree atrioventricular block, the P-P and R-R intervals are regular (constant) but firing at different rates.

How the Patient Is Affected and What You Should Know

With complete heart block, the atria and the ventricles are electrically separated from one another. This is often referred to as AV dissociation. As a result of this condition, the atria and ventricles are firing at different rates because different pacemaker sites are initiating depolarization of those areas of the heart. This condition results in a loss of atrial kick. Along with the loss of atrial kick and reduced ventricular rate, the patient will often exhibit signs and symptoms of low cardiac output. The slower ventricular rate increases the likelihood that the patient will be unconscious and require immediate medical intervention.

In a situation where the patient is in third degree AV block, your first responsibility is to observe the patient for signs and symptoms of low cardiac output. If the patient displays any signs and symptoms, notify a licensed practitioner immediately.

It may be necessary to initiate a cardiac arrest, rapid response, or Code Blue alarm. A temporary pacemaker should be available and ready for application as deemed necessary by the licensed practitioner. All rhythm strips should be mounted and identified in the patient's medical record as documentation of the dysrhythmia.

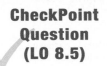

CheckPoint Question (LO 8.5)

Using the criteria for classification, select the rhythm that most closely resembles third degree AV block (complete heart block).

A.

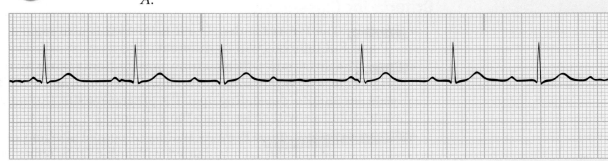

B.

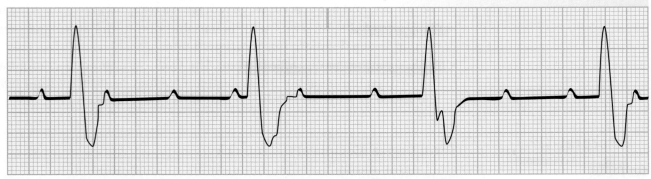

(Continued)

1. Which unique feature(s) led you to make the selection?

_____

_____

_____

Chapter Summary

Learning Outcomes	Summary	Pages
8.1 Describe the various heart block dysrhythmias.	In heart block rhythms, the electrical current has difficulty traveling along the normal conduction pathway, causing a delay in or absence of ventricular depolarization. The degree of blockage is dependent on the area affected and the cause of the delay or blockage. The P-P interval is regular with all heart blocks. There are three levels of heart blocks.	187
8.2 Identify first degree heart block using the criteria for classification, and explain how the rhythm may affect the patient, including basic patient care and treatment.	First degree AV block is a delay in electrical conduction from the SA node to the AV node, usually around the AV node, which prevents an electrical impulse from traveling to the ventricular conduction system.	188–189
8.3 Identify second degree atrioventricular (AV) block, Mobitz I using the criteria for classification, and explain how the rhythm may affect the patient, including basic patient care and treatment.	Second degree heart block type I has some blocked or nonconducted electrical impulses from the SA node to the ventricles at the atrioventricular junction. The impulses coming from the atria are regular, but the conduction through the AV node gets delayed where the impulse does not get to the ventricles, and becomes blocked.	189–192
8.4 Identify second degree atrioventricular (AV) block, Mobitz II using the criteria for classification, and explain how the rhythm may affect the patient, including basic patient care and treatment.	Second degree atrioventricular block, Mobitz II, is often referred to as the "classical" heart block. The atrioventricular node selects which electrical impulses it will block. No pattern or reason for the dropping of the QRS complex exists. Frequently this dysrhythmia will progress to third degree atrioventricular block.	192–194
8.5 Identify third degree atrioventricular (AV) block using the criteria for classification, and explain how the rhythm may affect the patient, including basic patient care and treatment.	Third degree atrioventricular block is also known as _third degree heart block_ or _complete heart block_ (CHB). All electrical impulses originating above the ventricles are blocked and prevented from reaching the ventricles. There is no correlation between atrial and ventricular depolarization. In third degree atrioventricular block, the P-P and R-R intervals are regular (constant) but firing at different rates.	194–197

Chapter Review

Multiple Choice

Circle the correct answer.

1. Which heart block rhythm is the one with the distinguishing feature of a PR interval that measures greater than 0.20 second and measures the same duration each time? (LO 8.2)
   a. First degree heart block
   b. Second degree type I
   c. Second degree type II
   d. Third degree heart block

2. Which of the following heart block dysrhythmias is identified by a repetitious prolonging PR interval pattern after each blocked QRS complex? (LO 8.3)
   a. First degree heart block
   b. Second degree type I
   c. Second degree type II
   d. Third degree heart block

3. Which of the following heart block dysrhythmias is identified by missing QRS complexes and a consistent PR interval measurement? (LO 8.4)
   a. First degree heart block
   b. Second degree type I
   c. Second degree type II
   d. Third degree heart block

4. Which of the following heart block dysrhythmias is identified by regular P-P and R-R intervals that are firing at two distinctly different rates? (LO 8.5)
   a. First degree heart block
   b. Second degree type I
   c. Second degree type II
   d. Third degree heart block

5. P-P intervals measure as _____ with all heart block dysrhythmias. (LO 8.2–8.5)
   a. irregular
   b. absent
   c. regular
   d. no P waves with heart blocks

6. QRS complexes that measure 0.12 second or greater with a rate between 20 and 40 beats per minutes indicate the impulses causing ventricular depolarization are coming from the _____. (LO 8.5)
   a. SA node
   b. interatrial pathways
   c. AV node
   d. Purkinje fibers (ventricles)

7. What is the typical heart rate range for first degree heart block? (LO 8.2)
   a. 20–40 beats per minute
   b. 40–60 beats per minute
   c. 60–100 beats per minute
   d. 100–150 beats per minute

8. Frequent nonconducted QRS complexes are likely to cause signs of _____. (LO 8.3, 8.4, 8.5)
   a. high cardiac output
   b. low cardiac output
   c. paranoia
   d. none of the above

9. Which heart block dysrhythmia has regular P-P and R-R intervals with both having the same rate? (LO 8.2)
   a. First degree heart block
   b. Second degree type I
   c. Second degree type II
   d. Third degree heart block

10. Which heart block dysrhythmia is known as the "classical" heart block? (LO 8.4)
    a. First degree heart block
    b. Second degree type I
    c. Second degree type II
    d. Third degree heart block

Short Answer

11. Name the heart block rhythms described in this section. Which one is most serious? (LO 8.2 to 8.5)
    _____
    _____

12. How can you tell the difference between a Mobitz I and Mobitz II heart block? (LO 8.3, 8.4)
    _____
    _____

13. What should you do if the patient has a third degree heart block? (LO 8.5)
    _____
    _____

Critical Thinking Application *Rhythm Identification*

Review the dysrhythmias pictured here and, using the criteria for classification provided in the chapter as clues, identify each rhythm and provide what information you used to make your decision. (LO 8.2–8.5)

14.

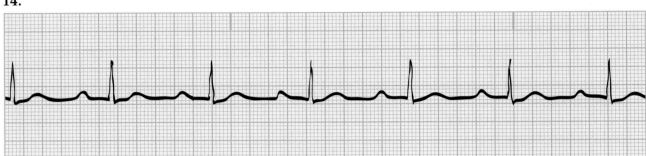

Rhythm (Regular or Irregular): _____ PR interval: _____

Rate: _____ QRS: _____

P wave: _____ Interpretation: _____

15.

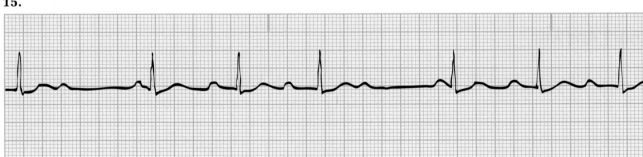

Rhythm (Regular or Irregular): _____ PR interval: _____

Rate: _____ QRS: _____

P wave: _____ Interpretation: _____

16.

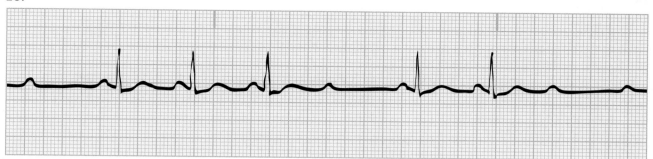

Rhythm (Regular or Irregular): _____ PR interval: _____

Rate: _____ QRS: _____

P wave: _____ Interpretation: _____

17.

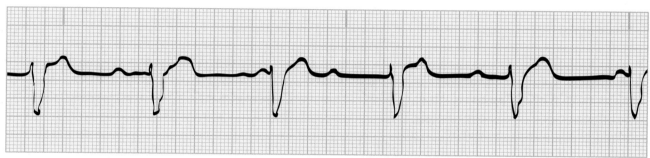

Rhythm (Regular or Irregular): _____ PR interval: _____

Rate: _____ QRS: _____

P wave: _____ Interpretation: _____

18.

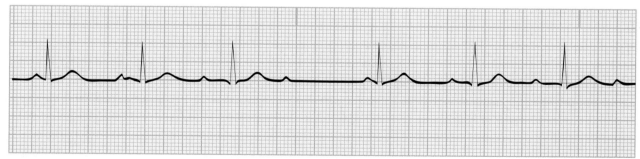

Rhythm (Regular or Irregular): _____ PR interval: _____

Rate: _____ QRS: _____

P wave: _____ Interpretation: _____

19.

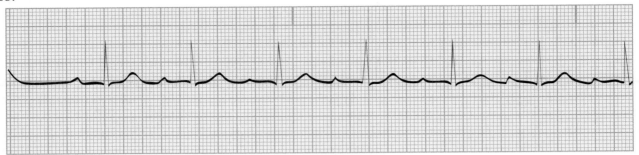

Rhythm (Regular or Irregular): _____ PR interval: _____

Rate: _____ QRS: _____

P wave: _____ Interpretation: _____

20.

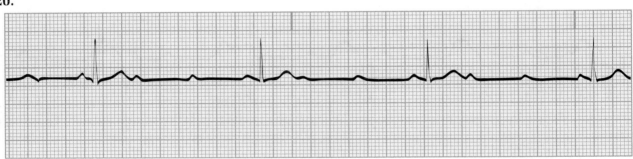

Rhythm (Regular or Irregular): _____ PR interval: _____

Rate: _____ QRS: _____

P wave: _____ Interpretation: _____

21.

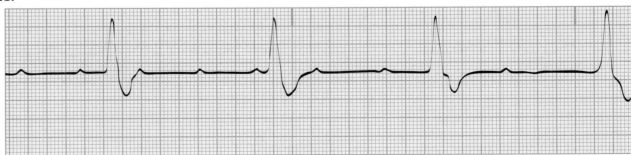

Rhythm (Regular or Irregular): _____ PR interval: _____

Rate: _____ QRS: _____

P wave: _____ Interpretation: _____

22.

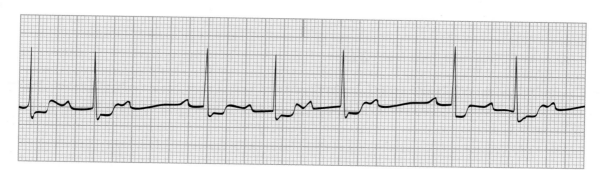

Rhythm (Regular or Irregular): _____ PR interval: _____

Rate: _____ QRS: _____

P wave: _____ Interpretation: _____

23.

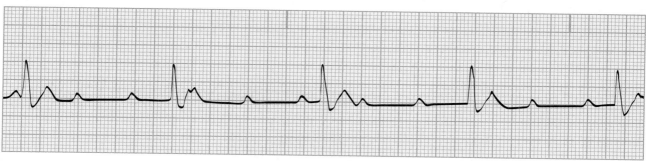

Rhythm (Regular or Irregular): _____ PR interval: _____

Rate: _____ QRS: _____

P wave: _____ Interpretation: _____

24.

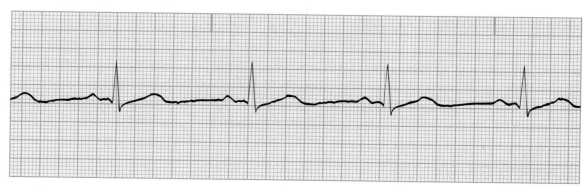

Rhythm (Regular or Irregular): _____ PR interval: _____

Rate: _____ QRS: _____

P wave: _____ Interpretation: _____

25.

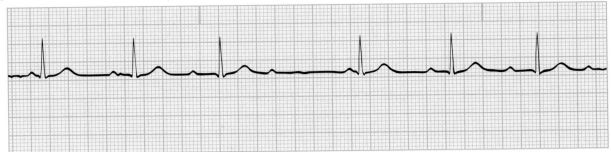

Rhythm (Regular or Irregular): _____ PR interval: _____

Rate: _____ QRS: _____

P wave: _____ Interpretation: _____

26.

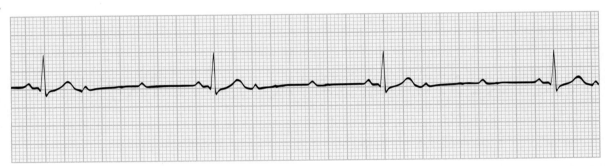

Rhythm (Regular or Irregular): _____ PR interval: _____

Rate: _____ QRS: _____

P wave: _____ Interpretation: _____

Get Connected *Internet Activity*

Visit the McGraw-Hill Higher Education Online Learning Center *Electrocardiography for Healthcare Professionals* Web site at **www.mhhe.com/boothecg3e** to complete the following activity.

1. Practice and review common heart block dysrhythmias using the dynamic rhythm simulator found at the following Web site: http://skillstat.com/Flash/ECG_Sim_2004.html

 ## Using the Student CD

Now that you have completed the material in the chapter text, return to the student CD and complete any chapter activities you have not yet done. Practice your terminology with the "Key Term Concentration" game. Review the chapter material with the "Spin the Wheel" and "ECG Challenge" game. Take the final chapter test, and complete the troubleshooting question; email or print your results to document your proficiency for this chapter.

Rhythms Originating from the Ventricles

9

Chapter Outline

- Introduction to Ventricular Dysrhythmias (p. 206)
- Premature Ventricular Complexes (PVCs) (p. 207)
- Agonal Rhythm (p. 210)
- Idioventricular Rhythm (p. 211)
- Accelerated Idioventricular Rhythm (p. 213)
- Ventricular Tachycardia (p. 215)
- Ventricular Fibrillation (p. 217)
- Asystole (p. 219)

Learning Outcomes

9.1 Describe the various ventricular dysrhythmias.

9.2 Identify PVCs using the criteria for classification, and explain how the rhythm may affect the patient, including basic patient care and treatment.

9.3 Identify agonal rhythm using the criteria for classification, and explain how the rhythm may affect the patient, including basic patient care and treatment.

9.4 Identify idioventricular rhythm using the criteria for classification, and explain how the rhythm may affect the patient, including basic patient care and treatment.

9.5 Identify accelerated idioventricular rhythm using the criteria for classification, and explain how the rhythm may affect the patient, including basic patient care and treatment.

9.6 Identify ventricular tachycardia using the criteria for classification, and explain how the rhythm may affect the patient, including basic patient care and treatment.

9.7 Identify ventricular fibrillation using the criteria for classification, and explain how the rhythm may affect the patient, including basic patient care and treatment.

9.8 Identify asystole using the criteria for classification, and explain how the rhythm may affect the patient, including basic patient care and treatment.

Key Terms

advanced cardiac life support (ACLS)
apnea
bigeminy
coupling
crash cart
frequent PVC
interpolated PVC
multifocal

occasional PVC
quadgeminy
R on T PVCs
trigeminy
unifocal

9.1 Introduction to Ventricular Dysrhythmias

As discussed in Chapter 2, the ventricle pacemaker cells are found at the Purkinje fibers (see Figure 2-9). This pacemaker is the last of the group of inherent pacemaker cells within the heart. The rate of automaticity is between 20 and 40 beats per minute. Current is initiated within the Purkinje fibers and spreads the electrical stimulation from one ventricular cell to the next. Since current is not traveling down the normal ventricular conduction pathway to activate both the right and left ventricles simultaneously, it will take longer than normal to depolarize the ventricles. A QRS duration and configuration measurement of 0.12 second or greater suggests that this cell-by-cell stimulation of electrical current is occurring to depolarize the ventricles. Ventricular rhythms occurring within the range of the Purkinje network (20 to 40 beats per minute) are occasionally referred to as ventricular escape rhythms. Ventricular rhythms either occur as a result of:

1. failure of the higher pacemaker sites within the heart, or
2. the rate of automaticity from this portion of the heart is faster, and it takes over as the primary pacemaker within the heart.

Remember, the fastest electrical activity in the heart will control the heart rate.

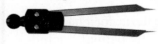

Interpret-TIP

Ventricular Complexes and Rhythms

They share a conspicuous morphologic similarity—missing P waves and "wide and bizarre" QRS complexes that measure 0.12 or greater.

Checkpoint Question (LO 9.1)

1. Why does it take longer than normal to depolarize the ventricles during a ventricular dysrhythmia?

_____

_____

9.2 Premature Ventricular Complexes (PVCs)

A premature ventricular complex (PVC) is caused by an ectopic impulse that occurs early in the cycle and originates from the ventricles (Figure 9-1). These ectopic events are often caused by an ischemic region within the ventricles. Ischemia increases excitability (irritability) of the ventricular myocardium. Table 9-1 shows the various types of premature ventricular complexes.

Figure 9-1   Premature ventricular complexes.

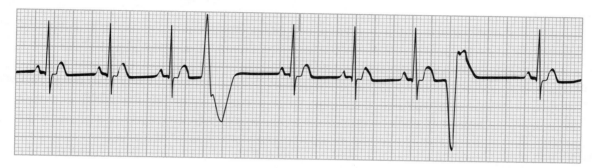

Criteria for Classification

- *Rhythm:* The P-P and R-R intervals will be regular with early QRS complexes. Every early complex has a full compensatory pause, meaning that two R-R interval periods are required before another electrical impulse can be conducted. These two R-R intervals are placed on the beat before the early complex and evaluated with the following complex if the QRS complex falls after the second point of the calipers.
- *Rate:* The atrial and ventricular rates will be the same as for the underlying rhythm, but the early complexes will provide a faster ventricular rhythm than the normal rhythm.
- *P wave configuration:* The P wave assumes the shape of the underlying rhythm. P waves are not identified on the early ventricular complex.
- *PR interval:* The PR interval measurement follows the underlying rhythm, but in the early complex there is no P wave present.
- *QRS duration and configuration:* The QRS morphology and duration must be analyzed for both the underlying rhythm and the premature complexes. Typically, the QRS complexes of the underlying rhythm will measure within the normal range (0.06–0.10). The QRS morphology of the premature complexes may be of different shapes, but will share the descriptive characteristic "wide and bizarre," measuring 0.12 seconds or greater. The T wave will be in the opposite direction of the ventricular depolarization.

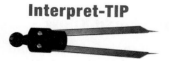

Interpret-TIP

Premature Ventricular Complexes

A PVC is an early QRS complex that measures 0.12 second or greater and has a wide and bizarre appearance. There is no P wave.

TABLE 9-1 Types and Patterns of Premature Complexes

Unifocal		Early complex (has similar shape, suggesting only one irritable focus present)
Multifocal		Varied shapes and forms of the PVCs
Interpolated PVC		PVC occurs during the normal R-R interval without interrupting the underlying rhythm
Occasional PVC		More than one to five PVCs per minute
Frequent PVC		Six or more PVCs per minute
Bigeminy		Every other complex is a PVC
Trigeminy		Every third complex is a PVC
Quadgeminy		Every fourth complex is a PVC
R on T PVCs		PVC occurs on the downslope of the T wave or the vulnerable period of the ventricular refractory period
Coupling		Two PVCs that occur back to back (Multifocal couplet pictured)

How the Patient Is Affected and What You Should Know

The clinical significance of the PVCs will depend on their frequency and the amount of decrease in cardiac output that occurs with each PVC. Since PVCs can occur in normal hearts, patients may tolerate PVCs without a noticeable change in their cardiac output and have no obvious symptoms. In fact, they may be unaware they are having PVCs. Other patients may complain of the "thump or skipping" sensation with each PVC. They may also experience dizziness and other symptoms of low cardiac output. More complex PVCs, such as frequent, multifocal, R-on-T PVCs, and coupling, indicate an increased risk of developing a more serious ventricular dys-rhythmia (see Table 9-1).

Observe the patient for symptoms of low cardiac output. If symptoms exist, a licensed practitioner should be notified to begin appropriate treatment. Patients are provided oxygen, since PVCs often occur because of hypoxic states (suffering from lack of oxygen). Blood samples are drawn to evaluate the hypoxic state as well as electrolyte values, specifically potassium and calcium levels.

Checkpoint Question (LO 9.2)

Using the criteria for classification, select the rhythm that most closely resembles a rhythm containing a premature ventricular complex (PVC).

A.

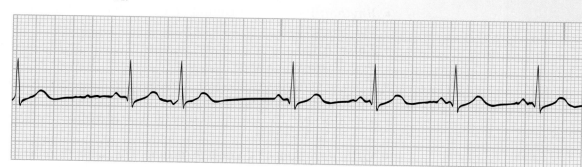

B.

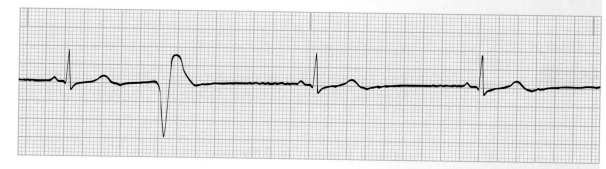

1. Which unique feature(s) led you to make the selection?

_____

_____

_____

9.3 Agonal Rhythm

Agonal rhythms occur when essentially all of the pacemakers in the heart have failed. This is the last semblance of ordered electrical activity in the heart. The heart is dying. The impulses showing on the monitor are ventricular but firing at a rate of less than 20 beats per minute. This dysrhythmia presents with "wide and bizarre" QRS (0.12 second or greater) complexes, and an absence of P waves (Figure 9-2).

Figure 9-2 Agonal rhythm.

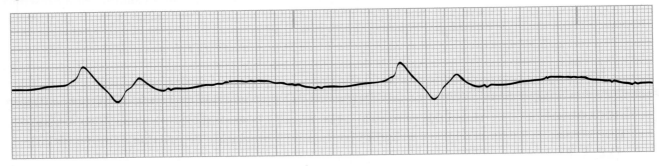

Criteria for Classification

- *Rhythm:* P-P interval cannot be determined. R-R interval may or may not be regular.
- *Rate:* Atrial rate cannot be determined due to the absence of atrial depolarization. The ventricular rate is less than 20 beats per minute.
- *P wave configuration:* The P wave is absent; therefore, no analysis of the P wave can be done.
- *PR interval:* The PR interval cannot be measured because the P wave cannot be identified.
- *QRS duration and configuration:* The QRS duration and configuration measures 0.12 second or greater and will have a "wide and bizarre" appearance.

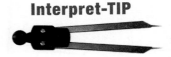

Interpret-TIP

Agonal Rhythm

The agonal rhythm has an absence of P waves, a ventricular rate of less than 20 beats per minute, and wide and bizarre QRS complexes.

How the Patient Is Affected and What You Should Know

The patient has a profound loss of cardiac output due to the loss of atrial kick and the slow ventricular rate. The patient will be unconscious. You must notify a licensed healthcare practitioner immediately. This is a medical emergency that will likely require both basic life support and advanced cardiac life support interventions. ECG strips must be saved and added to the patient's medical record.

Using the criteria for classification, select the rhythm that most closely resembles agonal rhythm.

A.

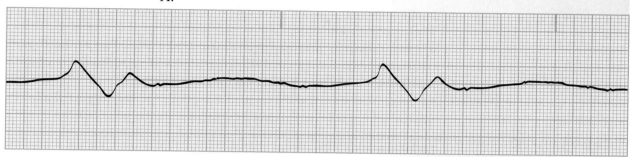

B.

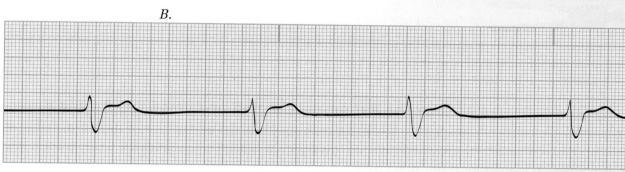

1. Which unique feature(s) led you to make the selection?

_____

_____

9.4 Idioventricular Rhythm

Idioventricular rhythms occur when the sinoatrial and junctional pacemakers fail to initiate an impulse and all that is remaining is the slow ventricular pacemaker (20 to 40 beats per minute). This dysrhythmia presents with the classic "wide" QRS (0.12 second or greater), a slow ventricular rate (20 to 40), and an absence of P waves (Figure 9-3).

Figure 9-3   Idioventricular rhythm.

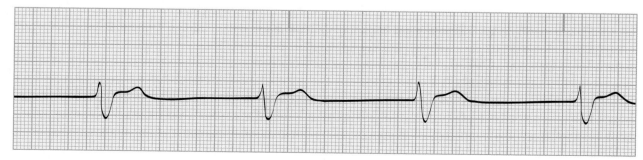

Criteria for Classification

- **Rhythm:** P-P interval cannot be determined. R-R interval is regular.
- **Rate:** Atrial rate cannot be determined due to the absence of atrial depolarization. The ventricular rate is 20 to 40 beats per minute.
- **P wave configuration:** The P wave is usually absent; therefore, no analysis of the P wave can be done.
- **PR interval:** The PR interval cannot be measured because the P wave cannot be identified.
- **QRS duration and configuration:** The QRS duration and configuration measures 0.12 second or greater and will have the classic ventricular "wide and bizarre" appearance.

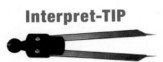

Interpret-TIP

> **Idioventricular Rhythm**
>
> An idioventricular rhythm has an absence of P waves, slow ventricular rate of 20 to 40 beats per minute, and wide and bizarre QRS complexes.

How the Patient Is Affected and What You Should Know

The patient has a profound loss of cardiac output due to the loss of atrial kick and the slow ventricular rate. The patient will likely be unconscious. You must notify a licensed healthcare practitioner immediately. This is a medical emergency that will likely require treatment with cardiac medications and/or pacing. ECG strips obtained must be saved and mounted in the patient's medical record.

Checkpoint Question (LO 9.4)

Using the criteria for classification, select the rhythm that most closely resembles idioventricular rhythm.

A.

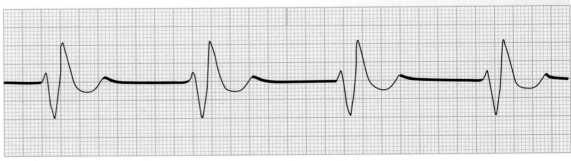

(Continued)

B.

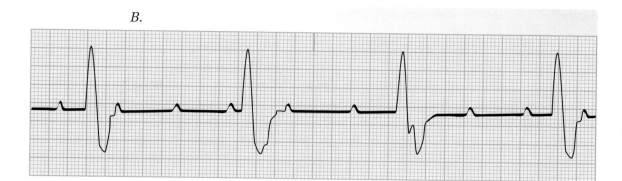

1. Which unique feature(s) led you to make the selection?

_____

_____

_____

9.5 Accelerated Idioventricular Rhythm

Accelerated idioventricular rhythms occur when the sinoatrial and junctional pacemakers fail to initiate an impulse and all that is remaining is the slow ventricular pacemaker. The primary difference between accelerated idioventricular and idioventricular dysrhythmias is the heart rates. This dysrhythmia still presents with the classic "wide" QRS (0.12 second or greater) complex and an absence of P waves. The impulse rate for this dysrhythmia is 40 to 100 beats per minute. It is simply a faster idioventricular rhythm (Figure 9-4).

Criteria for Classification

- *Rhythm:* P-P interval cannot be determined. R-R interval is regular.
- *Rate:* Atrial rate cannot be determined due to the absence of atrial depolarization. The ventricular rate is 40 to 100 beats per minute.
- *P wave configuration:* The P wave is usually absent; therefore, no analysis of the P wave can be done.
- *PR interval:* The PR interval cannot be measured because the P wave cannot be identified.
- *QRS duration and configuration:* The QRS duration and configuration measures 0.12 second or greater and will have the classic ventricular "wide and bizarre" appearance.

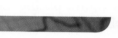

Interpret-TIP

Accelerated Idioventricular Rhythm

The accelerated idioventricular rhythm has an absence of P waves, a ventricular rate of 40 to 100 beats per minute, and wide and bizarre QRS complexes.

Figure 9-4 Accelerated idioventricular rhythm.

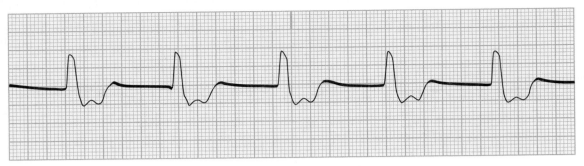

How the Patient Is Affected and What You Should Know

The patient may or may not be able to tolerate this dysrhythmia due to the decrease of cardiac output as a result of the loss of atrial kick and the slower ventricular rate. The patient may or may not be unconscious. You must notify a licensed healthcare practitioner immediately. This patient may require treatment with cardiac medications and/or pacing. ECG strips must be saved and mounted in the patient's medical record.

Checkpoint Question (LO 9.5)

Using the criteria for classification, select the rhythm that most closely resembles accelerated idioventricular rhythm.

A.

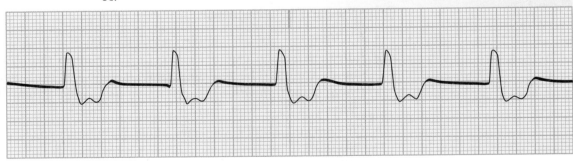

B.

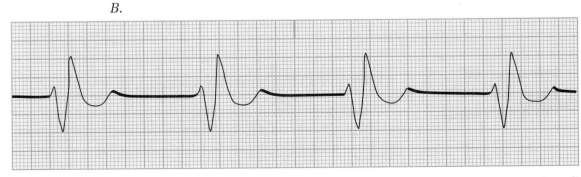

(Continued)

1. Which unique feature(s) led you to

_____

_____

_____

9.6 Ventricular Tachycard

Ventricular tachycardia occurs wh
and the ventricular rate is greater than
The ventricles are essentially in a continuous
pattern, and no period of delay exists between depolarization (cont

Figure 9-5   Ventricular tachycardia.

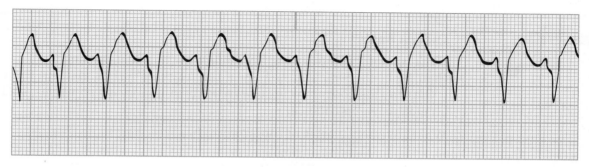

Criteria for Classification

- **Rhythm:** The P-P interval is usually not identifiable due to the large ventricular activity recorded. The R-R interval is usually regular, but it may be slightly irregular at times.
- **Rate:** Atrial rate cannot be determined because the P-P interval cannot be recognized. The ventricular rate is between 100 and 200 beats per minute.
- **P wave configuration:** The P wave is usually absent; therefore, no analysis of the P wave can be done.
- **PR interval:** The PR interval cannot be measured because the P wave is not able to be identified.
- **QRS duration and configuration:** The QRS duration and configuration measures greater than 0.12 second and will have a "wide and bizarre" appearance with an increase in amplitude. The T wave will be in the opposite direction (usually downward) from that of the QRS complex.

Interpret-TIP

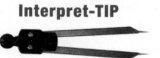

Ventricular Tachycardia

Ventricular tachycardia has wide and bizarre QRS complexes with a classic "sawtooth" appearance, a rate in excess of 100 beats per minute, and no P waves.

How the Patient Is Affected and What You Should Know

The patient will have a decrease in cardiac output due to the decrease in ventricular filling time and the loss of the atrial kick. Some patients can tolerate the dysrhythmia for a short time and will have a pulse and remain conscious, whereas other patients will be unresponsive immediately. About 50% of the patients will become unconscious immediately, with no pulse or respiration.

As soon as you recognize ventricular tachycardia on the monitor or ECG equipment, you should notify a licensed practitioner as the patient will need to be assessed for unresponsiveness. If the patient is unresponsive, an emergency protocol is initiated, sometimes called a Code Blue, then CPR is initiated. Emergency equipment such as a defibrillator, medications, and intubation equipment are necessary. Rhythm strips are saved to document the changes in rhythm that have occurred and should be mounted in the patient's medical record. If the patient is responsive, the licensed practitioner may initiate a treatment plan of medications and electrical treatments.

Troubleshooting

Escape Beats

PVCs, called "escape beats," can often occur when the heart rate is less than 60 beats per minute. This is the heart's effort to pick up the rate. PVCs may also occur because of hypoxia or abnormal lab values, such as an electrolyte imbalance.

What are likely causes of PVCs?

_____

_____

Checkpoint Question (LO 9.6)

Using the criteria for classification, select the rhythm that most closely resembles ventricular tachycardia rhythm.

A.

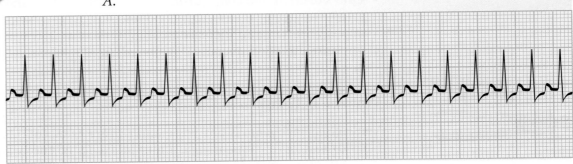

(Continued)

B.

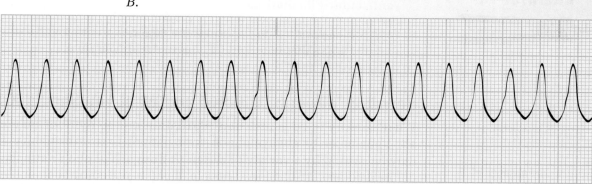

1. Which unique feature(s) led you to make the selection?

_____

_____

_____

9.7 Ventricular Fibrillation

Ventricular fibrillation is chaotic asynchronous electrical activity within the ventricular tissue. The ventricle walls are quivering, due to small, isolated portions of the ventricles depolarizing. There is no classic, uniform depolarization causing a true contraction. This prevents any ejection of blood out of the ventricles so results in no cardiac output (Figure 9-6). The entire myocardium is quivering similar to a bowl of Jell-O™ when shaken.

Figure 9-6 Ventricular fibrillation.

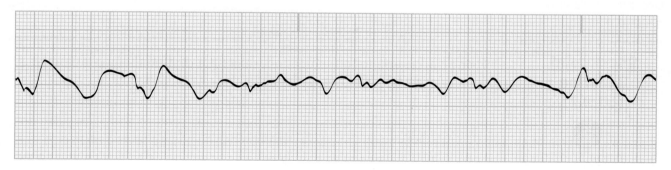

Criteria for Classification

- *Rhythm:* The P-P and R-R intervals cannot be determined because their waveforms are irregular and chaotic on the rhythm strips.
- *Rate:* The atrial and ventricular rate cannot be determined or identified.
- *P wave configuration:* The P wave configuration is not identifiable.
- *PR interval:* The PR interval cannot be identified.
- *QRS duration and configuration:* The QRS duration and configuration cannot be determined because only fibrillatory waves are present. No uniform depolarization of the ventricle occurs.

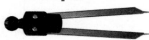

Interpret-TIP

Ventricular Fibrillation

Ventricular fibrillation is the absence of organized electrical activity. The tracing is disorganized or chaotic in appearance.

How the Patient Is Affected and What You Should Know

What appears to be ventricular fibrillation on the monitor may not be it at all. Remember to always check your patient first. Fibrillatory waveforms may be caused by a variety of different things, like poorly attached or dried out electrodes, broken lead wires, excessive patient movement, etc. If your patient is talking to you, they are *not* in ventricular fibrillation.

In true ventricular defibrillation, patients will be unresponsive when the ventricles are quivering without contracting. *This will always be a Code Blue situation, in which immediate intervention is necessary to prevent biological death.* Every patient experiencing ventricular fibrillation will be unconscious, apneic (**apnea** means not breathing), and pulseless. CPR and emergency measures should begin immediately. It is recommended that appropriate personnel begin the **advanced cardiac life support (ACLS)** to regain normal cardiac function. Rhythm strips are maintained and used as documentation in the patient's medical record.

apnea The absence of breathing.

advanced cardiac life support (ACLS) A set of clinical interventions for the urgent treatment of cardiac arrest and other life threatening medical emergencies, as well as the knowledge and skills to deploy those interventions.

Safety & Infection Control

crash carts A cart or tray used during emergencies containing medication/equipment at site of medical/surgical emergency for life support.

Crash Cart

Emergency equipment found on the "crash cart" must be ready when a code situation occurs. It is important that the cart be well stocked and the emergency equipment functioning properly. Each facility has a policy that requires regular checking and documentation of all emergency equipment and "**crash carts.**"

Checkpoint Question (LO 9.7)

Using the criteria for classification, select the rhythm that most closely resembles ventricular fibrillation.

A.

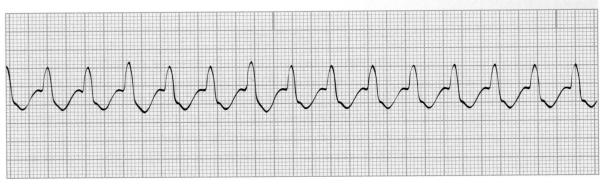

(Continued)

B.

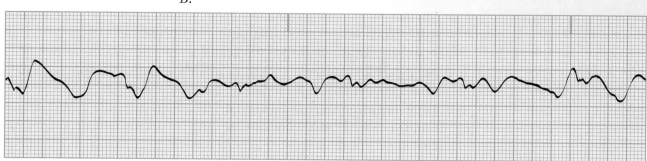

C.

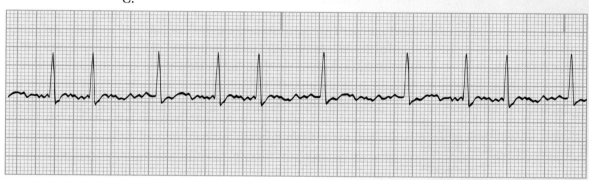

1. Which unique feature(s) led you to make the selection?

_____

_____

_____

9.8 Asystole

Asystole is absence of ventricular activity and depolarization. Often this is called "the straight or flat line" of rhythms. No electrical activity is present in the myocardium (Figure 9-7).

Note: Asystole is always confirmed in at least two different leads to rule out "fine" ventricular fibrillation.

Figure 9-7 Asystole.

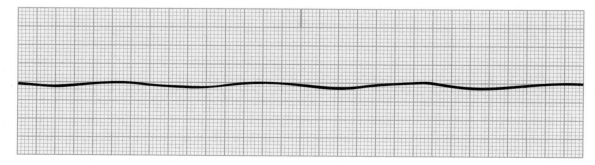

Criteria for Classification

- **Rhythm:** Since no waveforms are present, there are no P-P or R-R intervals.
- **Rate:** No atrial or ventricular rates are present.
- **P wave configuration:** No P waves are present.
- **PR interval:** The PR interval is unable to be measured because no waveforms are being recorded.
- **QRS duration and configuration:** The QRS duration and configuration is not measurable because no QRS waveform is observed.

How the Patient Is Affected and What You Should Know

This rhythm is associated with life-threatening conditions. The patient will display no pulse and no cardiac output, as evidenced by unconsciousness and apnea. The patient is in cardiac arrest, and emergency procedures must be initiated immediately. Emergency care includes immediate CPR and advanced cardiac life support measures.

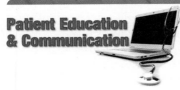

Handling Emergency Situations

During an emergency, family, friends, and other patients will be apprehensive and curious regarding the situation. You should calmly explain that there is an emergency and escort individuals out of the immediate area and view of the situation. Explain to any family members that a licensed practitioner will speak to them concerning their loved one as soon as possible.

Your local protocol may be different. Remember to follow the rules of your organization.

Checkpoint Question (LO 9.8)

Using the criteria for classification, select the rhythm strip that most closely resembles asystole.

A.

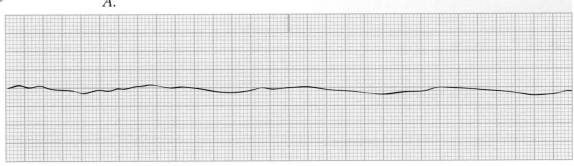

(Continued)

B.

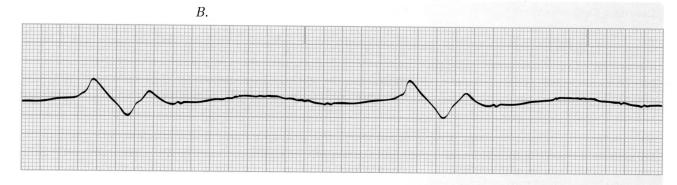

1. Which unique feature(s) led you to make the selection?

_____

_____

_____

Chapter Summary

Learning Outcomes	Summary	Pages
9.1 Describe the various ventricular dysrhythmias	Ventricular complexes and rhythms share a conspicuous morphologic similarity: missing P waves and "wide and bizarre" QRS complexes (measure 0.12 second or greater)	206
9.2 Identify PVCs using the criteria for classification, and explain how the rhythm may affect the patient, including basic patient care and treatment.	A premature ventricular complex (PVC) is caused by an ectopic complex that occurs early in the cycle and originates from the ventricles.	207–209
9.3 Identify agonal rhythm using the criteria for classification, and explain how the rhythm may affect the patient, including basic patient care and treatment.	Agonal rhythms occur when essentially all of the pacemakers in the heart have failed. This is the last semblance of ordered electrical activity in the heart. The heart is dying. The impulses showing on the monitor are ventricular but firing at a rate of less than 20 beats per minute.	210–211
9.4 Identify idioventricular rhythm using the criteria for classification, and explain how the rhythm may affect the patient, including basic patient care and treatment.	Idioventricular rhythms occur when the sinoatrial and junctional pacemakers fail to initiate an impulse and all that is remaining is the slow ventricular pacemaker (20 to 40 beats per minute).	211–213

(Continued)

Learning Outcomes	Summary	Pages
9.5 Identify accelerated idioventricular rhythm using the criteria for classification, and explain how the rhythm may affect the patient, including basic patient care and treatment.	Accelerated idioventricular rhythms occur when the sinoatrial and junctional pacemakers fail to initiate an impulse and all that is remaining is the slow ventricular pacemaker. The primary difference between accelerated idioventricular and idioventricular dysrhythmias is the faster heart rate (40–100 beats per minute).	213–215
9.6 Identify ventricular tachycardia using the criteria for classification, and explain how the rhythm may affect the patient, including basic patient care and treatment.	Ventricular tachycardia occurs when three or more PVCs occur in a row and the ventricular rate is greater than 100 beats per minute.	215–217
9.7 Identify ventricular fibrillation using the criteria for classification, and explain how the rhythm may affect the patient, including basic patient care and treatment.	Ventricular fibrillation is chaotic asynchronous electrical activity within the ventricular tissue. The ventricle walls are quivering due to small, isolated portions of the ventricles depolarizing. P-P and R-R intervals cannot be determined because only chaotic waveforms are recorded on the rhythm strips.	217–219
9.8 Identify asystole using the criteria for classification, and explain how the rhythm may affect the patient, including basic patient care and treatment.	Asystole is absence of ventricular activity and depolarization. Often this is called "the straight or flat line" of rhythms. No electrical activity is present in the myocardium.	219–221

Chapter Review

Multiple Choice

Circle the correct answer.

1. Which ventricular dysrhythmia has no P waves? (LO 9.2–9.8)
   a. Accelerated idioventricular
   b. Idioventricular
   c. Accelerated idioventricular
   d. Ventricular tachycardia
   e. Ventricular fibrillation
   f. All are correct responses

2. Which ventricular dysrhythmia has a heart rate between 40 and 100 beats per minute? (LO 9.5)
   a. Asystole
   b. Idioventricular
   c. Accelerated idioventricular
   d. Ventricular tachycardia
   e. Ventricular fibrillation
   f. Agonal

3. Which ventricular dysrhythmia has a heart rate less than 20 beats per minute? (LO 9.3)
   a. Idioventricular
   b. Accelerated idioventricular
   c. Ventricular tachycardia
   d. Ventricular fibrillation
   e. Agonal

4. Which ventricular dysrhythmia has a heart rate between 20 and 40 beats per minute? (LO 9.4)
   a. Asystole
   b. Idioventricular
   c. Accelerated idioventricular
   d. Ventricular tachycardia
   e. Ventricular fibrillation
   f. Agonal

5. What is unique about ventricular dysrhythmias with regard to the P-P intervals? (LO 9.1).
   a. They are irregular.
   b. They are biphasic.
   c. They are regular.
   d. There is no P waves so no measure P-P interval.

6. QRS complexes that measure 0.12 seconds or greater with a rate between 20 and 40 beats per minutes indicate the impulses causing ventricular depolarization are coming from the _____. (LO 9.1)
   a. SA node
   b. interatrial pathways
   c. AV node
   d. Purkinje fibers (ventricles)

7. Ventricular fibrillation is typically described as "_____." (LO 9.7)
   a. regular
   b. absent
   c. chaotic
   d. none of the above

8. Which of the following dysrhythmias is not considered to be a medical emergency? (LO 9.2)
   a. Agonal
   b. Asystole
   c. Ventricular fibrillation
   d. Occasional PVCs

Short Answer

9. What is the difference between idioventricular rhythm and accelerated idioventricular rhythm? (LO 9.4, 9.5)

   _____

   _____

10. How are agonal rhythm and asystole the same? (LO 9.3, 9.8)

   _____

   _____

11. What is the difference between ventricular tachycardia and ventricular fibrillation? (LO 9.6, 9.7)

   _____

   _____

Matching

Identify each of the following types or patterns of premature complexes. Answers may be used more than once. (LO 9.1, 9.2)

_____ 12. bigeminy   a

_____ 13. coupling   b

(Continued)

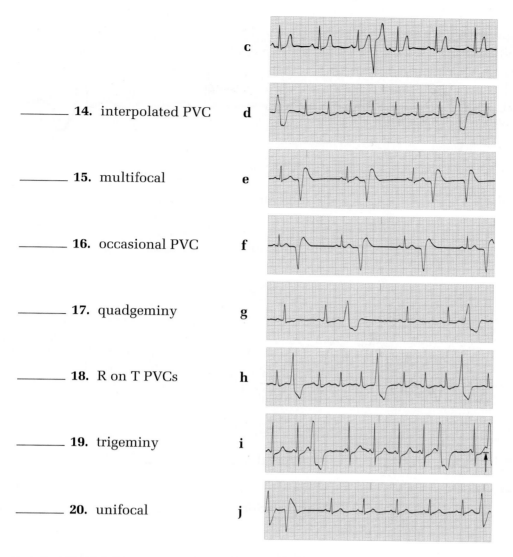

c

_____ **14.** interpolated PVC   d

_____ **15.** multifocal   e

_____ **16.** occasional PVC   f

_____ **17.** quadgeminy   g

_____ **18.** R on T PVCs   h

_____ **19.** trigeminy   i

_____ **20.** unifocal   j

Critical Thinking Applications *Rhythm Identification*

Review the dysrhythmias pictured here. Using the criteria for classification provided in the chapter as clues, identify each rhythm, and provide what information you used to make your decision. (LO 9.2–9.8)

21.

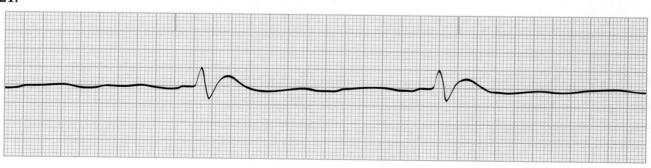

Rhythm (Regular or Irregular): _____   PR interval: _____

Rate: _____   QRS: _____

P wave: _____   Interpretation: _____

22.

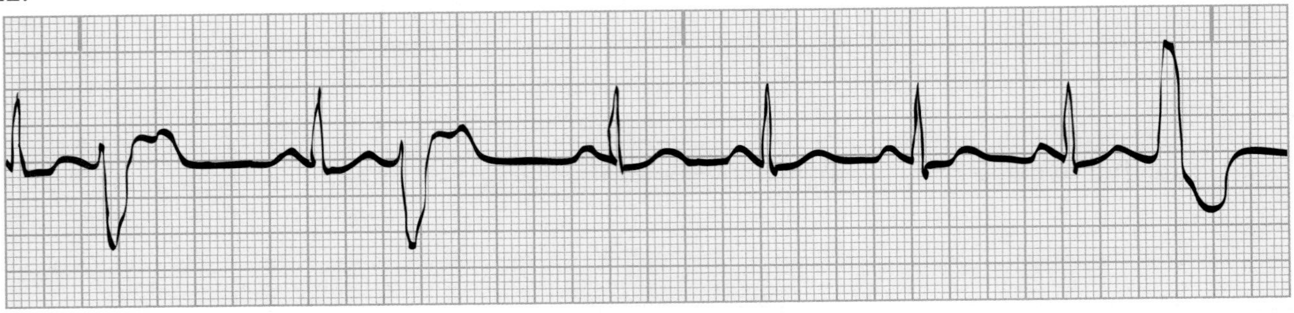

Rhythm (Regular or Irregular): _____ PR interval: _____

Rate: _____ QRS: _____

P wave: _____ Interpretation: _____

23.

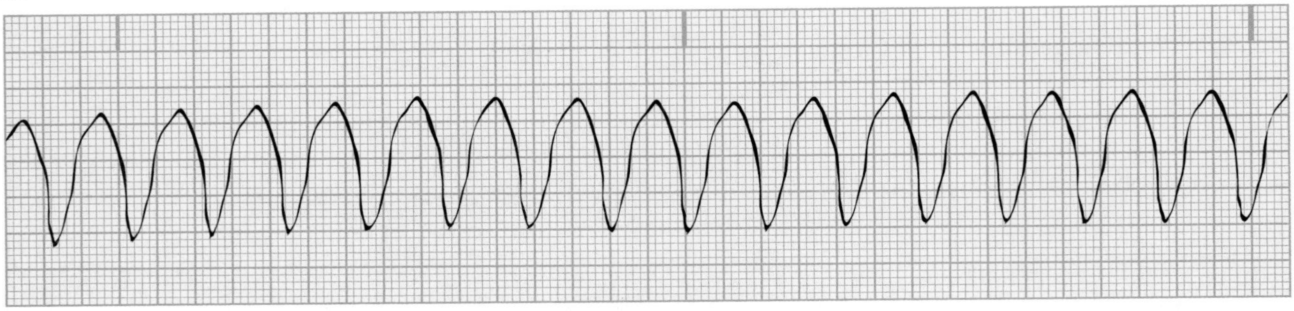

Rhythm (Regular or Irregular): _____ PR interval: _____

Rate: _____ QRS: _____

P wave: _____ Interpretation: _____

24.

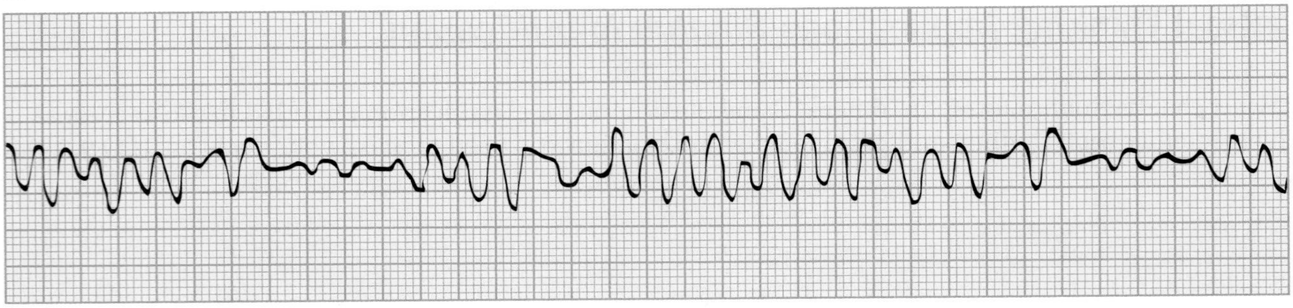

Rhythm (Regular or Irregular): _____ PR interval: _____

Rate: _____ QRS: _____

P wave: _____ Interpretation: _____

25.

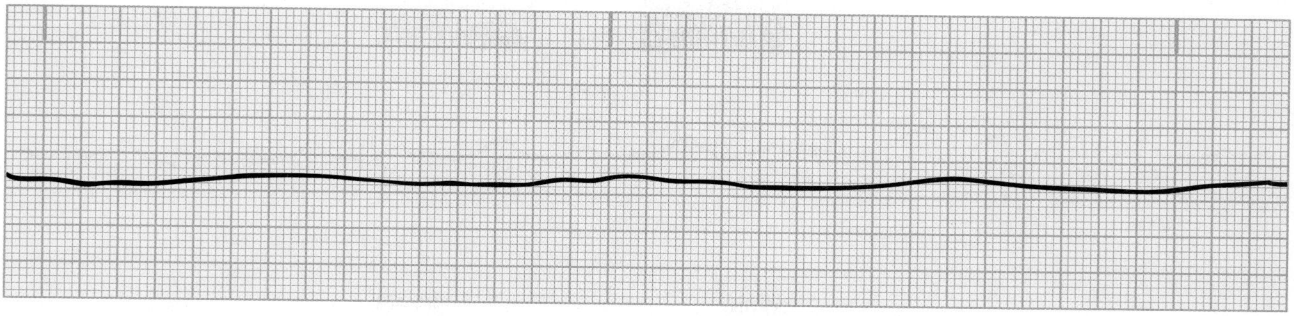

Rhythm (Regular or Irregular): _____ PR interval: _____

Rate: _____ QRS: _____

P wave: _____ Interpretation: _____

26.

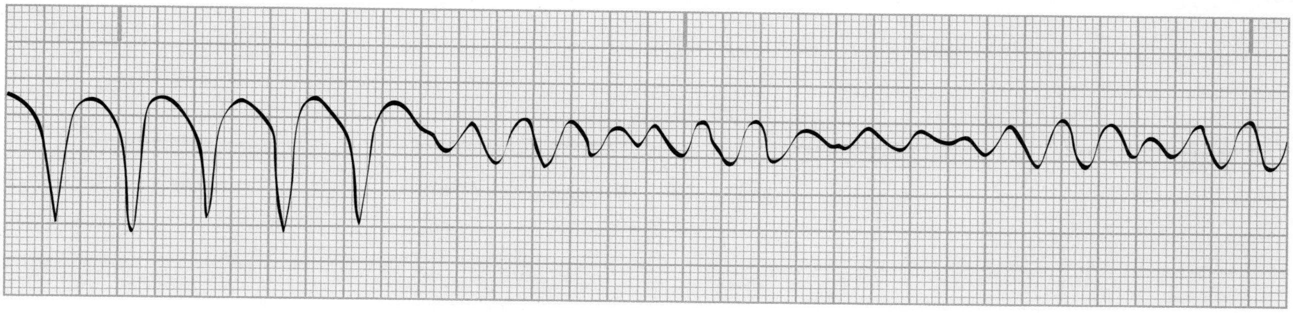

Rhythm (Regular or Irregular): _____ PR interval: _____

Rate: _____ QRS: _____

P wave: _____ Interpretation: _____

27.

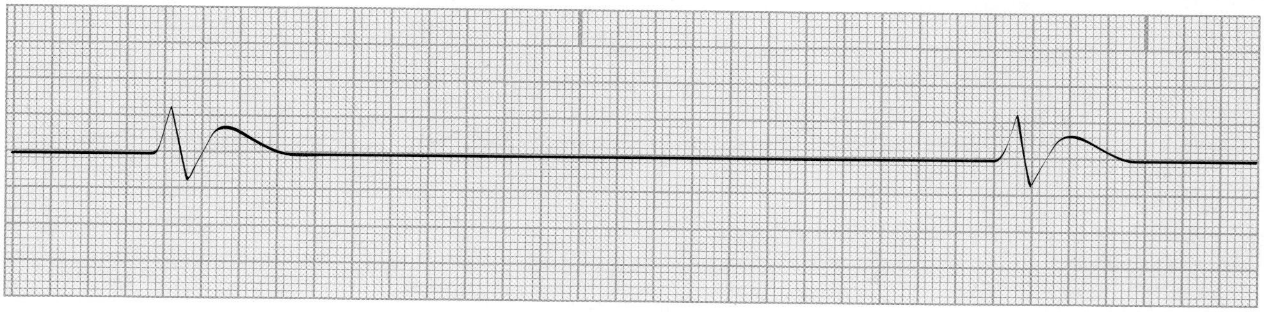

Rhythm (Regular or Irregular): _____ PR interval: _____

Rate: _____ QRS: _____

P wave: _____ Interpretation: _____

28.

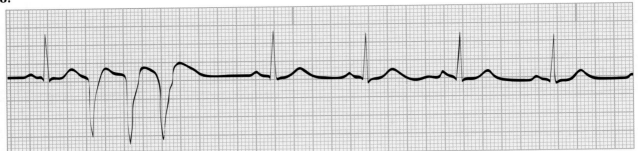

Rhythm (Regular or Irregular): _____   PR interval: _____

Rate: _____   QRS: _____

P wave: _____   Interpretation: _____

29.

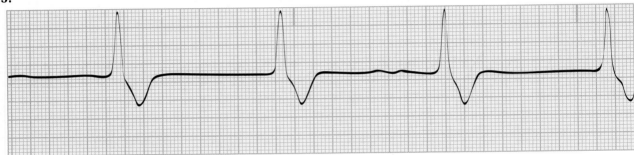

Rhythm (Regular or Irregular): _____   PR interval: _____

Rate: _____   QRS: _____

P wave: _____   Interpretation: _____

30.

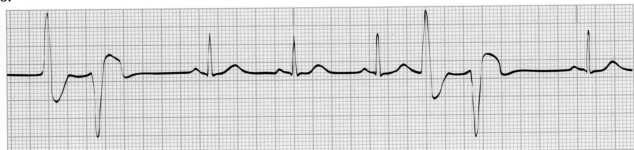

Rhythm (Regular or Irregular): _____   PR interval: _____

Rate: _____   QRS: _____

P wave: _____   Interpretation: _____

31.

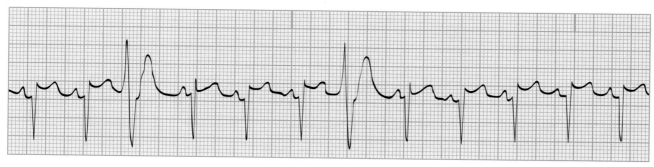

Rhythm (Regular or Irregular): _____ PR interval: _____

Rate: _____ QRS: _____

P wave: _____ Interpretation: _____

32.

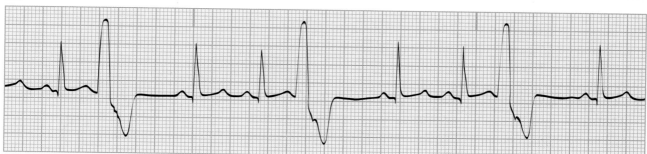

Rhythm (Regular or Irregular): _____ PR interval: _____

Rate: _____ QRS: _____

P wave: _____ Interpretation: _____

33.

Rhythm (Regular or Irregular): _____ PR interval: _____

Rate: _____ QRS: _____

P wave: _____ Interpretation: _____

34.

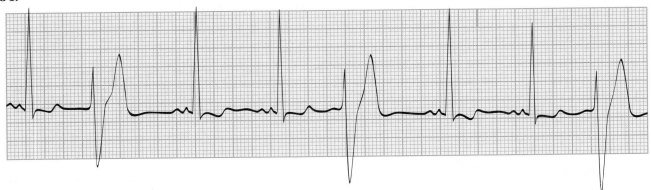

Rhythm (Regular or Irregular): _____   PR interval: _____

Rate: _____   QRS: _____

P wave: _____   Interpretation: _____

35.

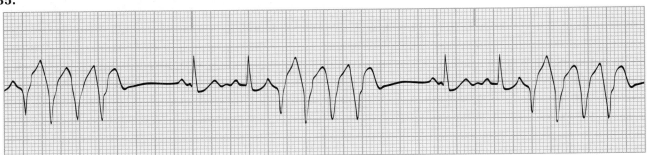

Rhythm (Regular or Irregular): _____   PR interval: _____

Rate: _____   QRS: _____

P wave: _____   Interpretation: _____

36.

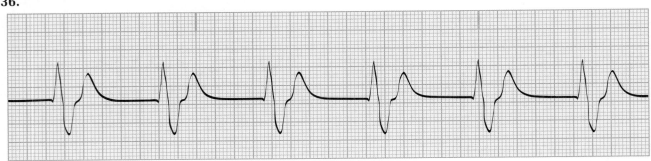

Rhythm (Regular or Irregular): _____   PR interval: _____

Rate: _____   QRS: _____

P wave: _____   Interpretation: _____

37.

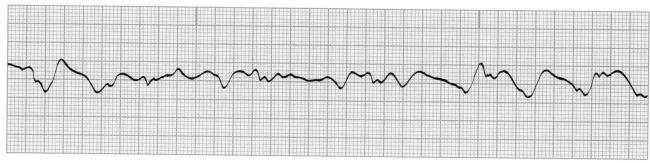

Rhythm (Regular or Irregular): _____ PR interval: _____

Rate: _____ QRS: _____

P wave: _____ Interpretation: _____

38.

Rhythm (Regular or Irregular): _____ PR interval: _____

Rate: _____ QRS: _____

P wave: _____ Interpretation: _____

39.

Rhythm (Regular or Irregular): _____ PR interval: _____

Rate: _____ QRS: _____

P wave: _____ Interpretation: _____

40.

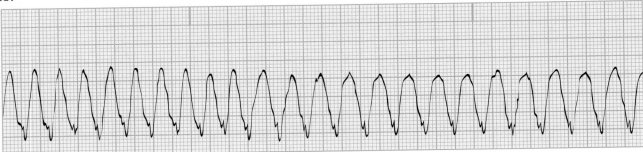

Rhythm (Regular or Irregular): _____ PR interval: _____

Rate: _____ QRS: _____

P wave: _____ Interpretation: _____

Get Connected *Internet Activity*

Visit the McGraw-Hill Higher Education Online Learning Center *Electrocardiography for Healthcare Professionals* Web site at **www.mhhe.com/boothecg3e** to complete the following activity.

1. Practice and review common ventricular dysrhythmias using the dynamic rhythm simulator found at the following Web site: http://skillstat.com/Flash/ECG_Sim_2004.html

 ## Using the Student CD

Now that you have completed the material in the chapter text, return to the student CD and complete any chapter activities you have not yet done. Practice your terminology with the "Key Term Concentration" game. Review the chapter material with the "Spin the Wheel" and "ECG Challenge" games. Take the final chapter test, and complete the troubleshooting question; email or print your results to document your proficiency for this chapter.

Pacemaker Rhythms and Bundle Branch Block

10

Chapter Outline

- Introduction to Pacemaker Rhythms (p. 233)
- Evaluating Pacemaker Function (p. 235)
- Pacemaker Complications Relative to the ECG Tracing (p. 240)
- Introduction to Bundle Branch Block Dysrhythmias (p. 242)

Learning Outcomes

10.1 Describe the various pacemaker rhythms.

10.2 Identify pacemaker rhythms using the criteria for classification and explain how the rhythm may affect the patient, including basic patient care and treatment.

10.3 Summarize pacemaker complications relative to the ECG tracing.

10.4 Identify bundle branch block using the criteria for classification and explain how the rhythm occurs and may affect the patient.

Key Terms

atrial kick
atrioventricular delay
bundle branch block
capture
electronic pacemaker
inherent rhythm
loss of capture (failure to depolarize)

malfunction (failure to pace)
malsensing (failure to sense)
oversensing
pacemaker competition
pacing spike
triggered

10.1 Introduction to Pacemaker Rhythms

electronic pacemaker
Refers to a natural or man-made source of electrical current causing depolarization of the myocardium; artificial pacemakers are electronic.

Electronic pacemakers, also known as artificial pacemakers, are devices that deliver an electrical impulse to the myocardium to cause the cells to depolarize. This electrical generator will provide small amounts of electrical current in a predetermined interval to mimic the normal pacemaker of the heart. Pacemakers have the capability to pace the atria, ventricles, or both sets of chambers. They are sometimes temporary but are usually implanted under the skin (Figure 10-1) to correct dysrhythmias. Although many different types of electronic pacemakers are implanted, the mode in which they function varies in only a few ways. Because of

Figure 10-1 Implanted pacemaker.

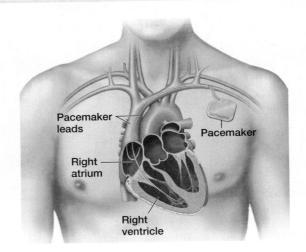

Pacemaker leads

Pacemaker

Right atrium

Right ventricle

the variety of pacemakers available on the market, it is recommended that you check in advance regarding the proper procedure for performing an ECG on a patient with a pacemaker.

The fastest pacemaker (electrical activity) in the heart controls the heartbeat, whether it is an inherent pacemaker, such as the SA node, or an artificial one. Electronic pacemakers work based on this principle. For example, when a patient is experiencing a bradycardic dysrhythmia, an artificial pacemaker is used and typically set at a rate of between 70 to 72 beats per minute. This artificial pacemaker will be the fastest pacemaker in the heart and thus will control the heart rate for the myocardium.

Pacemakers can stimulate several different cardiac functions. The stimulation may be for the atria, the ventricles, or both. The function will depend on the reason the pacemaker is inserted. For example, if the patient is experiencing problems with the conduction system in the ventricles, a ventricular pacemaker is inserted to deliver direct stimulation to the ventricles and produce a ventricular contraction. Atrial pacing is used alone when the conduction system from the atrioventricular node through the ventricles is intact and functioning.

Atrioventricular pacing provides direct stimulation of the atria and ventricles in a sequence pattern known as atrioventricular sequential pacing. This pacing option mimics the normal cardiac conduction system. It allows the atria to contract completely prior to the ventricles to allow an atrial kick. (*Remember that the* **atrial kick** *provides the extra blood supply needed for approximately 10% to 30% of the normal cardiac output.*) This pacing function is being used more when pacemakers are inserted because

atrial kick When blood is ejected into the ventricles by the atria immediately prior to ventricular systole.

it will mimic normal cardiac function and provide the atrial kick needed. A newer type of atrioventricular sequential pacing is atriobiventricular pacing used commonly in patients with heart failure. This atriobiventricular pacing stimulates both ventricles to contract instead of the typical stimulation of only the lower portion of the right ventricle.

Checkpoint Questions (LO 10.1)

1. When is a ventricular pacemaker used?
   _____
   _____

2. When is an atrial pacemaker used alone?
   _____
   _____

3. What is the advantage of atrioventricular pacing?
   _____
   _____

10.2 Evaluating Pacemaker Function

Pacemaker function can be evaluated based on the ECG tracings. Several different ECG characteristics must be identified prior to evaluating the pacemaker function. The most important aspect of care is to verify the effectiveness of the pacemaker and determine the presence of a pulse with each captured beat. (**Capture** refers to the ability of the heart muscle to respond to electrical stimulation and depolarize the myocardial tissue.) Electrically, this capture is represented by a pacing spike immediately prior to the waveform.

capture The ability of the heart muscle to respond to electrical stimulation and depolarize the myocardial tissue.

pacing spike Indicates the stimulation of electrical current from the pacemaker generator. The current is a quick delivery and is reflected as a thin spike on the ECG tracing.

Pacing Spike

The **pacing spike** or artifact indicates the stimulation of electrical current from the pacemaker generator. The current is a quick delivery and is reflected as a thin spike on the ECG tracing (Figure 10-2). After the pacing spike, a tracing of either a P wave or a wide QRS complex or both will appear, depending on which chamber is being paced.

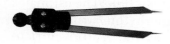

Interpret-TIP

> **Pacemaker Rhythms**
>
> The conspicuous presence of a spike prior to the waveform of the intended portion of the heart to be paced, i.e., a spike before the "P" wave, indicates the pacemaker has been implanted with the intention of pacing the atrial portion of the depolarization.

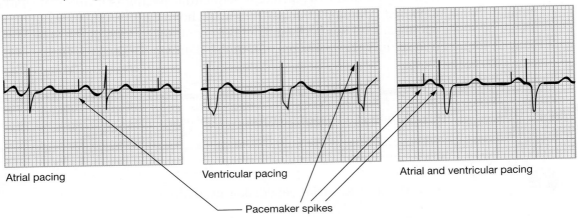

Atrial pacing   Ventricular pacing   Atrial and ventricular pacing

Pacemaker spikes

Chamber Depolarization Characteristics

If the pacemaker delivers atrial pacing, the pacing spike will be followed by a P wave. When the pacemaker delivers ventricular pacing, the pacing spike will be followed by a wide QRS complex, which looks similar to a left bundle branch block (LBBB, see page 242) pattern. The ventricles are stimulated low in the right ventricle, causing the myocardium to depolarize slowly. The complex is wide and shaped differently from a natural QRS complex. It is similar to the LBBB since the left ventricle takes longer than the right to depolarize because of its size.

AV Delay

atrioventricular delay
The measurement from the atrial spike to the ventricular spike, or from the beginning of the P wave to the ventricular spike on a pacemaker tracing.

The AV sequential pacemaker tracing will have an **atrioventricular delay.** An atrioventricular delay is similar to the measurement of the PR interval on a normal rhythm tracing. It is measured from the atrial spike to the ventricle spike. Usually this programmed time frame is somewhere between 0.12 to 0.20 second, similar to a normal PR interval.

If the patient has a normal P wave and a pacer-induced ventricular complex, the atrioventricular delay is determined from the beginning of the P wave to the ventricular spike. If the patient has a pacer-induced atrial complex and a normal QRS measurement, the measurement from the pacing spike to the beginning of the QRS complex should be less than the set atrioventricular delay time frame.

Evaluating a Pacemaker ECG Tracing

inherent rhythm The patient's own heart rhythm.

Evaluating a pacemaker rhythm involves seven steps, which are similar to those used to evaluate a nonpaced rhythm. If a patient does not have an atrioventricular sequential pacemaker, steps 3 through 5 can be eliminated. In addition, it is important to estimate the frequency of the pacemaker initiating the rhythm compared to the patient's **inherent rhythm.** The estimates are usually referred to in 25% intervals. If the entire rhythm strip displays an atrioventricular paced rhythm, it is referred to as 100% atrioventricular pacing (1:1). (*When less than 100% paced rhythm occurs, identify the patient's* inherent rhythm, *and then include the estimate of paced beats and the type of pacing function as seen on the rhythm strip.*)

Step 1. *What are the rate and regularity of the paced rhythm?*

The regularity of the pacemaker spikes should be exactly the same. Only if the patient's own rhythm becomes faster than the pacemaker will the regularity be different. The rate of the pacemaker rhythm should be exactly the number at which the pacemaker was set. Often the rate is set at 70 beats per minute.

Step 2. *What are the rate and regularity of the intrinsic rhythm (the patient's own rhythm)?*

When the patient's own heart rate beats faster than the pacemaker rhythm, the patient's intrinsic rhythm will control the heart rate. The patient's own rhythm should be noted on the ECG tracing. The rate and regularity will depend on the patient's inherent rhythm.

Step 3. (for AV sequential pacemakers only) *Is the atrial lead sensing appropriate?*

The ECG tracing needs to be evaluated for the presence of atrial spikes with the P wave following the spike. Occasionally, the patient's own SA node or atrial ectopic focus will initiate atrial contraction as evidenced by a P wave without an atrial spike.

Step 4. (for atrial, AV sequential, and atriobiventricular pacemakers) *Is atrial capture present?*

Every atrial spike should have a P wave after it to indicate that the electrical current is causing the cells to depolarize. The P wave after the spike indicates that the atrial capture occurred.

Step 5. (for atrioventricular sequential and atriobiventricular pacemakers) *Is atrioventricular delay appropriate?*

Measuring from the atrial spike to the ventricular spike, or from the beginning of the P wave to the ventricular spike, will give you the atrioventricular delay interval. This time frame should be the same as the atrioventricular delay set on the pacemaker program. This information should be available on the patient's medical record or pacemaker information card.

Step 6. *Is ventricular sensing appropriate?*

The ECG tracing needs to be evaluated for the presence of ventricular spikes with the wide QRS complex following the spike. Occasionally the patient's own conduction system will work appropriately, as evidenced by a normal P wave and/or QRS complex. If the ventricular contraction occurred normally before the time interval of when the pacemaker would send a ventricular impulse, the pacemaker generator will be inhibited, or stopped. This is evidenced by the absence of a ventricular spike.

Step 7. *Is ventricular capture present?*

Every ventricular spike should have a wide QRS complex after it to indicate that the electrical current caused the cells to depolarize. Appearance of the QRS complex after the spike indicates that ventricular capture occurred.

1. Using the criteria for classification, select the rhythm that most closely resembles atrial pacemaker rhythm.

A.

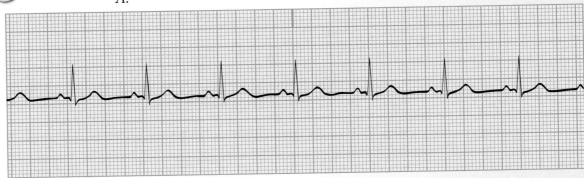

B.

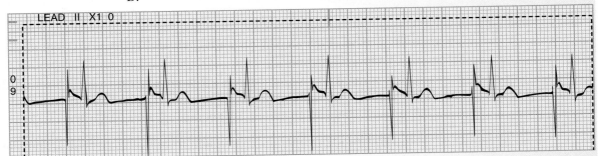

Which unique feature(s) led you to make the selection?

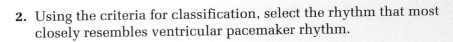

_____

_____

_____

2. Using the criteria for classification, select the rhythm that most closely resembles ventricular pacemaker rhythm.

A.

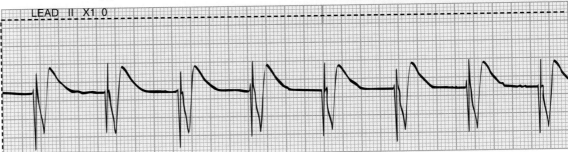

(Continued)

B.

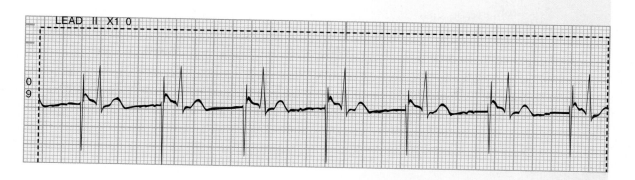

Which unique feature(s) led you to make the selection?

_____

_____

_____

3. Using the criteria for classification, select the rhythm that most closely resembles atrioventricular (AV sequential) pacemaker rhythm.

A.

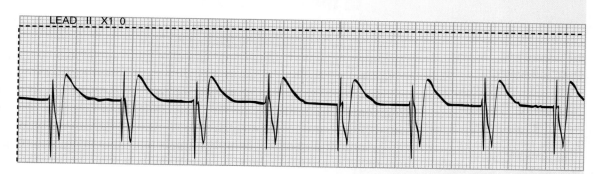

B.

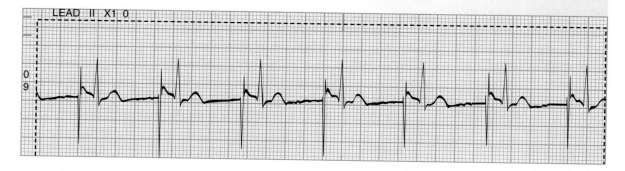

(Continued)

C.

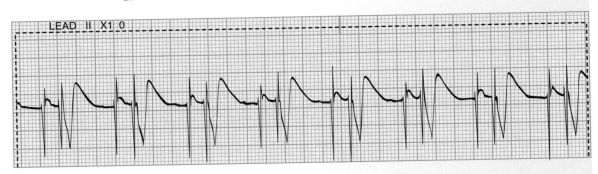

Which unique feature(s) led you to make the selection?

_____

_____

_____

triggered Electrical current is sent from the pacemaker generator to the myocardium to cause the depolarization of the myocardial tissue.

10.3 Pacemaker Complications Relative to the ECG Tracing

Pacemaker generators use lithium batteries to create an electrical impulse. As with any battery, the charge of the battery will decrease to the point at which the battery needs to be replaced. If a pacemaker is losing its ability to function properly, this failure will be evident on the ECG tracings. These changes in rhythms are often referred to as *complications* of the pacemaker. Complications include slower firing rates than set, less effective sensing capabilities, and lower electrical current than predetermined.

Another pacemaker complication is related to the functioning of the pacemaker generator when the sensing capability is too low. If sensing capability is low, the pacemaker will not be able to "see" the normal contractions occurring in the sensing chamber. Therefore, electrical impulses will not only be inhibited but may actually be **triggered,** sending an impulse to the myocardium because the normal electrical current of the heart's conduction system was not "seen."

There are several different reasons for pacemaker complications, but only four basic dysrhythmias are evident on the ECG tracing from these complications: **malfunctioning** (failure to pace), **malsensing** (failure to sense), **loss of capture** (failure to depolarize), and **oversensing** (perceiving electrical current from sources other than the heart) (Table 10-1).

Responsibility in caring for patients with pacemakers requires recognizing normal pacemaker rhythms and possible complications. When you are performing an ECG or monitoring a patient with a pacemaker, you should be aware of the differences in the ECG waveforms, including the presence of a pacing spike, chamber depolarization characteristics, and atrioventricular delay. If you observe complications of a pacemaker rhythm, immediately notify licensed personnel for appropriate treatment and interventions.

malfunctioning The pacemaker fails to send an electrical impulse to the myocardium

malsensing The pacemaker does not recognize or sense the patient's own inherent heartbeats.

loss of capture The pacing activity continues to occur without evidence that the electrical activity has depolarized or captured the myocardium.

oversensing The pacemaker senses electrical current from other muscle movements or electrical activity outside of the body as the patient's heart electrical current.

pacemaker competition Competition between the pacemaker generator and the heart's inherent rate over control of the myocardium.

TABLE 10-1 Pacemaker Complications

Complication	Cause	What Occurs	Patient Symptoms
Malfunctioning (failure to pace)	Pacemaker does not send electrical impulse to the myocardium.	Pacemaker intervals are irregular and impulse is slower than set rate. No pacemaker spike is seen.	Patient will most often experience hypotension, lightheadedness, and blackout periods due to bradycardia conditions.
Malsensing (failure to sense)	Pacemaker does not sense the patient's own inherent rate.	May send current to heart during relaxation (repolarization) phase; also known as **pacemaker competition** with the patient's own heart	With atrial pacing, atrial fibrillation can occur; with ventricular pacing, ventricular tachycardia or ventricular fibrillation can occur.
Loss of capture (failure to depolarize)	Pacing activity occurs, but myocardium is not depolarized.	Pacing spikes will occur without capture waveform, such as P wave or QRS complex (see first figure, below).	Symptoms depend on the basic dysrhythmia and the patient's condition prior to the pacemaker insertion.
Oversensing	Pacemaker perceives electrical current from sources other than the heart.	Either (1) the patient's own heart rate is recorded and is slower than the set rate of the pacemaker or (2) the pacemaker spikes and captures at a slower rate than set (see second figure, below).	Patient may have signs and symptoms of low cardiac output.

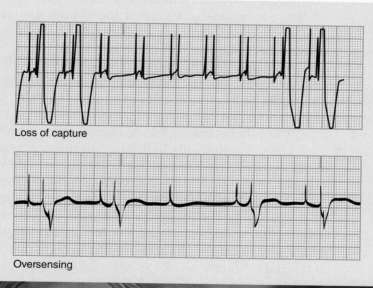

Loss of capture

Oversensing

Checkpoint Question (LO 10.3)

1. Name and describe four different reasons for pacemaker complications.

_____

_____

10.4 Introduction to Bundle Branch Block Dysrhythmias

bundle branch block
Impulse is delayed or blocked within the bundle branches of the normal conduction pathway.

Bundle branch blocks occur when one or both of the ventricular pathways are damaged or delayed due to cardiac disease, drugs, or other conditions. When an area of one of the bundle branches is damaged, electrical current will not be able to travel through that tissue to reach the myocardial tissue in its usual fashion. Current will travel down the good bundle and will activate the myocardial tissue in that corresponding ventricle only. The other ventricle must then receive the impulse as current travels from one cell to the next until the entire myocardial contraction occurs. It is similar to the knocking down of a line of dominoes where each domino represents a cardiac cell. The cell will not contract until the next cell delivers the energy.

Current traveling via the abnormal pathways will take longer to achieve the full ventricular contraction. This longer time frame is similar to driving a car to a specific destination and having to find an alternate route or detour when the road is closed. This is what happens to the current traveling through the heart's conduction pathway when it has a blocked bundle branch. The increased length of time is reflected in a wider than normal QRS. Remember that the QRS duration is a measurement of just how long it takes for current to travel through ventricular myocardial tissue.

When a patient has a right bundle branch block (RBBB), the impulse will travel down the conduction pathway normally until after the bundle of His. Since the right side of the conduction pathway is blocked, current must travel down the left bundle branch to activate the ventricles (Figure 10-3*A*).

The left bundle branch block (LBBB) will have the left conduction pathway blocked. Current travels down the right bundle branch to cause the right ventricle, the septum, then the left ventricle to contract (Figure 10-3*B*).

The bundle branch block classification provides additional information about another dysrhythmia. Information regarding a bundle branch block is extra data included with the basic rhythm classification. Typically the basic rhythm will be a rhythm that originates from above the ventricles. The rhythm has all the basic properties of sinus rhythms or atrial dysrhythmias with the exception of a wide QRS complex. The discovery of a wide QRS complex is the clue to further investigate for the bundle branch block. For example, the patient may be experiencing sinus rhythm with a left bundle branch block (SR with LBBB). The basic rhythm must always be determined with the distinction of a right bundle branch block or left bundle branch block present (see Figure 10-4).

Criteria for Classification

Characteristics of the right and left bundle branch block will be similar over monitoring leads I, II, and III. Specific characteristics of the right or left bundle branch will be present when monitoring with leads V1 to V6. Although bundle branch block (BBB) is seen in the precordial leads, to distinguish RBBB from LBBB, lead VI is referenced. If the QRS is positively deflected, it is an RBBB. If the QRS is negative, it is an LBBB.

Figure 10-3   Right and left bundle branch block ventricular conduction

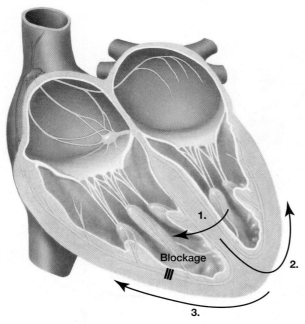

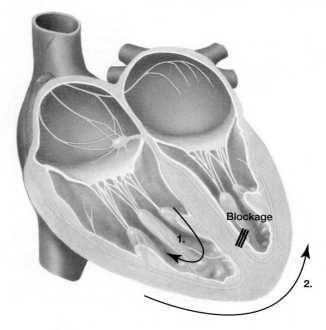

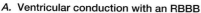

A. Ventricular conduction with an RBBB
  1. The septum is depolarized normally.
  2. The left ventricle is activated.
  3. The current travels to the right ventricle until there is complete ventricular contraction.

B. Ventricular conduction with an LBBB
  1. Current travels down the right bundle branch to cause right ventricle contraction.
  2. The current moves to the left ventricle causing the septum to be activated abnormally in a right-to-left fashion.

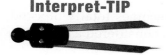

Interpret-TIP

Branch Bundle Blocks

The rhythm has a P wave, and the QRS complex measures 0.12 second or greater.

- ***Rhythm:*** The regularity or irregularity will depend on the underlying rhythm. Sinus or atrial is usually the underlying rhythm, with both regular and irregular rhythm patterns possible.
- ***Rate:*** The atrial and ventricular rates will depend on the basic rhythm.
- ***P wave configuration:*** The shape, configuration, deflection, and coordination with the QRS complex will depend on the basic rhythm.
- ***PR interval:*** The PR interval will be a normal measurement of 0.12 to 0.20 second.
- ***QRS duration and configuration:*** The QRS measurement will be 0.12 second or greater in length. The widening of the QRS duration indicates the presence of a bundle branch block (see Figure 10-4).

How the Patient Is Affected and What You Should Know

The patient will exhibit the normal effects of the basic rhythm he or she is experiencing. For example, if the rhythm is sinus tachycardia, the patient will exhibit the signs and symptoms of a fast heart rate. A bundle branch block condition can further deteriorate to the development

Figure 10-4 The presence of a P wave preceding each QRS complex indicates the rhythm is arising from the SA node. The wide QRS complexes result from a conduction defect through the ventricles indicating a bundle branch block.

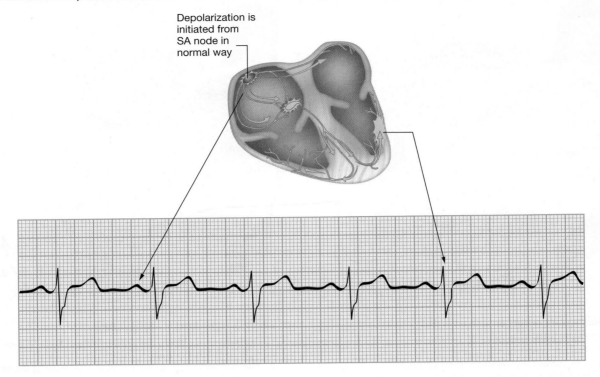

Depolarization is initiated from SA node in normal way

of another bundle branch block. If the current becomes totally blocked and current cannot reach the myocardium, this is considered a complete heart block.

Bundle branch block in and of itself is not considered to be life threatening, but what causes bundle branch block (e.g., a myocardial infarction) can be life threatening. Initially, you will observe a widening of the QRS complex, which indicates the presence of a bundle branch block. This should be reported to a licensed practitioner immediately. The patient will need to be monitored further by the licensed practitioner to determine whether an RBBB or LBBB pattern is present, and the patient's condition should be observed for deterioration. All patients must have a 12-lead ECG to document the bundle branch block. If further degeneration of the conduction system occurs, treatment may be a pacemaker. Pacemakers are applied to the external skin for a temporary condition for only 24 hours at a time. The patient may end up in a Code Blue situation and/or needing a permanent pacemaker.

Checkpoint Questions (LO 10.4)

1. What happens when one or both of the ventricular pathways are not functioning properly due to damage or a delay from cardiac disease, drugs, or other conditions?

_____

_____

2. Describe the electrical conduction for the RBBB and an LBBB.

_____

_____

3. Using the criteria for classification, select the rhythm that most closely resembles a rhythm containing bundle branch block.

A.

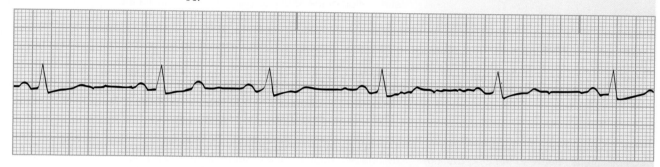

B.

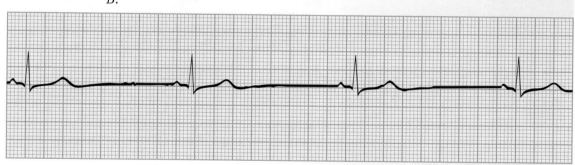

Which unique feature(s) led you to make the selection?

_____

_____

_____

Chapter Summary

Learning Outcomes	Summary	Pages
10.1 Describe the various pacemaker rhythms.	Electronic pacemakers, also known as artificial pacemakers, are devices that deliver an electrical impulse to the myocardium to cause the cells to depolarize. Pacemakers can stimulate several different cardiac functions. Atrial pacing is used alone when the conduction system from the atrioventricular node through the ventricles is intact and functioning. Ventricular pacemakers are inserted to deliver direct stimulation to the ventricles and produce a ventricular contraction. Atrioventricular pacing provides direct stimulation of the atria and ventricles and mimics the normal cardiac conduction system.	232–234
10.2 Identify pacemaker rhythms using the criteria for classification and explain how the rhythm may affect the patient, including basic patient care and treatment.	Pacemaker function can be evaluated based on the ECG tracings. The most important aspect of care is to verify the effectiveness of the pacemaker and determine the presence of a pulse with each captured beat. If a pacemaker is losing its ability to function properly, this failure will be evident on the ECG tracings.	234–239
10.3 Summarize pacemaker complications relative to the ECG tracing.	Caring for patients with pacemakers requires recognizing normal pacemaker rhythms and possible complications. When performing an ECG or monitoring a patient with a pacemaker, you should be aware of the differences in the ECG waveforms, including the presence of a pacing spike, chamber depolarization characteristics, and atrioventricular delay	239–240
10.4 Identify bundle branch block using the criteria for classification and explain how the rhythm occurs and may affect the patient.	Bundle Branch Blocks occur when one or both of the ventricular pathways are damaged or delayed due to cardiac disease, drugs, or other conditions. Current will travel down the good bundle and will activate the myocardial tissue in that corresponding ventricle only. An increased length of time of cell to cell conduction is reflected in a wider than normal QRS complex. The rhythm has all the basic properties of sinus rhythms, atrial dysrhythmias, or junctional dysrhythmias with the exception of a wide QRS complex. The patient will exhibit the normal effects of the basic rhythm he or she is experiencing. BBB should be reported to a licensed practitioner immediately. The patient will need to be monitored further to determine whether an RBBB or LBBB pattern is present, and the patient's condition should be observed for deterioration.	241–244

Chapter Review

Multiple Choice

Circle the correct answer.

1. Which pacemaker rhythms have a pacing spike before P waves? (LO. 10.1)
   a. Atrial pacemaker rhythm
   b. Ventricular pacemaker
   c. Atrioventricular pacemaker
   d. Normal sinus rhythm

2. Which pacemaker rhythms have a pacing spike before QRS complexes? (LO. 10.1)
   a. Atrial pacemaker rhythm
   b. Ventricular pacemaker
   c. Atrioventricular pacemaker
   d. Normal sinus rhythm

3. Which pacemaker rhythm has a pacing spike before P waves and QRS complexes? (LO. 10.1)
   a. Atrial pacemaker rhythm
   b. Ventricular pacemaker
   c. Atrioventricular pacemaker
   d. Wandering atrial pacemaker

4. Which pacemaker complication shows a pacing spike, but no waveform immediately following it? (LO. 10.2)
   a. Failure to sense
   b. Failure to capture
   c. Oversensing
   d. Normal sinus rhythm

5. You observe a wide QRS complex while continuously monitoring a patient in lead II. Which lead placement is necessary to evaluate the location of blockage in the bundle branch system? (LO. 10.4)
   a. Lead I
   b. Lead V4
   c. Lead III
   d. Lead VI

6. The labeling of the ECG rhythm strip for documentation of the bundle branch block should include what other information besides which bundle is being blocked? (LO. 10.4)
   a. Symptoms the patient is experiencing
   b. Blood pressure reading
   c. Presence of an MI diagnosis
   d. Patient's inherent rhythm pattern

7. When the QRS complex measures _____, bundle branch block must be considered? (LO. 10.3)
   a. 0.06 to 0.10 second
   b. 0.04 to 0.08 second
   c. Less than 0.06 second
   d. 0.12 second or greater

8. Which of the following is not one of the components to be evaluated on a pacemaker tracing? (LO. 10.2)
   a. The presence of atrial and/or ventricular spikes
   b. The QT interval
   c. The characteristic patterns of the chambers captured after the spikes
   d. The atrioventricular delay period

Matching

Match the following terms related to electronic (artificial) pacemakers to their definitions. (LO 10.2)

9. pacemaker competition
10. pacemaker (electronic)
11. loss of capture
12. malsensing
13. malfunctioning
14. oversensing
15. triggered
16. capture

a. electrical current causes the myocardial tissue to depolarize (contract)
b. heart muscle responds to electrical stimulation and depolarizes (contracts)
c. device that delivers electrical energy to cause depolarization (contractions)
d. pacing activity occurs but is not captured by the myocardium
e. pacemaker does not recognize the patient's inherent heart rate
f. electrical current from muscle movements or other activities are sensed by the pacemaker
g. pacemaker fails to send electrical impulse to the heart
h. patient's own heart and the electronic pacemaker

Critical Thinking Application *Rhythm Identification*

Review the dysrhythmias pictured next and, using the criteria for classification provided in the chapter as clues, identify each rhythm and provide what information you used to make your decision. (LO 10.2, 10.4)

17.

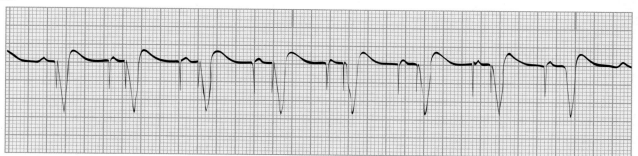

Rhythm (Regular or Irregular): _____ PR interval: _____

Rate: _____ QRS: _____

P wave: _____ Interpretation: _____

18.

Rhythm (Regular or Irregular): _____ PR interval: _____

Rate: _____ QRS: _____

P wave: _____ Interpretation: _____

19.

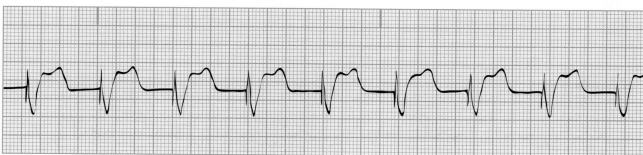

Rhythm (Regular or Irregular): _____ PR interval: _____

Rate: _____ QRS: _____

P wave: _____ Interpretation: _____

20.

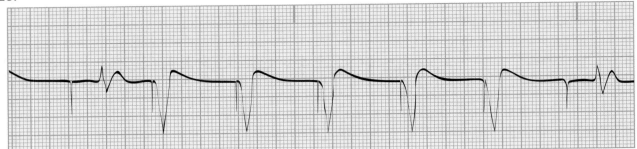

Rhythm (Regular or Irregular): _____ PR interval: _____

Rate: _____ QRS: _____

P wave: _____ Interpretation: _____

21.

Pacemaker
spike

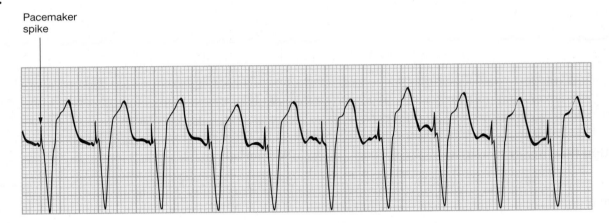

Rhythm (Regular or Irregular): _____ PR interval: _____

Rate: _____ QRS: _____

P wave: _____ Interpretation: _____

22.

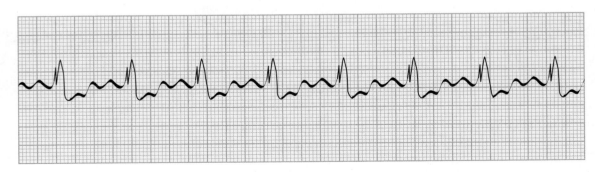

Rhythm (Regular or Irregular): _____ PR interval: _____

Rate: _____ QRS: _____

P wave: _____ Interpretation: _____

23.

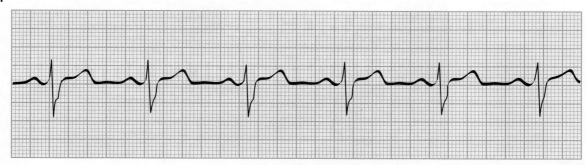

Rhythm (Regular or Irregular): _____ PR interval: _____

Rate: _____ QRS: _____

P wave: _____ Interpretation: _____

Get Connected *Internet Activity*

Visit the McGraw-Hill Higher Education Online Learning Center *Electrocardiography for HealthCare Professionals* Web site at **www.mhhe.com/boothecg3e** to complete the following activities.

1. The Alan E. Lindsay ECG Learning Center in Cyberspace is an excellent resource for more ECG learning and practice. Visit this link from the Online Learning Center and review images of rhythms, then test your knowledge. Challenge yourself and then print your scores for your instructor.

2. The 12-Lead ECG Library is also a useful site for reviewing ECGs. Go to this site from the Online Learning Center and practice before completing the rhythm identification section of this chapter.

3. Practice and review common pacemaker rhythms using the dynamic rhythm simulator found at the following Web site: http://skillstat.com/Flash/ECG_Sim_2004.html

 ## Using the Student CD

Now that you have completed the material in the chapter text, return to the student CD and complete any chapter activities you have not yet done. Practice your terminology with the "Key Term Concentration" game. Review the chapter material with the "Spin the Wheel" and "ECG Challenge" games. Take the final chapter test and complete the troubleshooting question and email or print your results to document your proficiency for this chapter.

11 Exercise Electrocardiography

Chapter Outline

- What Is Exercise Electrocardiography? (p. 253)
- Why Is Exercise Electrocardiography Used? (p. 255)
- Variations of Exercise Electrocardiography (p. 256)
- Preparing the Patient for Exercise Electrocardiography (p. 257)
- Providing Safety (p. 261)
- Performing Exercise Electrocardiography (p. 263)
- Common Protocols (p. 265)
- Following Exercise Electrocardiography (p. 268)

Learning Outcomes

11.1 Describe exercise electrocardiography and identify its other names.

11.2 Identify uses of exercise electrocardiography.

11.3 Describe variations of exercise electrocardiography.

11.4 Prepare a patient for exercise electrocardiography.

11.5 Summarize safety measures that are used before, during, and after exercise electrocardiography.

11.6 Explain the responsibilities of a healthcare professional during exercise electrocardiography.

11.7 Compare common protocols followed in exercise electrocardiography.

11.8 Explain the responsibilities of a healthcare professional after exercise electrocardiography.

Key Terms

angina	hypertension
angiogram	hyperventilation
beta blockers	invasive
cardiologist	maximal exercise
chemical stress test	noninvasive
congestive heart failure	pharmacologic stress test
coronary vascular disease (CVD)	skin rasp
echocardiogram	submaximal exercise
false positive	target heart rate (THR)

11.1 What Is Exercise Electrocardiography?

Often a patient has symptoms of cardiac problems that do not show up on a resting ECG. In order to determine the problems and to obtain an accurate diagnosis, the physician may order an exercise electrocardiograph. Exercise electrocardiography has been used for more than 50 years. This test is known by many names, such as an exercise tolerance test, a treadmill stress test, a cardiac stress test, a stress ECG, or an exercise treadmill test. It is most commonly known as a treadmill stress test because the exercise is usually performed on an exercise treadmill (Figure 11-1). This **noninvasive** procedure—meaning that it does not require entrance into a body cavity, tissue, or blood vessel—is an effective means of diagnosing cardiac disorders. The procedure is performed with a cardiologist or other physician present. The patient is carefully monitored throughout the testing.

During exercise electrocardiography, the patient is asked to walk on a treadmill (Figure 11-2). While the person is exercising, his or her ECG is continuously monitored. The person is asked to increase the level of exertion of exercise as the test progresses. In addition to monitoring the ECG, the blood pressure, heart rate, skin temperature, oxygen level, and physical appearance are also assessed. The monitoring may be measured using a ergometer which is part of the stress testing equipment. Toward the end of each exercise stage, a blood pressure and a 12-lead ECG are obtained. The patient is asked to report any chest pain, dizziness, shortness of breath, or any other symptoms. Abnormalities, physical changes, or complaints could indicate a problem that requires treatment.

As a healthcare professional, you may be responsible for providing patient instructions and monitoring the patient during the procedure by taking the blood pressure and other measurements (see Appendix F). You will also be observing for pain, discomfort, fatigue, or difficulty breathing;

noninvasive Procedure that does not require entrance into a body cavity, tissue, or blood vessel.

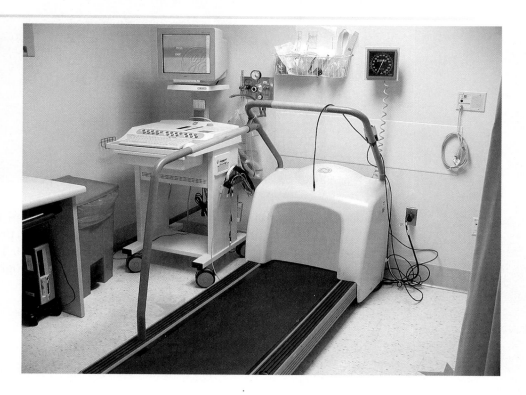

Figure 11-1 Common exercise electrocardiography equipment includes a treadmill, an ECG machine, and a monitor.

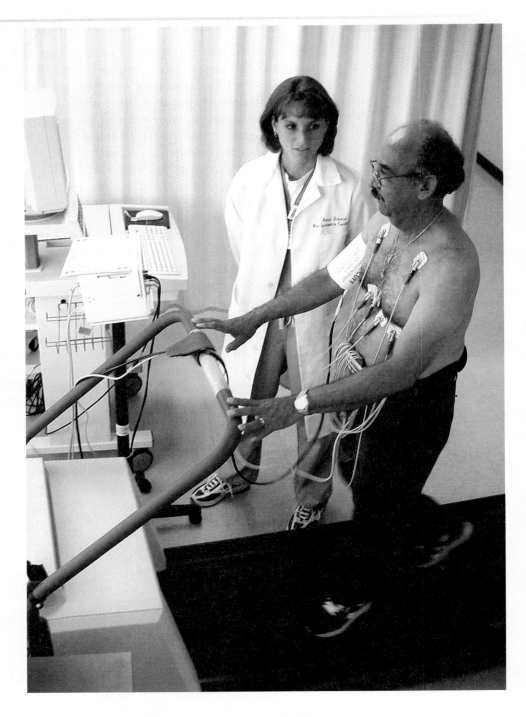

Figure 11-2 The goal during the treadmill test is to exercise the heart and evaluate how it responds to the stress of exercise.

and applying and removing the electrodes. The most important responsibilities of the health care professional is to provide for safety and to be prepared in case an emergency should arise. The following is a list of responsibilities during an exercise electrocardiograph.

- Provide for safety.
- Prepare the patient prior to the procedure.
- Attach the electrodes properly.
- Instruct the patient to report symptoms.
- Monitor the patient, including blood pressure and 12-lead ECG.

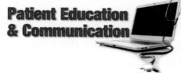
Report Abnormal Blood Pressure

Failure to report an abnormal blood pressure or other complications such as tachycardia or increased respiration rate during exercise electrocardiography could lead to severe patient problems and inaccurate test results.

Checkpoint Questions (LO 11.1)

1. Why is exercise electrocardiography considered noninvasive?

   _____

   _____

2. Name at least three responsibilities you will have during exercise electrocardiography.

   _____

   _____

11.2 Why Is Exercise Electrocardiography Used?

Coronary vascular disease (CVD) Narrowing of the arteries surrounding the heart, causing a reduction in the blood flow to the heart.

Exercise electrocardiography is used to evaluate how the heart and blood vessels respond to physical activity. Treadmill stress testing is typically performed when the physician suspects a cardiac problem, most commonly coronary vascular disease. **Coronary vascular disease (CVD)** is usually due to atherosclerosis, which occurs when plaque forms in the blood vessels from an accumulation of excess fat. When the heart is exercised, it requires additional blood to provide oxygen to the myocardium (heart muscle). The exercise increases the myocardial oxygen demand. If a patient has narrowed or obstructed arteries due to CVD, blood flow to the heart will not increase in response to the exercise. This additional workload may change the ECG tracing. One such change in the ECG tracing is ST segment depression, as shown in Figure 11-3. ST depression may indicate a myocardial ischemia. Certain medications, such as digitalis, may also cause

Figure 11-3 ST segment depression is depression of the ST segment below the normal baseline of the ECG. It may indicate myocardial ischemia, which can occur during exercise electrocardiography.

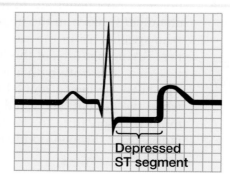

Depressed ST segment

angina An oppressive pain or pressure in the chest when the heart muscle does not receive enough oxygen due to partial or complete blockage of a coronary artery.

ST segment depression. The exercise may also produce symptoms of chest pain (**angina**), weakness, shortness of breath, palpitations, or dizziness.

Exercise electrocardiography is used for other reasons as well. The physician may want to assess how well the patient's blood pressure is maintained during exercise. Exercise electrocardiography may be used to evaluate exercise-induced symptoms such as palpitations or angina or to determine the patient's risk of a myocardial infarction. After an MI or cardiac surgery, the treadmill stress test is frequently used to evaluate the functioning of the heart. It may be used to evaluate the effectiveness of cardiac medications, identify arrhythmias that occur during exercise, and aid in the development of an exercise program. The following is a list of uses for exercise electrocardiography.

- Helps diagnose cause of chest pain
- Determines functional capacity of the heart after surgery or myocardial infarction
- Screens for heart disease (particularly in men over age 35) when no symptoms are present
- Helps set limitations for an exercise program
- Identifies cause of abnormal heart rhythms that develop during physical exercise
- Evaluates effectiveness of heart medications

Checkpoint Question (LO 11.2)

1. What does exercise electrocardiography help identify?

_____

_____

11.3 Variations of Exercise Electrocardiography

chemical stress test An invasive type of exercise electrocardiography in which thallium and/or another a radiopaque substance (one that is visible with an x-ray machine), is injected into the body to permit viewing the vessels around the heart.

cardiologist A physician who specializes in the study of the heart.

One variation of exercise electrocardiography is a **chemical stress test.** A chemical stress test is similar to a treadmill stress test. The exercise and monitoring portion are the same; however, during a chemical stress test, the patient is injected intravenously with thallium or other nuclear isotopes such as Cardiolite 1 to 2 minutes before the end of the exercise period. Thallium and Cardiolite are radiopaque substances, which means they do not let x-rays penetrate so they can be traced by an x-ray machine. As the chemical flows into the heart it is viewed by the **cardiologist,** a physician who specializes in the study of the heart, using a special camera or scanner. Taking pictures of the heart lasts about 10 to 20 minutes. The patient lies on a table with both arms above the head and the scanner above them. The heart is viewed immediately after the test as well as 3 to 4 hours later, when the patient has rested. The cardiologist studies the pictures to determine if blood flow to the heart improves with rest. The chemicals flow more easily through nondiseased arteries. The purpose of the procedure is

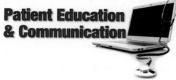
Complete Explanation Is Necessary

Patient education brochures are valuable to help the patient understand the procedure. However, they may not be enough. The physician should explain the purpose for the test, but it is your responsibility to ensure that the patient understands what will occur during the test and what the patient should report to the physician while the test is in progress.

invasive Procedure that requires entrance into a body cavity, tissue, or blood vessel.

pharmacologic stress test Other medications may also be injected if the patient is unable to exercise. These medications cause the heart rate to increase or the coronary blood vessels to dilate.

to determine if exercise causes a decrease in blood flow to any area of the heart. This procedure is considered **invasive** since the patient is injected with thallium.

Another variation of the exercise electrocardiography is a **pharmacologic stress test**. This test is given to patients who, for some reason, should not exercise. It is similar to a chemical stress test except instead of actual exercise the patient is given medication to induce cardiovascular stress similiar to exercise. These cardioactive medications include adenosine, dipyridamole (Persantine), dobutamine, or regadenoson (Lexiscan). During this test, the physician or nurse administers one of these medications, which causes the heart to exercise artificially. The medication is injected over time to stimulate the heart to exercise throughout the testing. This test requires the patient to have intravenous injections of both an imaging agent, such as thallium and one of the cardioactive drugs.

Checkpoint Question (LO 11.3)

1. Why would it be necessary to use chemical stress testing?

_____

_____

11.4 Preparing the Patient for Exercise Electrocardiography

When scheduling a patient for exercise electrocardiography, you will need to make sure the patient comes prepared for the test (Table 11-1). Describe the procedure, and ensure that the patient understands what will happen. The patient should not smoke or drink alcohol or caffeine 3 hours prior to the test. He or she should also be advised not to eat for at least 2 hours before the test. The patient should be instructed to bring or wear comfortable clothing and shoes. Tennis shoes and loose pants will make the exercise portion of the test easier for the patient.

TABLE 11-1 The Stress Test Procedure

Before the Test

- Verify that the medical history is complete.
- Explain the procedure, including the reason for test, possible complications, and *safety* measures that will be followed during procedure.
- Explain "Informed Consent," and ask the patient to sign consent form.
- Inform patients that on the day of the test they should wear comfortable clothing (shorts, tennis shoes, etc.). Female patients should not wear an underwire bra. Refrain from use of tobacco, caffeine, or alcohol for *at least 3 hours* prior to test. The patient should eat a light meal 2 hours prior to the test.
- Check the physician's orders against the patient medication list to provide information as to what medications the patient should *not* take the day of the test.
- Go over all instructions and information with the patient. Encourage questions; make sure the patient fully understands the procedure.
- Provide a detailed list of instructions, making sure that your facility telephone number and your name appear on the list. Encourage patients to call if they have any questions prior to test day.

Day of Appointment

- Verify that equipment is in working order and supplies are on hand. (Ensure plenty of tracing paper is available, inspect cables, check that treadmill is working, and verify computer setup and correct protocol.)
- Gather supplies—electrodes, alcohol, gauze sponges, razor, adhesive tape, blood pressure cuff, and so on.
- Check that the *crash cart* is ready and fully supplied and the defibrillator is working.
- Verify the physician's order, that the medical history is complete, and that the informed consent is signed.
- Bring the patient into the room.
- Verify with the patient that he or she has complied with all instructions.
- Provide the patient with privacy to change into gown with the opening to the front unless the patient needs assistance. Female patients should not wear an underwire bra.
- *Remember: During all aspects of the procedure, always provide for safety of the patient!*
- Assist the patient to lie down on the table. Prep the patient's skin and apply electrodes as indicated by the protocol of the facility or the equipment manual.
- Connect cables, apply the blood pressure cuff, and check the ECG tracing for artifact. Check and set the artifact filters as necessary.
- Obtain the patient's blood pressure and ECG in the following positions (assist the patient as necessary and provide for safety):
  - Supine
  - Sitting
  - Sitting, post 30-second hyperventilation
  - Standing

(Make sure you change the resting position in the stress test machine and enter a new blood pressure for each tracing.)

- Demonstrate the treadmill (posture, hand grip, etc.).
- Explain the test protocol, making sure the patient understands that the speed and incline will increase every 3 minutes during the test phase.
- *Be sure the patient understands that he or she is to report any pain, shortness of breath, faintness, tingling sensations, numbness, or extreme fatigue immediately! Monitor patient closely during the test looking for visual signs of any of the above. Ask the patient repeatedly during the procedure how he or she feels. Providing for patient safety is your number one priority!*
- Explain again that the test will be completed when the target heart rate is reached [(220 − age) × 0.85] or when the patient cannot continue due to fatigue or other symptoms.
- Inform the physician that the patient is ready to begin the test. The physician should be present and immediately available.
- When the physician is in the room, assist the patient to the treadmill, making sure the patient's feet are not on the belt. Start the belt; tell patient to get used to the speed and then to step onto the belt. Ask the patient if he or she is ready to begin, explaining again that the belt speed and incline will increase. Begin the test phase.

- At the 2½-minute mark of each phase, take the patient's blood pressure and enter the data into the computer. Remind the patient before every transition to a new phase. *Be ready* to assist the patient as needed.
- When the treadmill phase of the test is complete (the target heart rate is reached or the patient cannot continue), assist the patient to a waiting chair.

Posttest

- Continue to monitor and observe the patient's condition closely, taking the patient's blood pressure, entering data, and then taking an ECG tracing every 3 to 5 minutes for 10 to 15 minutes.
- When the cooldown period is completed, remove the cables and electrodes; wipe off any remaining gel or adhesive.
- Allow the patient to dress (assist if needed).
- Explain to the patient that he or she should avoid tobacco, caffeine, and alcohol for at least 3 hours. The patient should avoid extreme temperature changes, including hot showers or baths for 2 hours. The patient should rest and recuperate after the test.
- Explain that the physician will have the results of the test in 10 days. Thank the patient for his or her cooperation.
- File your report per the protocol of the facility.
- Make sure all information from the patient chart is returned to its proper place.
- Prepare for the next patient.

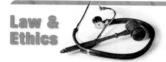

Law & Ethics

Informed Consent

Informed consent is required for surgery, HIV testing, and other procedures, including exercise electrocardiography. Informed consent implies that the patient understands the treatment, why it is being performed, any risks to the patient, alternative treatments and their risks, and the risk involved if the patient refuses treatment. Table 11-2 lists the typical reasons patients refuse the test and suggestions for resolving the problem.

What happens when you ask the patient to sign an informed consent form and he or she refuses?

_____

_____

TABLE 11-2 Handling a Patient's Refusal to Grant Consent

Reason for Refusal	Possible Solution
Patient does not understand why the consent form is necessary.	Explain the legal requirement of an informed consent, and refer the patient to the physician for questions, if necessary.
Patient does not understand the procedure.	Notify the physician, and provide a brochure for the patient to review while he or she is waiting for the physician to explain the procedure.
Patient is illiterate and unable to sign his or her name.	Have a witness present (preferably a family member), and have the consent form marked with an X by the patient and signed by the witness and yourself.
Patient is unable to sign because glasses are not available.	Make every attempt to obtain the glasses and then have the patient sign; if this is not possible, have the patient sign to the best of his or her ability. Be certain to have a witness (preferably a family member) sign the form as well.

Sometimes certain medications should not be taken prior to the test. The patient may need instruction regarding medications that can affect the test results and should not be taken. Always check the physician's order. If it is not written on the chart or order, ask the physician. When asking, have a list of the patient's current medications or the patient's chart available for the physician to review. Medications commonly known as beta blockers— drugs used to treat hypertension—are frequently stopped prior to an exercise electrocardiography test because this type of medication could affect the test results or delay the test. See Appendix A for more information about common cardiovascular medications. Remember, your responsibility is to ensure that the patient comes to the office or clinic properly prepared for the exercise electrocardiography test.

Diaforeus (w.r.) -excessive sweating

beta blockers Drugs used to treat hypertension.

Figure 11-4   Your patient must sign an informed consent for exercise electrocardiography. Most facilities use a standardized form such as the one pictured here.

Consent Form for Exercise/Chemical Stress Testing

A Stress Test is being performed to provide information about the blood supply to your heart, as well as to assess your ability to do various activities.

In order to determine an appropriate plan of medical management, I hereby consent to voluntarily engage in a myocardial stress test to determine the state of my heart and circulation.

The information obtained will help my physician recommend treatment options regarding my cardiovascular health. The test that I will undergo will be performed on a treadmill with the amount of effort increasing gradually as the test progresses. This increase in effort will continue until either a predetermined heart rate is achieved or symptoms such as fatigue, shortness of breath, or chest discomfort appear, which indicate to me to stop. An alternative type of stress test may be administered where a medication may be used to "stress" or exercise the heart. During the performance of the test, trained staff will closely monitor my pulse, blood pressure, and electrocardiogram.

If performed as part of a nuclear myocardial perfusion study, I will be injected with a small amount of radioactive material (thallium) followed by imaging of the heart. The amount of radioactivity I will be exposed to is about equivalent to a chest x-ray.

There is always the possibility of certain changes occurring during the test. They include abnormal blood pressure, fainting, shortness of breath, abnormal heart rhythms (too rapid, too slow, or ineffective), and very rare instances of heart attack. Every effort will be made to minimize them by the preliminary examination and by observations during and immediately after testing. Emergency equipment and highly trained personnel are available to manage any unusual situations that may arise.

I have read the above information and understand the procedures, as well as any possible complications or risks. I understand that in rare instances, heart attack or stroke has been reported. I acknowledge that my physician has explained my condition and the nature and purpose of this test, as well as alternative tests, and that all questions asked about my care and its attendant risks have been answered in a satisfactory manner. I understand that any question(s) I still may have can be answered by my physician or clinic staff members at any time. I hereby accept the risk of harm, if any, in hopes of obtaining the desired beneficial diagnostic information.

Signed:

_____   _____
Patient   Date

_____   _____
Patient Name Printed   Witness

_____
Physician Supervising Test

A complete history of the patient may need to be recorded before beginning the test. A standard form should be used. The information you need to obtain from the patient includes the medical history, medications currently being taken, cardiovascular risk factors (see Table 1-1 in Chapter 1), and the reason for this examination. Much of this information may already be on the patient's chart. In addition, an informed consent form must be signed and witnessed (Figure 11-4). The patient should understand the procedure, its risks, and the reason the test has been ordered before signing the informed consent form.

The patient should be informed that exercise electrocardiography is not a "timed" test. The length of time the test takes depends on several factors, including the patient's age, degree of conditioning or health status, other medical problems, and medications. You should inform the patient that the test will take approximately 45 minutes to an hour. Carefully explain the safety precautions provided during the procedure to help alleviate any fears the patient may have.

Checkpoint Questions (LO 11.4)

1. Stress testing is a noninvasive procedure. Why is informed consent necessary?

   _____

   _____

2. Why should you obtain a list of the current medications the patient is taking before the stress test procedure?

   _____

   _____

11.5 Providing Safety

Exercise electrocardiography is done on patients who are already at risk. At-risk patients may have just recently had a myocardial infarction or may currently be experiencing some type of chest pain or other symptoms, or they may have a history of coronary vascular disease. Exercise electrocardiography does place stress on the patient's heart. There is some risk of a heart attack or stroke during the procedure that should be considered. You should follow the safety measures and be prepared for emergencies (Table 11-3).

In order to provide for safety, certain rules must be followed. A physician should always be present during the procedure. Emergency equipment should be in the room or nearby, including a crash cart with emergency medications and supplies. You must know the location of this equipment. In addition, the patient should be monitored at all times, and he or she must understand the need to report any abnormal symptoms when they occur.

TABLE 11-3 Preparing for Emergencies During Exercise Electrocardiography

- Inform the patient how he or she can expect to feel during the test, including mild fatigue, increased heart rate, perspiration, and increased respiratory rate.
- Explain to the patient the need to report signs and symptoms such as chest or other pain, dizziness, weakness, or extreme fatigue.
- Make sure the patient knows to stop the exercise if any pain or extreme fatigue is felt.
- *Make sure the physician is present during the entire procedure.*
- Check to see that emergency equipment is close by, including a code or crash cart with defibrillator.
- Observe and monitor the patient, and report any symptoms to the physician.

Some health conditions prevent patients from participating in exercise electrocardiography. These conditions include but are not limited to

- A change in the resting ECG
- Abnormal heart rhythms, including uncontrolled ventricular or atrial dysrhythmia or a third degree AV block
- Recent myocardial infarction or unstable angina
- Inflammation surrounding the heart or heart muscle (pericarditis or myocarditis)
- Uncontrolled **hypertension** (high blood pressure)
- Certain cardiovascular conditions such as severe aortic stenosis, aneurysm, thrombophlebitis, and systemic or pulmonary embolism
- **Congestive heart failure** (the heart's failure to pump an adequate volume of blood)
- Acute infection
- Significant emotional stress (psychosis)

The physician should be aware of any of these conditions. Make sure that the health history is current and complete for the physician to review.

hypertension High blood pressure.

congestive heart failure (CHF) Failure of the heart to pump an adequate amount of blood to the body tissue.

Safety & Infection Control

hyperventilation To breathe at an increased rate and depth of inspiration and expiration.

Observe Patients Carefully

Observe your patient carefully when he or she changes position and during **hyperventilation** for dizziness and potential for a syncopal (fainting) episode. Many of your patients will have cardiac and/or vascular disease that increases the chances for these symptoms.

Checkpoint Question (LO 11.5)

1. Can everyone have a standard stress test? Why or why not?

_____

_____

11.6 Performing Exercise Electrocardiography

Assemble and prepare the equipment before the patient's arrival. You will need:

- Blood pressure equipment
- Shaving equipment, abrasive skin cleaner, skin rasp
- Skin prep solution
- 2 × 2 or 4 × 4 gauze
- Chest electrodes
- Stress test unit
- Lead wires
- Treadmill or stationary bicycle
- Adhesive tape belt (used to attach monitoring unit) or mesh vest
- Crash cart

Safety & Infection Control

CPR Required

As a healthcare professional you should know cardiopulmonary resuscitation (CPR) and be prepared to respond to cardiac or respiratory emergencies.

When the patient arrives for the test, you should verify that he or she has come properly prepared by making sure the patient has not had alcohol, caffeine, or tobacco for at least 3 hours or food for 2 hours prior to the test. Verify that medications were stopped, if required. Complete the patient's medical history, and make sure the informed consent form has been signed.

Next, prepare the electrode sites for placement. If the sites are hairy, dry shave the skin. Rub the site with skin prep solution, and let it dry. Abrade the skin using a special prep pad, dry 4 × 4 gauze, **skin rasp,** or other type of abrasive cleaner. Abrading the skin consists of rubbing firmly and briskly at each of the sites where the electrodes will be placed to ensure that they will adhere better to the skin.

Attach the blood pressure cuff and electrodes. Check the manufacturer's instructions for the system you are using and the policy at your facility for correct placement of the electrodes (Figure 11-5). Many exercise electrocardiography monitors include leads for both chest and back.

Check and set the artifact filters before running the stress test. These filters help reduce small signals caused by muscle movements from the ECG tracing during the test. Review the manufacturer's instructions to ensure the proper setting.

Prior to the exercise test, a series of blood pressures and 12-lead ECGs will be obtained with the patient in different positions. The following is a common example. Your facility may or may not use each of these pretest steps. Check the policy where you are employed.

First: A resting ECG and blood pressure (see Appendix F) are obtained while the patient is supine.

Second: The patient is asked to sit up, and another blood pressure and ECG are obtained.

skin rasp A rough piece of material used to abrade (scrape) the skin prior to electrode placement.

Figure 11-5 Standard placement of electrodes for exercise electrocardiography is usually the same as for a 12-lead ECG. Since machines may vary, check the manufacturer's instructions for proper placement of the electrodes for the exercise electrocardiograph machine you are using.

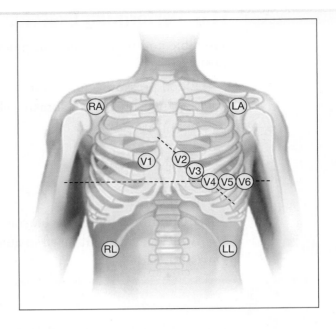

Third: The patient is asked to breathe quickly and deeply to produce a state of hyperventilation for about 30 seconds. Then another blood pressure and ECG are taken. This ECG is done to identify ECG changes caused by breathing. These changes could be misinterpreted as being related to heart disease if they occurred during the stress test.

Fourth: The patient is asked to stand, and the final preexercise blood pressure and ECG are obtained.

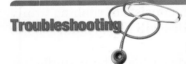

Troubleshooting

Reporting Problems

If your patient has any complaints or problems during exercise electrocardiography, you should be prepared to respond. Keep in mind that while the physician should be in the room, he or she may not always be aware of the patient's complaints or problems. Any symptom that the patient reports, such as extreme fatigue, dizziness, shortness of breath, or chest pain, should be immediately reported to the physician.

What should you do if the patient collapses?

_____

_____

1. What equipment must be assembled for exercise electrocardiography to be performed?

_____

_____

11.7 Common Protocols

The stress test is divided into stages of 2 or 3 minutes each. Each stage is based upon stress test protocols. The protocols include the length of time of exercise and the incline of the treadmill. The physician determines the protocol or length and incline of each stage of exercise (Table 11-4 and Figure 11-6).

TABLE 11-4 Common Stress Testing Protocols

Bruce Protocol: Most commonly utilized stress test. Uses 3-minute stages.

Stage	Speed (mph)	Grade (%)
1	1.7	10
2	2.5	12
3	3.4	14
4	4.2	16
5	5.0	18
6	5.5	20
7	6.0	22

"Modified" Bruce Protocol: Most often used in older individuals or those whose exercise capacity is limited by cardiac disease. Uses 3-minute stages.

Stage	Speed (mph)	Grade (%)
1	1.7	0
2	1.7	5
3	1.7	10
4	2.5	12
5	3.4	14
6	4.2	16
7	5.0	18
8	5.5	20

(Continued)

TABLE 11-4 Common Stress Testing Protocols *(Continued)*

Naughton Protocol: Better suited for sicker patients, more gradual increase in intensity. Speed stays at 2 mph. Uses 2-minute stages.

Stage	Grade (%)
1	0.0
2	3.5
3	7.0
4	10.5
5	14.0
6	17.5
7	21.0

Figure 11-6 During this Bruce Protocol Stress test, ECG recordings are made continuously during and after exercise. This image shows ST segment depression and depicts a positive test (identifies a problem). This result coupled with any patient complaints would support the diagnosis.

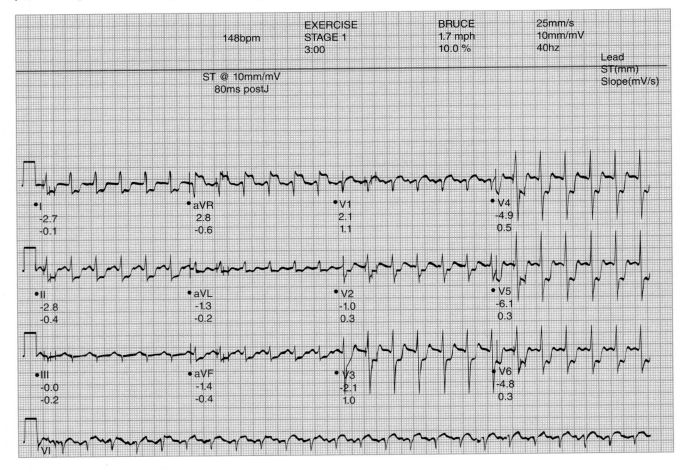

Patient Education & Communication

Reducing the Patient's Fears

You can help reduce the patient's fears by maintaining a sense of confidence, answering questions, and following safety precautions during exercise electrocardiography.

The entire exercise period lasts up to 15 minutes. The time may vary based on the patient's cardiac risk factors and ability. Toward the end of each stage, the patient's blood pressure is checked, the ECG is repeated, and the level of exercise is increased.

Most people exercise to the point of fatigue or symptoms of chest discomfort or shortness of breath. The supervising physician may halt the test because of blood pressure, ECG, or heart rhythm changes that are not perceived by the patient. In other words, though the patient may not complain of any symptoms, the physician may identify changes in the blood pressure, heart rate, or ECG tracing that may lead to complications and may order that the test be stopped.

During the test, the goal is to achieve the **target heart rate (THR)** without symptoms or complications such as a dysrhythmia (abnormal heart rhythm). The target heart rate is 220 minus the patient's age multiplied by a percentage that ranges between 60 and 85, depending upon which testing protocol is being followed (often referred to as **submaximal exercise**). This is different from the target heart rate for aerobic exercise, which is simply 220 minus the age of the person without using an additional multiplier (often referred to as **maximal exercise**).

The THR is the rate that the patient should not be allowed to exceed during the test. Achieving the THR without symptoms or abnormalities is a good indication that the heart is functioning well. Generally, the closer the patient is to the target heart rate, the more reliable the test results.

Instruct the patient to report any symptoms such as shortness of breath, chest pain, dizziness, or weakness he or she experiences during the procedure because you are responsible for monitoring and recording this information. You will need to monitor blood pressure, pulse, and any signs of cardiac distress. You may also be monitoring the patient's blood oxygen level on the monitor screen.

Rate pressure product (RPP) or double product is a measurement that may be asked for by the doctor. It is as simple as multiplying the systolic blood pressure times the patient's heart rate. This is one technique used to estimate oxygen utilization or myocardial work. For example:

$$\text{Systolic blood pressure (SYS BP)} = 118$$
$$\text{Heart rate (HR)} = 88$$
$$\text{SYS BP} \times \text{HR} = \text{RPP}$$
$$118 \times 88 = \text{RPP}$$
$$10{,}384 = \text{RPP}$$

During exercise, the heart rate and systolic blood pressure are the two main factors determining the workload on the heart. If these factors increase, the heart has to work harder and will require more oxygen and nutrients to keep going, thus putting stress on the heart. The response

target heart rate (THR) Heart rate measurement needed to truly exercise the heart.

maximal exercise Target heart rate of 220 minus the age of the patient.

submaximal exercise Target heart of 220 minus the age multiplied by a percentage between 60 and 85.

of the heart rate and blood pressure to a fixed level of exercise tends to decrease with regular exercise. So a person with good blood supply and a strong heart muscle should have a lower RPP than a person who has a disruption of the blood supply to the heart muscle and a weaker heart muscle.

Thus the RPP is an index of the myocardial oxygen requirement and helps determine the work placed on the heart, as well as the heart's response.

Watch the patient closely, including skin color, breathing pattern, amount of perspiration, and facial expressions. Many times a patient is hesitant to report a symptom. If you suspect a problem, ask the patient and then report your suspicion to the supervising physician.

Checkpoint Questions (LO 11.7)

1. Identify which stress-test protocol would most likely be used for each of the following patients.

   a. A 76-year-old, 285 pound man who has recently had a heart attack.
   b. A 46-year-old airline pilot during a yearly physical.
   c. A 65-year-old patient with hypertension and complaints of chest pain.

2. What is the target heart rate of a patient who is 49 years old?

_____

_____

11.8 Following Exercise Electrocardiography

When the patient has completed the exercise portion of the test, monitoring will continue during a "cooling off" period. This will last from 6 to 15 minutes, depending upon the protocol at your place of employment and the physician's preference. You will need to stay with the patient and continue to monitor the patient for any changes.

Many factors are used to interpret the results of exercise electrocardiography. The most important factors are the presence of ECG changes and symptoms. Other factors include heart rate and rhythm, blood pressure, and changes in oxygen consumption. If a patient has no abnormal ECG changes or unusual elevations in blood pressure, this usually means

Patient Education & Communication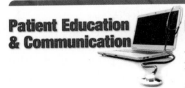

Exercise Electrocardiography Results

As a healthcare professional, you are not responsible for reporting the results of exercise electrocardiography to the patient. Should a question arise, refer the patient to the physician.

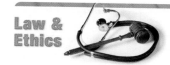
Secure Patient Testing Information

Remember to save and secure all patient testing information upon completion.

the risk for coronary vascular disease is low. If the test is stopped early because of ECG or blood pressure changes or patient symptoms, this is a sign of abnormal test results. When the results of the test are inconclusive or abnormal, additional tests may be performed. An inconclusive test is one with questionable results, meaning it does not necessarily show an abnormality or eliminate the potential for an abnormality. Additional testing is needed to either identify or eliminate any abnormalities. These additional tests may include an **echocardiogram,** which uses sound to study the heart and blood vessels (also known as ultrasound), or a coronary **angiogram,** involving x-rays following injection of a radiopaque substance.

After exercise electrocardiography, the patient should be given some instructions. These include the following:

- Rest for several hours.
- Avoid extreme temperature changes.
- Avoid stimulants, such as caffeine, tobacco, or alcohol, for at least 3 hours.
- Do not take a hot shower or bath for at least 2 hours.
- When to expect the test results.
- The results should be discussed with the physician.

Stress testing is considered a good method to detect early coronary artery disease and delay its progression. However, it is interesting to note that approximately 5% of healthy adults may have **false positive** results, meaning that the test may indicate that disease is present when it is not. Research has shown that false positives occur more frequently in females than in males, though researchers are not sure why. False positives can cause unnecessary fears and the need for additional expensive tests. As a healthcare professional you should be aware of this problem and be sensitive to the patient when concerns arise. However, the physician is responsible for providing additional information to the patient regarding false positive test results and any additional testing that may be required.

echocardiogram Noninvasive diagnostic test that uses sound to study the heart and blood vessels; also known as an ultrasound.

angiogram An invasive procedure during which x-rays are taken of a blood vessel after injection of a radiopaque substance.

false positive When a diagnostic test indicates that disease is present, but in reality, the test result is negative and no disease is present.

Checkpoint Question (LO 11.8)

1. Name at least three instructions you would give a patient after exercise electrocardiograpy.

_____

_____

Chapter Summary

Learning Outcome	Summary	Pages
11.1 Describe exercise electrocardiography, and learn its other names (synonyms).	Exercise electrocardiography is the recording of an ECG and monitoring of a patient during active or medication-induced exercise to diagnose problems that do not occur when the patient is at rest.	253–255
11.2 Identify uses of exercise electrocardiography.	Exercise electrocardiography is used to diagnose the cause of chest pain, determine the capacity of the heart, screen for heart disease, set limits for exercise, identify abnormal heart rhythms, and evaluate the effectiveness of heart medications.	255–256
11.3 Describe variations of exercise electrocardiography.	Chemical stress tests are variations of exercise electrocardiography that include the injection of medications before the procedure.	256–257
11.4 Prepare a patient for exercise electrocardiography.	To prepare a patient for exercise electrocardiography, you must schedule the appointment, prepare the patient, obtain a consent form, and document what you have completed. The patient needs to be taught about the procedure, its complications, what to wear, what medications or other substances they can and cannot take, and what to report during the procedure itself.	257–261
11.5 Summarize safety measures that are used before, during, and after exercise electrocardiography.	Providing for safety before, during, and after exercise electrocardiography, including following standard precautions, preparing the crash cart, monitoring the patient, providing complete patient instructions, and making sure the physician is present during the entire exercise portion of the procedure.	261–262
11.6 Explain the responsibilities of a healthcare professional during exercise electrocardiography.	As an assistant during the procedure, you may be responsible for safety, education, and preparation of the patient, attachment of the electrodes, instructions on reporting symptoms, and monitoring the patient, including taking the blood pressure.	263–265
11.7 Compare common protocols followed in exercise electrocardiography.	Common protocols for exercise electrocardiography include Bruce, modified Bruce, and Naughton.	265–268
11.8 Explain the responsibilities of a healthcare professional after exercise electrocardiography.	After exercise electrocardiography, the patient will need to be monitored during the cooling off period, and provided with additional education and information about when the results will be ready.	268–269

Chapter Review

Multiple Choice

Circle the correct answer for each of the following.

1. What is your most important responsibility during exercise electrocardiography? (LO 11.5)
   a. Providing for safety
   b. Applying the leads
   c. Monitoring the ECG tracing
   d. Taking the patient's blood pressure

2. Which of the following conditions would be a reason that a patient should not perform exercise electrocardiography? (LO 11.5)
   a. Coronary vascular disease
   b. Previous heart attack
   c. Congestive heart failure
   d. Previous symptoms of angina

3. What type of test would be performed on a patient who is unable to stand or exercise? (LO 11.3)
   a. Chemical stress test
   b. Blood pressure test
   c. Treadmill stress test
   d. Cardiac stress test

4. During exercise electrocardiography, your patient appears to be short of breath. After informing the physician of your suspicions, what would you do? (LO 11.6)
   a. Continue the test.
   b. Take the patient's blood pressure.
   c. Ask the patient to stop the exercise portion of the test.
   d. Without the patient's knowledge, count the respiratory rate and compare to the previous rate.

5. Mr. Jones is on several medications and is scheduled for an exercise electrocardiography test tomorrow. What should you do first to determine if he should take his medications prior to the test? (LO 11.5)
   a. Check the chart or order.
   b. Ask the physician.
   c. Instruct the patient not to take his beta blocker medications.
   d. Mr. Jones should take all of his medications since they are necessary for his treatment.

6. A beta blocker is: (LO 11.5)
   a. a protocol for exercise electrocardiography.
   b. a medication for hypertension.
   c. necessary when performing exercise electrocardiography.
   d. a medication for heart disease.

7. Which of the following is measured during exercise electrocardiography? (LO 11.6)
    a. Blood pressure and temperature
    b. Blood pressure and weight
    c. 12-lead ECG and weight
    d. 12-lead ECG and blood pressure

8. When educating the female patient for exercise electrocardiography, you should instruct her *not* to wear: (LO 11.4)
    a. shorts.
    b. tennis shoes.
    c. an underwire bra.
    d. comfortable clothing.

Patient Education

You are assigned to teach Mr. Hussein about exercise electrocardiography. From the following list, determine which are correct patient instructions for exercise electrocardiography and which are not. Place a *C* beside the correct statements and an *I* beside the incorrect statements. For each of the incorrect (*I*) statements, write the correct instructions for the patient.

_____ 9. Patients should avoid alcohol, tobacco, and caffeine for at least 8 hours prior to exercise electrocardiography. (LO 11.4)

_____

_____

_____ 10. Patients should be encouraged to report any symptoms such as shortness of breath, weakness, dizziness, or fatigue during exercise electrocardiography. (LO 11.6)

_____

_____

_____ 11. After exercise electrocardiography, the patient should not take a hot bath or shower for at least 2 hours. (LO 11.8)

_____

_____

_____ 12. You should discuss the results of exercise electrocardiography with the patient as soon as the results are available. (LO 11.8)

_____

_____

_____ 13. Patients should wear comfortable, casual clothing on the day of the test, including tennis shoes and loose fitting pants. (LO 11.4)

_____

_____

_____ 14. You should attach the leads to the chest at the same sites as you would for an ambulatory monitor. (LO 11.6)

_____

_____

_____ **15.** Emergency equipment should be available in the room or nearby during exercise electrocardiography. (LO 11.6)

_____

_____

Lead Placement

16. Draw and label the electrodes for exercise electrocardiography on the figure below. (LO 11.6)

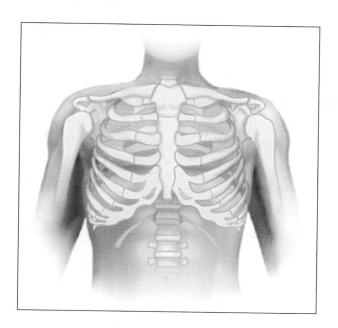

Matching

Match these terms with the correct definitions. Place the appropriate letter on the line to the left of each term.

_____ **17.** chemical stress test (LO 11.3)

_____ **18.** myocardium (LO 11.2)

_____ **19.** hypertension (LO 11.5)

_____ **20.** beta blocker (LO 11.4)

_____ **21.** angiogram (LO 11.8)

_____ **22.** angina (LO 11.2)

_____ **23.** dysrhythmia (LO 11.7)

a. medication used to treat hypertension

b. pain around the heart caused by lack of oxygen to the heart

c. failure of the heart to pump an adequate amount of blood to the tissue

d. loss of normal rhythm of the heart beat

e. a physician who specializes in the study of the heart

f. x-rays taken of the blood vessels after injection of a radiopaque substance

(Continued)

_____ 24. cardiologist (LO 11.3)

_____ 25. congestive heart failure (LO 11.5)

_____ 26. coronary vascular disease (LO 11.2)

_____ 27. echocardiogram (LO 11.8)

_____ 28. false positive (LO 11.8)

_____ 29. THR (LO 11.7)

g. accumulation of plaque and fatty deposits in the coronary arteries

h. noninvasive diagnostic test that uses ultrasound to study the heart and blood vessels

i. when a diagnostic test indicates that disease is present and in reality it is not

j. high blood pressure

k. middle layer of the heart composed of muscle tissue

l. calculated by subtracting your age from 220

m. exercise electrocardiography that is invasive because of injection of a radiopaque substance to view the vessels around the heart

True/False

Read each statement and determine if it is true or false. Circle the T or F. For false (F) statements, correct them to "make them true" on the lines provided.

T   F   30. A noninvasive procedure requires entrance into a body cavity, tissue, or blood vessel. (LO 11.1)

_____

_____

T   F   31. A Naughton protocol is most commonly utilized for a stress test. (LO 11.7)

_____

_____

T   F   32. A modified Bruce protocol is most often used during a stress test for patients with an exercise capacity limited by cardiac disease. (LO 11.7) _____

_____

T   F   33. A 12-lead ECG is obtained toward the beginning of each stage of exercise electrocardiography. (LO 11.7) _____

_____

T   F   34. After a stress test, the patient should avoid alcohol, tobacco, and caffeine for at least 3 hours. (LO 11.8) _____

_____

T   F   35. A patient should take all of his prescribed medications on the day of his stress test. (LO 11.1) _____

_____

Critical Thinking Application *What Should You Do?*

Read the following situations, and use your critical thinking skills to determine how you would handle each. Write your answer in detail in the space provided.

36. Your patient, Mr. Rollins, is scheduled for an exercise electrocardiography test on Friday. When scheduling the appointment, you notice he is taking several heart medications, including A tenolol. You check the patient's order, and it does not mention whether any of the medications should not be taken before the procedure. Mr. Rollins is getting ready to leave. What should you do? (LO 11.4)

_____

_____

37. During an exercise electrocardiography procedure, your patient complains of weakness and shortness of breath. He suddenly collapses on the treadmill and falls into the chair. What should you do? (LO 11.6)

_____

_____

38. Mrs. Annon just had an exercise electrocardiography procedure performed. You are responsible for providing instructions to her before she leaves. After you review the instructions, Mrs. Annon tells you she is going to go for a walk to have a cigarette while she waits for her husband to pick her up. It is about 97°F outside. What should you do? (LO 11.8)

_____

_____

39. Mr. Wong is required to have a thallium stress test at the outpatient clinic where you are employed. He is a very busy businessman and requests to have the test during his lunch hour. What would be your response? (LO 11.4)

_____

_____

Get Connected *Internet Activity*

Visit the McGraw-Hill Higher Education Online Learning Center *Electrocardiography for Healthcare Professionals* Web site at **www.mhhe.com/boothecg3e** to complete the following activity.

1. Patient Information for Exercise Electrocardiography. Go to the Online Learning Center that accompanies this book and visit the American Heart Association, the National Library of Medicine, and the Heart Health Center Online. Search these and other Web sites to research how frequently exercise electrocardiography is performed and its effectiveness. Be prepared to present your information to the class or prepare your own patient informational brochure.
2. Treadmill and Pharmacologic Stress Testing. Go to this emedicine from WebMD site to learn more about exercise electrocardiography. Review the article, including the list of absolute and relative contraindications to exercise stress testing. You can also search for stress test demonstration and view a short video of the procedure.

 ## Using the Student CD

Now that you have completed the material in the chapter text, return to the student CD and complete any chapter activities you have not yet done. Practice your terminology with the "Key Term Concentration" game. Review the chapter material with the "Spin the Wheel" and "ECG Challenge" games. Take the final chapter test and complete the troubleshooting question and email or print your results to document your proficiency for this chapter.

PROCEDURE CHECKLIST 11-1

Assisting with Exercise Electrocardiography (Stress Testing)

Procedure Steps (*Rationale*)	Practice Yes	No	Practice Yes	No	Performed Yes	No	Mastered
Before the Procedure							
1. Verify that the medical history is complete. (To ensure safety and accurate testing)							
2. Explain the procedure, including reason for test, possible complications, and all safety measures that will be followed during procedure.							
3. Explain "Informed Consent," and ask patient to sign consent form.							
4. Inform patient that on the day of test he or she should wear comfortable clothing (shorts or gym suit, tennis shoes). Refrain from use of tobacco, caffeine, or alcohol for *at least 3 hours* prior to test. Patient should eat a light meal 2 hours prior to test. (The effects of tobacco, caffeine, or alcohol could affect the results of the test.							
5. Check the physician's order against the patient medication list to provide information as to what medications patient should *not* take day of test. (Certain medications can affect the results of the test.)							
6. Go over all instructions and information with the patient. Encourage questions, and ask the patient to repeat important information back to you. (To make sure patient fully understands procedure)							
7. Provide a copy of the detailed list of instructions, making sure that facility telephone number and your name appear on list. Encourage patient to call if he or she has any questions prior to test day.							
Procedure: Day of Appointment							
1. Verify that the equipment is in working order and supplies are on hand, including plenty of tracing paper. Be certain to inspect the cables; make sure the treadmill and computer are working and the correct protocol is determined. (To prevent problems during the procedure when the patient and physician are present)							
2. Gather all supplies, including electrodes, alcohol, gauze sponges, razor, adhesive tape, and blood pressure cuff.							
3. Check that the crash cart is ready and fully supplied, with the defibrillator working.							

Procedure Steps (*Rationale*)	Practice Yes	No	Practice Yes	No	Performed Yes	No	Mastered
Procedure: Day of Appointment							
4. Verify the physician's order, that the medical history is complete, and that the informed consent is signed.							
5. Bring the patient into the room.							
6. Verify with the patient that he or she has complied with all instructions.							
7. Provide patient with privacy to change into gown with opening to front. Assist if necessary. (Opening needs to be in the front in order to place leads.)							
8. Assist patient to lie down on table. (Provides for safety)							
9. Prepare the skin, and apply electrodes as indicated by protocol of facility or equipment manual.							
10. Connect the cables, apply the blood pressure cuff, and check ECG tracing for artifact. (Ensures proper results during the examination.)							
11. Obtain blood pressure and ECG in the following positions. Assist as necessary. (Provides for safety of patient) • Supine • Sitting • Sitting, post 30-second hyperventilation • Standing							
12. Change the resting position in stress test machine, and enter new blood pressure for each tracing.							
13. Demonstrate the treadmill, including the proper posture and holding the hand grip. (Prevents falls)							
14. Explain the test protocol, making sure the patient understands that the speed and incline will increase every 3 minutes during test phase.							
15. Be sure patient understands that he or she is to report any pain, shortness of breath, faintness, tingling sensations, numbness, or extreme fatigue immediately. (Provides for safety of patient)							

(Continued)

Procedure Steps (*Rationale*)	Practice Yes	No	Practice Yes	No	Performed Yes	No	Mastered
Procedure: Day of Appointment							
16. Watch the patient closely during the test, looking for visual signs of any pain, shortness of breath, faintness, tingling sensations, numbness, or extreme fatigue. (Provides for safety of patient)							
17. Ask patient repeatedly during procedure how he or she feels. (Provides for safety of patient)							
18. Explain to the patient again that the test will be completed when target heart rate (THR) is reached [THR = (220 − age) × 0.85] or when the patient cannot continue due to fatigue or other symptoms.							
19. Inform the physician that the patient is ready to begin test. (The physician must be present during the procedure.)							
20. When the physician is in the room, assist patient to the treadmill, making sure patient's feet are not on the belt.							
21. Start the belt, tell patient to get used to speed and then to step onto the belt. Ask patient if he or she is ready to begin, explaining again that belt speed and incline will increase. Begin the test phase.							
22. At the two and one-half minute mark of each phase, take the blood pressure and enter the data into computer. Remind patient before every transition to new phase, and be ready to assist the patient as needed. (Provides for safety)							
23. When treadmill phase of test is complete by either the THR reached or the patient cannot continue, assist patient to waiting chair. (Provides for safety)							
Postprocedure Posttest							
1. Continue to monitor and observe the patient's condition closely, taking the blood pressure, entering the data, and then taking an ECG tracing every 3 to 5 minutes for 10 to 15 minutes. (Verifies the patient condition and tolerance of the testing procedure)							
2. After the 10-to-15-minute cooldown period, remove the cables and electrodes and wipe off any remaining gel or adhesive.							

Procedure Steps (*Rationale*)	Practice Yes	Practice No	Practice Yes	Practice No	Performed Yes	Performed No	Mastered
Postprocedure Posttest							
3. Allow patient to dress (assist if needed).							
4. Explain to patient that he or she should avoid tobacco, caffeine, and alcohol for at least 3 hours. Patient should avoid extreme temperature changes, including hot shower or bath for 2 hours. Patient should rest and recuperate after test. (Provides for safety)							
5. Explain that the physician will have the results of the test in 10 days. Thank the patient for his or her participation.							
6. File the results and report per the protocol of the facility.							
7. Make sure all information from patient chart is returned to its proper place. (Maintains HIPAA)							

Comments: _____

_____

_____

_____

Signed

Evaluator: _____

Student: _____

12 Ambulatory Monitoring

Chapter Outline

- What Is Ambulatory Monitoring? (p. 280)
- How Is Ambulatory Monitoring Used? (p. 282)
- Functions and Variations (p. 283)
- Educating the Patient (p. 288)
- Preparing the Patient (p. 292)
- Applying an Ambulatory Monitor (p. 292)
- Removing an Ambulatory Monitor and Reporting Results (p. 295)

Learning Outcomes

12.1 Identify the types of ambulatory monitors and their functions.

12.2 Explain why ambulatory monitoring is used in addition to the 12-lead ECG.

12.3 Summarize the common uses and variations of ambulatory monitoring.

12.4 Educate the patient about ambulatory monitoring.

12.5 Prepare a patient for application of an ambulatory monitor.

12.6 Describe the procedure for applying an ambulatory monitor correctly.

12.7 Describe the procedure for removing the ambulatory monitor and reporting the results.

Key Terms

ambulating	oscilloscope
anti-arrhythmic	palpitations
dysrhythmia	stress ECG
Holter monitor	syncope

12.1 What is Ambulatory Monitoring?

Ambulatory monitoring is the process of recording an ECG tracing for an extended period of time while a patient goes about his or her daily activities, including walking or **ambulating**. A typical ambulatory monitor is a small box that is strapped to the patient's waist or shoulder to

ambulating Walking.

Figure 12-1 An ambulatory monitor is attached to the shoulder or waist so the patient is free to move about during the 24- to 48-hour period while the electrical activity of the heart is being recorded.

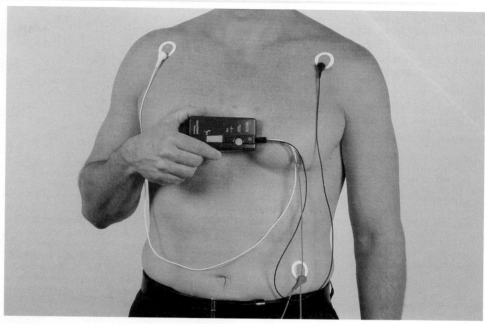

24-to-72 hours

record an ECG over a 24- to 48-hour period (Figure 12-1). Inside the box is a recording device; the entire device usually weighs less than 2 pounds. The most common type looks like a small tape recorder. Newer ambulatory monitors on the market are digital recorders, as seen in Figure 12-2. One type of ambulatory monitor is also known as a **Holter monitor**, named after its inventor, Norman Holter.

Holter monitor An instrument that records the electrical activity of the heart during a patient's normal daily activities; also known as an *ambulatory monitor*.

15 lead wires
Required to keep
Diary

During ambulatory monitoring, the patient has three to five leads attached to his or her chest, depending on the type of monitor used. The patient may move around and is encouraged to maintain his or her normal daily activities. While the monitor is in place and recording, the patient is asked to keep a diary to record all usual and unusual activities. Any symptoms or abnormal sensations such as chest pain, indigestion, or dizziness should be recorded. If symptoms do occur, the patient is asked to monitor the symptoms and what he or she was doing prior to and during the symptoms. When the monitoring is completed, the information from the monitor and diary must be interpreted. A computer is used to print and/or view the ECG tracing from the monitor. A computer may be used for analysis of the tracing. This computer analysis may be done within the facility, or the tracing may be sent to an outside laboratory, known as a reference laboratory. A physician, usually a cardiologist, does final interpretation of the results. If the results are sent to a reference laboratory, they are returned to the patient's physician.

As a healthcare professional, you may be responsible for applying and removing the ambulatory monitor, providing patient education, and ensuring that the results are placed in the patient's chart. Depending on your place of employment, you may be responsible for scanning the tape or digital disk. The scanner will analyze the data, highlighting any irregularities, or provide a printout for the physician to interpret. Part of your job may be to assist with distinguishing artifact from cardiac dysrhythmias.

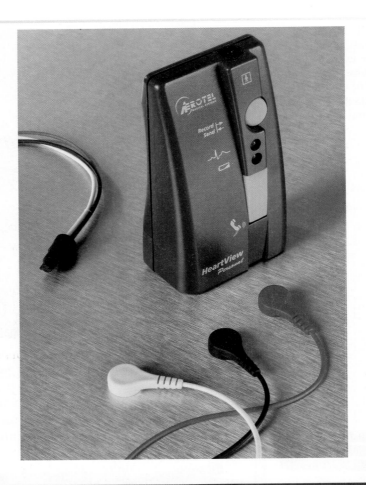

Figure 12-2 Digital ambulatory monitors record the electrical activity of the heart, which is transferred directly to a computer or over the Internet or phone line for interpretation.

Checkpoint Questions (LO 12.1)

1. How long does a typical ambulatory monitor record an ECG?

_____

_____

2. What responsibilities might you have for ambulatory monitoring?

_____

_____

12.2 How Is Ambulatory Monitoring Used?

syncope Condition when the patient loses consciousness (fainting).

palpitations Fast, irregular heartbeat sensation felt by the patient, which may or may not be associated with complaints of chest pain.

The purpose of ambulatory monitoring is to document the electrical activity in the heart and identify any abnormal heart behaviors such as dysrhythmias. Abnormal heart behaviors can occur randomly or spontaneously and may be sleep related, disease related, or diet or stress induced. As you have learned in previous chapters, abnormal electrical behavior of the heart can be life threatening.

The ambulatory monitor captures abnormal heart rhythms and correlates symptoms experienced by the patient. For example, a typical patient may be experiencing chest pain, lightheadedness, **syncope** (fainting spells), dizziness, or **palpitations** (rapid, irregular heartbeat). To find the cause of

stress ECG Another name for exercise electrocardiography.

anti-arrhythmic Type of medication given to prevent cardiac rhythm abnormalities.

these symptoms, the patient may have already had a 12-lead ECG and a cardiac **stress ECG** (exercise electrocardiography). However, the patient may not have experienced symptoms during these tests, so no abnormal rhythms would have been detected. If the patient is still having symptoms, an ambulatory monitor can be used. During the 24 to 48 hours (or in some case longer) that the monitor is in place, the patient records all daily activities, abnormal experiences, and symptoms in a diary. The ambulatory monitor provides an ECG tracing at the exact time the patient experiences any symptoms. The physician can interpret the results and evaluate the patient's symptoms based on the ECG tracing.

Ambulatory monitoring is used for other reasons as well. The physician may want to evaluate the effectiveness of cardiac medications such as **anti-arrhythmic** drug therapy (medication given to prevent cardiac rhythm abnormalities). Ambulatory monitoring is also used to evaluate artificial pacemaker functioning. Pacemaker functioning is evaluated after implantation or if problems arise. Ambulatory monitoring can also evaluate the function of the heart after a recent myocardial infarction.

As you can see, ambulatory monitoring is an effective tool to evaluate a wide variety of conditions and problems. However, the decision to use long-term ambulatory monitoring does not come without problems. Education of the patient is essential, as discussed throughout this chapter. The patient must have the ability to understand the process. For example, a patient with dementia would not be a good candidate for long-term ambulatory monitoring. Also, the equipment may fail, such as with a lead failure wherein the lead quits working during the monitoring process.

Checkpoint Question (LO 12.2)

1. Why is a diary a necessary part of Holter monitoring?

_____

_____

12.3 Functions and Variations

The two most common types of ambulatory monitoring are continuous and intermittent. Continuous monitoring provides a complete tracing of the ECG from the time the monitor is applied until it is removed. During continuous monitoring, the patient may be asked to press a button on the machine to mark the tracing whenever a symptom is felt. This is known as an "event marker." The marker marks the tracing at the exact time the event occurs. The monitor has an accurate clock that indicates the time the marker is applied. The clock is necessary for the physician to be able to correlate the diary entries with what is happening on the ECG tracing.

Intermittent recording records only while the patient is experiencing symptoms. The patient is instructed to press a button on the machine when symptoms occur to start the ECG tracing. The results from this type of tracing are shorter and can be evaluated more quickly than continuous monitoring. However, intermittent monitoring only shows the ECG tracing during the symptoms. Some abnormal rhythms can occur prior to symptoms, and an intermittent recording may not show these abnormalities.

Some ambulatory monitors can be voice activated. When the patient experiences an unusual symptom or changes in activity, he or she can speak into the recorder to describe each event. The event is timed for comparison to the ECG tracing during continuous monitoring. During intermittent monitoring, the ECG tracing may also be activated by the voice. (It is your responsibility to know the type and features of the monitor used in order to properly apply and remove the monitor and to instruct the patient.)

Two other variations of ambulatory monitoring include telemetry and transtelephonic monitoring. Telemetry monitoring is performed within a medical facility such as a hospital. Transtelephonic monitoring is performed outside the medical facility. Both of these types of monitoring are performed on patients who can ambulate.

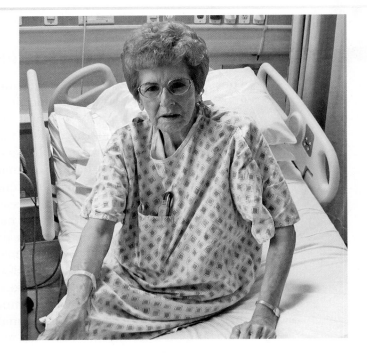

Safety & Infection Control

Handle Monitors Carefully

Ambulatory monitors are sensitive and can be very expensive. Be careful when handling an ambulatory monitor. Dropping or hitting the machine against something could cause permanent damage.

People with dementia

Telemetry monitoring is done with a small transmitting device attached to the chest with three or five electrodes (Figure 12-3). A continuous tracing of the heart is recorded and sent directly to a monitoring station. Telemetry monitors are only transmitting devices designed to send the electrical signal of the heart to a central location to be evaluated continuously. At this location, single or multiple patients may be monitored at the same time on multiple screens (Figure 12-4). There is no need for a patient diary since the patient is admitted to the facility and will be observed and monitored at all times. In a cardiac intensive care unit, your role as a healthcare professional may include observing the ECG tracings for abnormalities

Figure 12-3 At an in-patient facility, patients wear the telemetry monitor leads and the unit attached to the chest. The unit can be placed in the pocket of their gown or on their waist. This allows patients to ambulate and perform activities of daily living during their hospitalization.

Figure 12-4 Several patients can be monitored simultaneously at a central patient care station. In this picture of an electronic Intensive Care Unit (eICU) the patients being monitored are in another building.

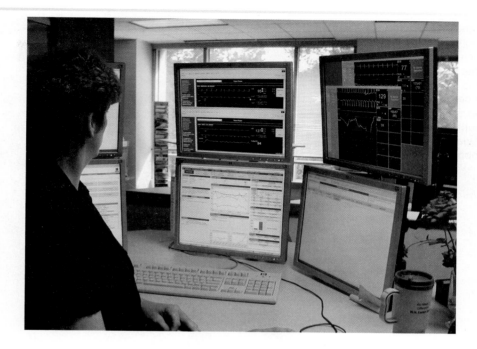

Figure 12-5 Multiple patients can be monitored on a single LCD display screen.

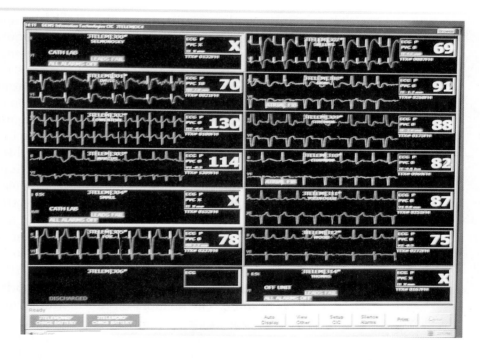

dysrhythmias Irregularity or loss of rhythm of the heart beat.

on a computer-type screen (Figure 12-5). You will need to be familiar with the dysrhythmias (irregularities in heart rhythm) presented in Chapter 5. In addition, you may also be required to pass a certification examination to work as a telemetry monitoring technician.

Transtelephonic monitoring was developed in the 1960s after Holter monitoring was developed. It is used mainly to evaluate pacemaker function but is also used for any patient requiring monitoring for longer than 24 to 48 hours. Patients with permanent pacemakers or certain cardiac dysrhythmias may require monitoring for 30 days or more. Transtelephonic monitors are small and portable. The information recorded is stored in the

Figure 12-6 Transtelephonic monitors such as this one includes a transmitting device that is attached to the patient and includes a carrying case. A cellular phone device picks up the ECG tracing from the patient transmitter and sends it via cell phone line to a monitoring location.

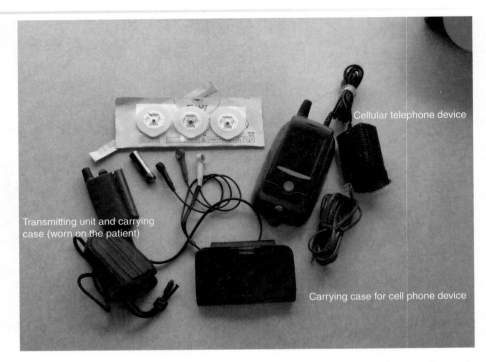

monitor and transmitted over the telephone line, either remotely through a cell phone type device or at the end of the monitoring period (Figure 12-6).

There are two types of transtelephonic monitors. One type is known as a postsymptom event monitor. This type is used when a patient is experiencing symptoms. It is worn like a wristwatch or it can be handheld. The handheld type should be kept in a convenient place by the patient and is activated when pressed onto the chest (Figure 12-7A and B). The patient should activate the monitor while experiencing symptoms. The electrode feet on the handheld monitor record a lead II tracing. The wristwatch type is worn at all times and records a two-directional or bipolar lead I tracing. Postsymptom event monitoring records the heart activity for short periods immediately after the patient experiences symptoms. It is used primarily to document dysrhythmias that last more than a few seconds, such as atrial fibrillation, atrial flutter, and supraventricular tachycardias.

Another type of transtelephonic monitor is a loop-memory monitor. This small device is attached to the chest with two lead wires. It remains in place continuously throughout the monitoring period, which may be 30 days or more. The memory on this monitor can hold up to 5 minutes of the ECG tracing and is programmed based on the patient's symptoms and complaints. For example, if a patient has a history of syncope (fainting spells), activating the monitor after an episode will lock the previous 5 minutes of ECG tracing into the memory for transmission over the telephone and evaluation. This provides the physician with an ECG tracing of the heart before, during, and after the episode and helps the physician determine the cause of the syncope (Figure 12-8).

A new "transtelephonic" capability is a 12-lead ECG. This 10-cable device is attached in the same manner and locations discussed in Chapter 4. The difference is that the patient can activate this device any place at any time and send the data to the doctor's office or monitoring facility for immediate interpretation. This transtelephonic device measures approximately 2½ by 5 inches and weighs only 6 ounces (Figure 12-9)!

Figure 12-7 The small Heart Card monitor is activated by the patient when pressed onto the chest.

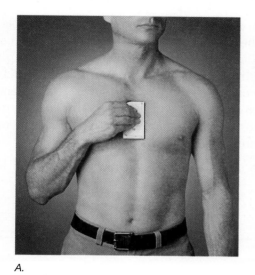

A.

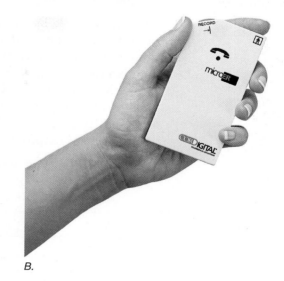

B.

Figure 12-8 The patient presses a button once symptoms begin in order to record all pre- and post- ECG segments.

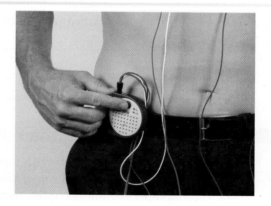

Figure 12-9 Twelve-lead transtelephonic monitor. A 12-lead ECG is produced with this 10-cable transtelephonic monitor.

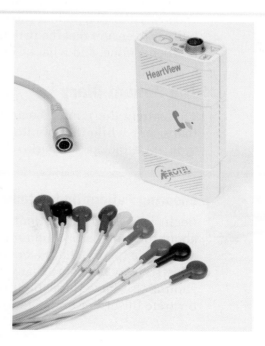

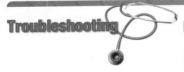

Patient Problems

Sometimes during ambulatory monitoring, the electrodes may become loose or disconnected, and the patient will need to know how to handle this situation. Check the policy of the facility where you are employed to give the patient correct instructions. Usually patients are instructed to press loose electrodes in the center to reapply. However, if the electrode comes off completely, the patient will need to report this and return to the facility for replacement. Information about how and when to contact your place of employment should be provided to the patient.

A patient asks you what he should do if an electrode becomes loose. What should you do?

_____

_____

Checkpoint Question (LO 12.3)

1. Why is a diary not necessary for telemetry patients?

_____

_____

12.4 Educating the Patient

Prior to having an ambulatory monitor, the patient must be thoroughly instructed on its proper use. Maintaining a diary is vital for accurate interpretation and evaluation of the results of the ECG tracing. The ECG tracing alone is not helpful unless the physician can correlate the results with the activities and symptoms the patient was experiencing during the tracing. Your responsibility is to ensure that the patient understands the monitoring procedure, why it is being done, and what he or she must do while the monitor is in place.

The Patient Diary

The patient diary must be an accurate record of the events and symptoms that occur while the monitor is in place (Figure 12-10). Most diaries provide time blocks to mark when activities and symptoms occur, making

Patient Education & Communication

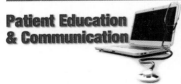

Ensuring Patient Understanding

Begin by asking the patient to tell you what he or she already knows about the ambulatory monitoring procedure. Based on the response, you can then explain what he or she does not know or understand. This is an effective way to ensure that your patient understands the procedure. You should also have the patient repeat the information back to you to demonstrate his or her understanding.

Figure 12-10 Explain the importance of the patient diary and the need for an accurate account of the patient's activities during the monitoring. Make sure the patient understands the diary's importance before he or she leaves with an ambulatory monitor.

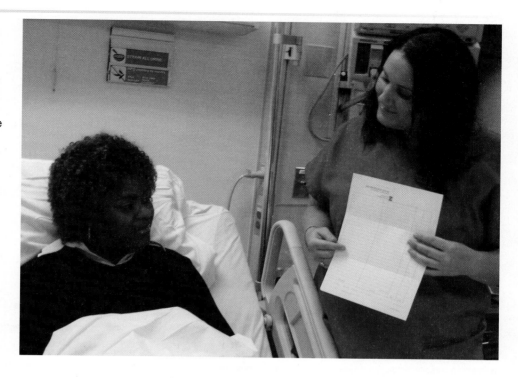

entry easy for the patient (Figure 12-11). The patient must record *all* activities, including physical and emotional stress and all usual and unusual daily events, such as urinating, bowel movements, sexual activities, walking, emotional upset, eating, and sleeping. You should emphasize the need for an accurate and complete diary. Make sure the patient knows not to change diet or daily activity during ambulatory monitoring.

To ensure that the patient understands the diary recording procedure, have him or her repeat your instructions back to you. You may want the patient to demonstrate his or her understanding by placing a sample entry into the diary. Provide the patient with a complete set of instructions with your name and the facility phone number in the event the patient has any questions or problems. If the patient does not understand how to maintain the diary correctly, the monitoring procedure may have to be repeated. This unnecessary time and expense can be avoided by properly instructing the patient.

As previously mentioned, ambulatory (Holter) monitoring may be done to evaluate the effectiveness of new cardiac medications or the patient's response to discontinuation of cardiac medications. In these circumstances, the physician may change the patient's heart medications prior to the monitoring, either adding a new medication or discontinuing one the

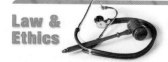

Scope of Practice

Licensed practitioners are responsible for educating the patient regarding actions, indications, side effects, and precautions of medications. When a question arises regarding this information, refer the patient to a licensed practitioner to avoid practicing outside the scope of your education and training.

Figure 12-11 Note the sample entries in this Holter monitoring patient diary. The patient should make entries into the diary frequently throughout the Holter monitoring period.

Sample Diary

A portion of a sample diary is shown below. Remember that the more complete your diary, the more valuable it is for your doctor. If in doubt, write it down. Please print clearly so that your doctor or technician will understand your comments.

TIME	ACTIVITY	SYMPTOM
11:30 am	walking in hall	dizzy
1:45 pm	BM	
2:30 pm	exercise class began	
3:45 pm	sitting watching TV	flutter
11:30	Bed	

Patient Instructions

Carry this diary and a pencil with you at all times and enter your activities, symptoms, and times they occur. Generally you should record:

Time of Day: For every entry in the diary.

Activities: Routine & strenuous exercise, bowel movements, taking medication, or emotional upsets, such as anger.

Symptoms: Chest, neck, arm or face pain, heart pounding, dizziness, nausea, shortness of breath or any other-whether or not you feel they are important. If in doubt, write it down.

Important:
1. Do not tamper with the recorder, electrodes, or electrode leads.
2. Do not get the recorder wet.
3. Your recorder is equipped with a digital clock display and an event marker button; activate it when symptoms occur.

Patient Activity Diary

( )hr   ( )12 hr   ( )24 hr

Patient's Name_____
Patient's Addr._____
_____

Age:_____ Sex:_____
Phone:_____
Medication:_____
_____

Hospital:_____
Room:_____
Date of Recording:_____
Started:_____am/pm
Connected by:_____
_____

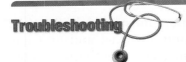

Troubleshooting

Patient Instructions

When reviewing the instructions for the diary with your patient, he asks you if he is allowed to do certain things during the monitoring, such as sleep on his stomach or dance at an upcoming dinner party. You should inform him that he is encouraged to participate in his normal daily activities during the monitoring, whatever they may be. Since there is a chance that some activities may cause the electrodes to become loose or disconnected, you should check to be sure he knows the procedure for correcting this situation. You should also explain that if the electrodes become loose or disconnected, it could interfere with the accuracy of the results.

Your patient wants to know if he can continue his daily bike ride while being monitored. What should you say?

_____

_____

patient is currently taking. It is your responsibility to remind the patient of medication changes prescribed by the physician.

It is best that the patient wear loose-fitting clothing during the monitoring procedure for comfort and convenience and to reduce artifact. A front-buttoning shirt is preferred because you can conveniently access the patient's chest and apply the electrodes. The patient must not tamper with the monitor or disconnect the lead wires or electrodes. While the monitor is in place, he or she may take only a sponge bath; no shower or tub bath is allowed during the monitoring because the equipment must not get wet. Patients may sleep in any position that does not apply tension on the lead

TABLE 12-1 Ambulatory Monitoring Checklist

A checklist such as this provides documentation for the medical record of patient instructions for the ambulatory monitoring procedure.

Ambulatory Monitoring—Checklist for Patient Education		
Patient Name		
Patient was able to	**YES**	**NO**
• Describe ambulatory monitoring.		
• Explain why he or she is having the test performed.		
• Know the length of time the monitor will be on and when to return the monitor and diary.		
• State where the leads are placed and what they will feel like.		
• Adjust the shoulder strap or waist belt.		
• Wear loose-fitting clothing for comfort and convenience.		
• Operate the event marker.		
• Replace loose electrodes and report loose or removed electrodes.		
• Avoid metal detectors, electric detectors, high-voltage wires, and magnets.		
• State required physical restrictions such as bathing, swimming, and daily activities.		
• Log usual and unusual activities and symptoms experienced.		
• Contact the facility when necessary.		
Signature	**Date**	**Initials**

wires or electrodes. Avoiding magnets, metal detectors, high-voltage areas, and electric blankets is necessary because these devices can interfere with the tracing. The patient should also know how the monitoring equipment works and be instructed to check that it is working properly during the procedure. Documentation of accurate patient education is necessary and must be included on the patient's chart. You may use a paper or electronic checklist similar to the one found in Table 12-1.

Checkpoint Question (LO 12.4)

1. Why should the patient wear loose-fitting clothing during ambulatory monitoring?

_____

_____

12.5 Preparing the Patient

Patients must be prepared for the ambulatory monitoring procedure both emotionally and physically. Many times the patient will be apprehensive. Children may be especially fearful. The first step in reducing the fear is to help them understand the procedure. Take time with the patient to explain each step of the procedure as you perform it. For children, be sure to explain in terms they can understand. Let the patient know it is normal to have some fear and allow the patient to express his or her feelings. Allow the patient to ask questions, and answer as completely as you can. If you do not know the answer, ask a licensed practitioner or your supervisor.

The patient should understand the physical requirements of the monitoring procedure. If the patient is male, he may have to have his chest shaved in order to place the electrodes. For both males and females, there may be some discomfort while the electrodes are in place. You should remind patients that during the procedure they should maintain all regular physical activities.

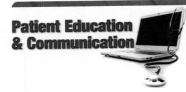

Patient Education & Communication

Pediatric Patients

Pediatric patients require special consideration when explaining the ambulatory monitoring procedure. Consider the child's age, and use terms that he or she will understand. To decrease the child's potential anxieties and fears, allow the patient to touch the equipment prior to applying it. Be sure to instruct the parent as well.

Checkpoint Question (LO 12.5)

1. While answering questions for a patient, she asks something and you do not know the answer. What would you say?

_____

_____

12.6 Applying an Ambulatory Monitor

Before the Procedure

Prepare for the procedure by gathering the necessary equipment (Figure 12-12). You will need the following:

- Monitor with holder and shoulder strap or belt
- New batteries and new tape or disk
- Electrodes (three to five, depending on the type of monitor used)
- Lead wires
- Alcohol and gauze
- Patient diary
- Skin preparation materials (prep pads, benzoin, abrasive cleaner, or skin rasp)
- Shaving equipment

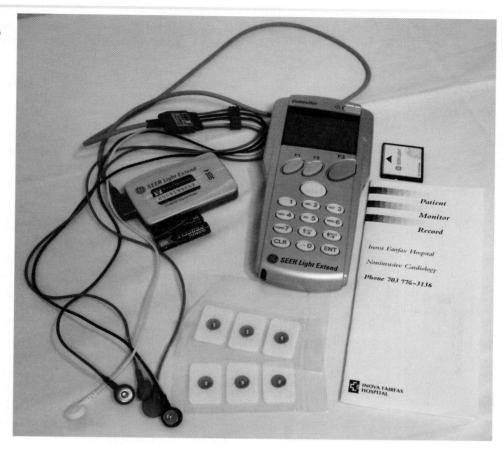

Figure 12-12 Gather all the necessary equipment prior to applying the ambulatory monitor.

- Tape
- Checklist for patient education
- Manufacturer's directions for specific monitor used
- Pen

Before entering the room to begin the procedure, you should prepare the monitor and review the manufacturer's instructions for the type of monitor you are using. Check to see that the monitor is adequately charged. You will need to insert new batteries to ensure that the monitor will not lose charge during the procedure. Insert a new blank tape or disk if required.

Placing the Electrodes

Have the patient remove his or her clothing from the waist up so you can position the electrodes. You should provide a drape, especially for female patients. Have the patient sit or lie down in a comfortable position on the bed or examination table. The patient should be relaxed.

Prepare the sites for electrode placement. Rub the site with an alcohol swab and let it dry. If the sites are hairy, dry shave the skin. Wet shaving is not done because soap film will interfere with electrode adhesion. Use the adhesive side of tape to remove any shaved hair remaining. Abrade the skin using a special prep pad, a dry 4 × 4 gauze, a skin rasp, or another type of abrasive cleaner. Abrading the skin consists of rubbing firmly and briskly at each of the sites where the electrodes will be placed so they will adhere to the skin better. Preparation of the electrode sites may vary depending on the type of ambulatory monitoring performed. For telemetry monitoring, it is recommended that the chest hair be *clipped* and not shaved. This prevents irritation and keeps the patient from scratching, which can cause artifact on the tracing. Check the manufacturer's instructions and the policy of your facility for proper electrode placement.

Place the electrodes on the chest at the proper sites. See Figure 12-13 for one example. Electrode placement depends on the number of lead wires, the type of monitor used, and the lead tracing to be produced. Check the manufacturer's instructions for accurate placement of the electrodes for the monitor you are using. If the leadwires are the "snap-on" type, you should attach the electrodes to the lead wires prior to placing them on the patient to reduce discomfort. Remove the backing from the adhesive, then apply each electrode to its proper position by pressing firmly at the center. Run your finger around the edge of each electrode to ensure firm attachment.

Attach the lead wires to the electrodes. Check the wire color and cable identification to ensure proper attachment to the electrode. Arrange the lead wires and cable comfortably on the patient. Tape each of the electrodes in place to reduce tugging and pulling on the electrodes during movement. Some electrodes include stress loops to reduce artifact (Figure 12-14).

Attach the cable to an electrocardiograph and run a baseline ECG tracing. Make sure the tracing is correct and that the machine is not malfunctioning. Have the patient put on his or her shirt and run the lead wire between the buttons or out the bottom of the shirt. Attach the cable to the monitor, place it in the carrying case, and attach it comfortably to the

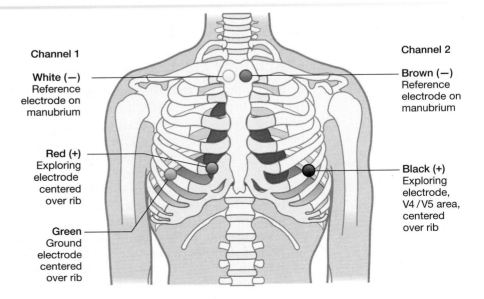

Figure 12-13 This is one example of 5-lead electrode placement for ambulatory monitoring. Lead placement may vary, so check the manufacturer's instructions for the correct placement for the monitor you wil be using.

Channel 1

White (−)
Reference electrode on manubrium

Red (+)
Exploring electrode centered over rib

Green
Ground electrode centered over rib

Channel 2

Brown (−)
Reference electrode on manubrium

Black (+)
Exploring electrode, V4/V5 area, centered over rib

Figure 12-14 Individual stress loops take up slack and prevent tension on the lead wires and electrodes during ambulatory monitoring.

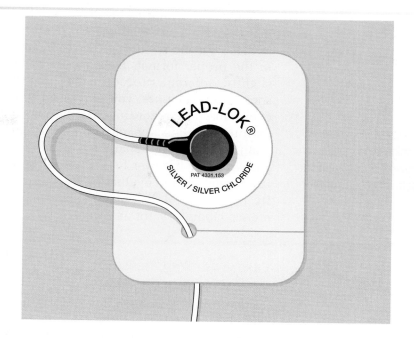

patient's waist or shoulder. Double-check the lead wires and electrodes to ensure that there is no tension on them.

Start the monitor and have the patient place the first entry into the diary. Make sure the beginning time is noted in the diary. Review all instructions with the patient, and set the date and time for him or her to return for removal. Make sure the patient knows how to get assistance in case problems arise.

Checkpoint Question (LO 12.6)

1. What kind of problems could the patient encounter during monitoring?

_____

_____

12.7 Removing an Ambulatory Monitor and Reporting Results

When the patient returns to have the monitor removed, briefly review the completed diary with him or her. Turn off the monitor and detach it from the lead wires, then detach the lead wires and cables from the patient. Remove the tape and electrodes from the patient's chest. Clean the skin where the electrodes had been placed. Record the removal procedure on the patient's chart.

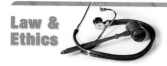

Law & Ethics

Document and Label

Carefully document and label the report, diary, and tape or digital disk with all required information as established by the facility protocol.

Once the monitoring is complete, your next responsibility is to see that the results are evaluated and a report is placed in the medical record. In order for the results of the recording to be evaluated, they must be put in the proper format. Each type and brand of ambulatory monitor has a slightly different procedure for preparing the recording for analysis. In some circumstances, you may need to attach the machine to a scanner or computer. The recording will be viewed on an output device such as a monitor, **oscilloscope,** or printer. The computer may provide an analysis as well. A physician, usually a cardiologist, must view the recording and the patient diary in order for a final interpretation to be completed. Computer interpretation and evaluation by a cardiologist may occur within your facility, or the digital disk may be sent to an outside laboratory, known as a reference laboratory, for analysis.

oscilloscope A monitor or television-type device that shows the tracing of the electrical activity of the heart.

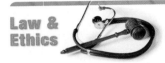

Law & Ethics

Ensure Accurate Results

You are assigned to apply a new type of Holter monitor that has a five-lead system. Since you have never used this type of five-lead system before, you should first check the manufacturer's instructions prior to placing the electrodes. Ambulatory monitors can vary, and correct placement of the electrodes is essential for accurate results. If you cannot locate the directions or still do not understand the correct placement, you should consult your supervisor.

Cassette recorder-type monitors are sometimes used and will need to be prepared for interpretation. This involves preparing the ECG tracing printout and computer analysis, along with the diary, for the physician to interpret. In other facilities, you may only have to remove the cassette and send it to a reference laboratory for interpretation. In either case, make sure the cassette or results are properly labeled with the patient's name, medical record number, date, physician's name, and any other identifying information. In addition, the patient's diary must be kept with the cassette or printed results. Check the manufacturer's information provided with the monitor and your supervisor for specific instructions.

Accurate results must be provided for correct interpretation of the ECG tracing. Many factors can affect these results such as improper lead attachment, incomplete patient diary, and failure of the patient to maintain a normal routine. You can reduce the chances of having to repeat the procedure by ensuring proper lead attachment, patient education, and recording of results. The test may need to be repeated if the results are inconclusive.

When the results are sent to an outside lab, it usually takes 7 to 10 days to get the report. The final report must be placed on the patient's chart for the physician to provide the patient with the results of the test. Abnormal results may indicate any of the following:

- Electrical-conduction defects in the heart's rate and rhythm-controlling system
- Rhythm abnormalities
- Premature atrial or ventricular contractions

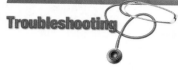

Troubleshooting

No Diary

When your patient returns to have his or her monitor removed, you should first ask for the patient diary. If the patient has forgotten to bring the diary, the results of the recording cannot be evaluated.

What do you think you should do if a patient arrives without the diary?

_____

_____

Advise your patient to discuss the results of the ambulatory monitoring with his or her physician. It is important to note that the ambulatory monitor is only part of the diagnostic process. Results of the Holter monitoring will correlate the patient's symptoms with changes on the ECG tracing. Additional tests may be required, depending on the patient's condition. Some examples of additional tests that may be needed include the following:

- Echocardiogram
- Coronary angiogram
- CT (computerized tomography) scan
- MRI (magnetic resonance imaging) scan
- PET (positron emission tomography) scan

Checkpoint Question (LO 12.7)

1. What factors can affect the results of ambulatory monitoring?

_____

_____

Chapter Summary

Learning Outcomes	Summary	Pages
12.1 Identify the types of ambulatory monitors and their functions.	The most common type of ambulatory monitor is the Holter monitor. Telemetry for inpatients and transtelephonic for outpatients monitoring are also common. Ambulatory monitoring can be either continuous or intermittent. Intermittent only records when the patient is experiencing symptoms and the tracing is shorter. During continuous monitoring the patient uses an event marker or voice activation.	280–282
12.2 Explain why ambulatory monitoring is used in addition to the 12-lead ECG.	Unlike an ECG, which evaluates the heart at one point in time, ambulatory monitoring is used to evaluate the ECG during a long period of time when symptoms or problems could occur.	282–283

(Continued)

Learning Outcomes	Summary	Pages
12.3 Summarize the common uses and variations of ambulatory monitoring.	Ambulatory monitoring is used to evaluate for dysrhythmias and correlate them to symptoms the patient is experiencing, to evaluate the effectiveness of cardiac medications, and to check the functioning of an artificial pacemaker.	283–288
12.4 Educate the patient about ambulatory monitoring.	The patient undergoing ambulatory monitoring must be educated about the procedure, its reasons, how long and when to return, the equipment, including marking the tracing during symptoms and electrode problems, the diary, and when and how to contact the medical facility.	288–291
12.5 Prepare a patient for application of an ambulatory monitor.	A patient must be prepared physically and emotionally before the ambulatory monitoring procedure. Reducing a patient's fear may help improve cooperation during the procedure.	292
12.6 Describe the procedure for applying an ambulatory monitor correctly.	After educating the patient, the equipment must be gathered and prepared, and the electrodes are placed on the patient's chest.	292–295
12.7 Describe the procedure for removing the ambulatory monitor and reporting the results.	Before removing the ambulatory monitor, the diary must be completed by the patient, then turn off the recording, remove the leads, clean the skin, and report the results. The ambulatory monitor recording must be prepared for review and evaluation. This process is based upon the type of equipment used.	295–297

Chapter Review

Ordering

The following is a list of steps for applying the ambulatory monitor. Number the steps in sequential order from 1 to 13. (LO 12.6)

_____ **1.** Prepare the chest for lead placement.

_____ **2.** Identify the patient.

_____ **3.** Remove the patient's clothes from the waist up, and use a drape for female patients.

_____ **4.** Explain the procedure.

_____ **5.** Record the procedure in the patient's chart.

_____ **6.** Attach the lead wires.

_____ **7.** Record the start time in the patient's diary.

_____ **8.** Start the monitor, and make sure that it is functioning correctly.

_____ **9.** Remove the adhesive backing, and apply the electrodes at the correct sites.

_____ **10.** Place the monitor in its holder, and strap it comfortably to the patient.

_____ **11.** Give the patient the diary, and review the instructions.

_____ **12.** Attach the cable to the monitor.

_____ **13.** Secure the lead wires to the electrodes with tape.

Matching

Match the key terms with their definitions. Place the correct letter on the line provided.

_____ **14.** Holter monitor (LO 12.1)

_____ **15.** palpitation (LO 12.2)

_____ **16.** stress ECG (LO 12.1)

_____ **17.** myocardial infarction (LO 12.3)

_____ **18.** syncope (LO 12.2)

_____ **19.** oscilloscope (LO 12.3)

_____ **20.** dysrhythmia (LO 12.3)

_____ **21.** ambulate (LO 12.3)

_____ **22.** anti-arrhythmic (LO 12.2)

a. walk

b. medication given to prevent arrhythmias

c. irregularity or loss of rhythm of the heartbeat

d. ambulatory monitor

e. heart attack

f. monitor or TV-type device used to view the ECG

g. fast, irregular heartbeat sensation felt by the patient

h. exercise electrocardiography

i. fainting

Patient Education

You are assigned to teach Mr. Booth about ambulatory monitoring. From the following list, determine which are correct patient instructions for ambulatory monitoring and which are not. Place a *C* beside the correct statements and an *I* beside the incorrect statements. For each of the incorrect (*I*) statements, write the correct instructions for the patient. (LO 12.4)

_____ 23. You should avoid alcohol and caffeine during ambulatory monitoring.

_____

_____

_____ 24. During ambulatory monitoring, you will need to record your activities and any symptoms in your diary.

_____

_____

_____ 25. Mr. Booth, you may take a tub bath as long as you do not let the monitor drop into the water.

_____

_____

_____ 26. Wear a loose-fitting shirt, preferably one that buttons down the front, and you will be more comfortable during the procedure.

_____

_____

_____ 27. Mr. Booth, you should not take your heart medications during the ambulatory monitoring procedure unless instructed to do so by the physician.

_____

_____

Multiple Choice

Circle the correct answer for each of the following.

28. Mr. Jones will be attached to a transtelephonic monitor. How long will he have the monitor in place? (LO 12.3)
    a. 2 to 4 hours
    b. 24 to 48 hours
    c. Up to 30 days
    d. Only during his hospital stay

29. Ms. Buckwalter is attached to a telemetry monitor. How long will she have the monitor in place? (LO 12.3)
    a. 2 to 4 hours
    b. 24 to 48 hours
    c. Up to 30 days
    d. Only during her hospital stay

30. Mr. Casler is having an ambulatory (Holter) monitor attached and asks you how long it will remain in place. Your answer would be (LO 12.4)
   a. "2 to 4 hours."
   b. "24 to 48 hours."
   c. "Up to 30 days."
   d. "Only during his hospital stay."

31. Your patient Mrs. Jackson asks, "Why am I having this ambulatory monitor attached when I just had an ECG the other day?" What would be your *best* answer? (LO 12.3)
   a. "Ambulatory monitors record your heart activity in a different way than an ECG does."
   b. "Your doctor wants to find out what is happening to your heart during a longer period of time than an ECG."
   c. "It is necessary to monitor your heart while you are walking. That is why it is called ambulatory monitoring."
   d. "I cannot answer that question. You should speak to your doctor."

32. Which of the following is *not* a common use of the ambulatory monitor? (LO 12.3)
   a. To monitor the heart during exercise
   b. To monitor the heart during a typical day
   c. To evaluate pacemaker function
   d. To correlate symptoms and heart activity

Lead Placement

Label the color and lead placement of the electrodes on the lines provided. (LO 12.6)

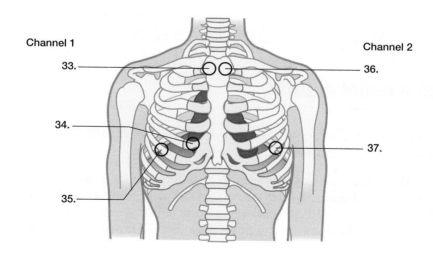

33. _____

34. _____

35. _____

36. _____

37. _____

Critical Thinking Application *What Should You Do?*

Read the following situations and use critical thinking skills to determine how you would handle each. Write your answer in detail in the space provided.

38. While working in an ambulatory care facility, you are preparing an ambulatory monitor for placement. You are about to insert the batteries when the monitor slips out of your hands. You are by yourself, and no one sees or hears you drop the monitor. What should you do? (LO 12.6)

_____

_____

39. When a patient returns to have his or her monitor removed, you check the patient's diary. You notice that many places have been left blank, and the diary does not appear complete. What should you do? (LO 12.7)

_____

_____

40. Mr. Hernandez, a 67-year-old man with a pacemaker, has just had his monitor applied. You ask Mr. Hernandez to enter the first entry into his diary before he leaves. He appears hesitant. You try to encourage him, and he flatly refuses. What should you do? (LO 12.4)

_____

_____

41. You are applying an ambulatory monitor to Ms. Lin. She states that she will be going into court tomorrow before she returns to have the monitor removed. Should this be a concern to you or Ms. Lin? How would you respond to her statement? Is there a reason why Ms. Lin should or should not go to court, and if so, what is it? (LO 12.7)

_____

_____

Get Connected *Internet Activity*

Visit the McGraw-Hill Higher Education *Electrocardiography for HealthCare Personnel* Web site at **www.mhhe.com/boothecg3e** to complete the following activity.

1. Visit the Web MD Internet site and/or perform a search to review patient information about the ambulatory monitoring. Consider how you might simplify the explanation of the ambulatory monitoring procedure to a child. What comparisons could you make? Write a paragraph explaining how you would describe the procedure to a 6-year-old, a 10-year-old, or 2-year-old.

Using the Student CD

Now that you have completed the material in the chapter text, return to the student CD and complete any chapter activities you have not yet done. Practice your terminology with the "Key Term Concentration" game. Review the chapter material with the "Spin the Wheel" and "ECG Challenge" game. Take the final chapter test, and complete the troubleshooting questions and E-mail or print your results to document your proficiency for this chapter.

PROCEDURES CHECKLIST 12-1

Applying and Removing an Ambulatory (Holter) Monitor

Procedure Steps (Rationale)	Practice Yes	No	Practice Yes	No	Test Yes	No
Preprocedure						
1. Gather supplies and equipment.						
• Prep razor						
• Alcohol						
• Electrodes						
• Gauze pads						
• Skin rasp						
• Tape						
• Holter unit with strap and case						
• Fresh batteries						
• New tape or digital disk						
• Pen and patient diary						
2. Review patient instructions per facility policy. (To ensure accuracy and prevent problems during the testing procedure.)						
• Documentation (diary), activities of daily living (ADLs), when symptoms occur						
• Medications						
• Physical restrictions such as new activities (should maintain normal routine), bathing, showers, swimming while wearing the device						
• How to operate the "event" marker						
• How to reapply electrode if one comes loose or falls off						
• Must return with the Holter and diary to complete the test						
• Must wear loose-fitting garments on the upper body to reduce artifact						
• Provide facility phone number, copy of instructions, and "point of contact" if the patient has questions, problems, or concerns.						
• Provide picture of electrode locations, extra electrodes, and adhesive tape per clinic policy.						

(Continued)

Procedure Steps (Rationale)	Practice Yes	No	Practice Yes	No	Test Yes	No
Procedure						
1. Electrode application						
• Using alcohol pads, gently rub and cleanse the patient's skin to obtain a good skin-to-electrode contact. (Reduces artifact.)						
• Dry each site completely by rubbing the skin with a gauze pad until it is dry.						
• Shave and/or clip any hair in the areas where the electrodes will be attached.						
• Wrap tape with adhesive side facing outward from hand, and pat gently to remove any loose hairs remaining on the patient's skin.						
• Remove the electrodes from their package and snap onto the patient leads. (Prevents pressure on the patient's chest caused by applying leads to electrodes after they are placed on the chest.)						
• Peel the protective backing off the electrodes one at a time as they are placed on the patient.						
2. Lead placement						
• Place electrodes in the appropriate position. (Follow the physician's preference or manufacturer's instructions.)						
• Try to center the electrodes over the ribs by gently setting the gelled center against the skin. (A wrinkled electrode or dispersed gel would cause an inaccurate tracing.)						
• If the electrode wrinkles or gel is dispersed, apply a new electrode.						
• Form a stress loop for each electrode and tape the cable, loop, and electrode to the skin.						
• Leave enough slack between the electrode and the stress loop to allow the patient to move without pulling or stressing the electrodes. Prevents inaccurate tracing						
• Verify that all leads are firmly inserted into the monitor.						
3. Prepare equipment						
• Insert the digital flashcard or tape into the recorder.						
• Insert appropriate number and size of new batteries into the recorder.						

Procedure Steps (Rationale)	Practice Yes	No	Practice Yes	No	Test Yes	No
Procedure *(continued)*						
• Once the batteries have been inserted, DO NOT remove the flashcard; doing so will render the flashcard unusable until it has been reinitialized by a scan technician.						
• Slide and secure the battery cover onto the recorder.						
• An LED may blink as the recorder performs an initialization sequence and self-diagnostics. This will take approximately 20 seconds.						
4. Starting the recording						
• Wait for the green LED to stop flashing and stay lit. This indicates the recorder is collecting ECG data and functioning properly.						
• Note start time on enrollment form and patient's diary.						
• Place recorder in pouch and review instructions with the patient.						
• Have patient sign the Patient Responsibility Statement on the enrollment form.						
• Complete paperwork.						
Postprocedure						
1. Ending the recording						
• Collect the patient diary—check to ensure entries were made.						
• Check with the patient to make sure no problems occurred during the recording procedure.						
• Report problems to the licensed practitioner per facility policy.						
• Turn off and disconnect the device per manufacturer's instructions.						
• Disconnect the cable from the Holter unit.						
• Remove the recorder from the pouch.						
• Carefully remove electrodes from patient. (Prevents irritation and tearing of the skin, especially for patient with paper-thin skin.)						

(Continued)

Procedure Steps (Rationale)	Practice Yes	No	Practice Yes	No	Test Yes	No
• Clean any residual electrode gel from the patient's skin, and assist the patient as necessary.						
• Remove and discard the batteries.						
• Remove the flashcard/tape from the recorder.						
• Remove excess tapes, and clean cables with a nonalcohol adhesive remover.						
• Turn in recording and diary for analysis per facility policy.						
• Document completed procedure according to your facility policy.						
• Explain to the patient that results may take 7 to 10 days and when he or she will be notified of the results.						

Comments: _____
_____
_____
_____
_____

Signed

Evaluator: _____

Student: _____

13

Clinical Management of the Cardiac Patient

Chapter Outline

- Coronary Arteries (p. 309)
- Cardiac Symptoms (p. 311)
- Atypical Patient Presentation (p. 313)
- Acute Coronary Syndrome (p. 315)
- Heart Failure (p. 316)
- Cardiac Patient Assessment and Immediate Treatment (p. 320)
- Further Treatment For The Cardiac Patient (p. 326)

Learning Outcomes

13.1 Identify the major coronary arteries, and describe the structure of arteries.

13.2 Describe typical cardiac symptoms and unstable angina.

13.3 Summarize atypical patient types and presentation.

13.4 Compare ST segment elevation and non-ST segment elevation.

13.5 Explain heart failure.

13.6 Identify assessment and immediate treatment needed for the cardiac patient.

13.7 Discuss continued treatment for the cardiac patient.

Key Terms

acute coronary syndrome (ACS)
angina
angioplasty
anorexia
ascites
atherosclerotic plaque
bolus
cardiac enzymes (cardiac markers or cardiac biomarkers)
cardiogenic shock
circumflex artery
collateral blood vessels
coronary angiography
coronary artery bypass graft (CABG) surgery

echocardiography
electrocardiogram (ECG)
enhanced external counter pulsation (EECP)
fibrinolytic agent
hypercoagulopathy
IV fluid challenge
left anterior descending artery
neuropathy
non-ST segment elevation MI (NSTEMI)
pallor
percutaneous coronary intervention (PCI)

percutaneous transluminal
   coronary angioplasty (PTCI)
posterior descending artery
pulmonary edema
rales (crackles)
stent

ST segment elevation MI (STEMI)
thrombolytic agent
unstable angina (pre-infarction
   angina)
volume expander
widow maker

13.1 Coronary Arteries

posterior descending artery One of the primary branches of the right main coronary artery providing blood to the posterior wall of the heart.

circumflex artery One of the primary branches of the left main coronary artery, which winds around, supplying blood to the lateral wall of the left ventricle.

Just as arteries carry oxygenated blood throughout the body, the heart is no different. It needs its own nutrition and oxygen supply in order to live and function the way that it should. Recall from Chapter 2, this is accomplished by arteries that supply blood to the heart (Figure 13-1). The first two branches of the aorta are the left and right coronary arteries. The right coronary artery passes along the atrioventricular sulcus (groove) between the right atrium and the right ventricle. It has two major branches. One is the **posterior descending artery** (posterior interventricular artery), which supplies blood to the walls of both ventricles. The other is the marginal artery, whose branches supply the walls of the right atrium and the right ventricle. One branch of the left coronary artery is the **circumflex artery.** This artery follows the atrioventricular sulcus between the left atrium and left ventricle. Its branches supply blood to the left atrium and left ventricle. Another branch of the left coronary artery is the

Figure 13-1 Blood vessels on the surface of the heart. *A.* Anterior view. *B.* Posterior view (next page).

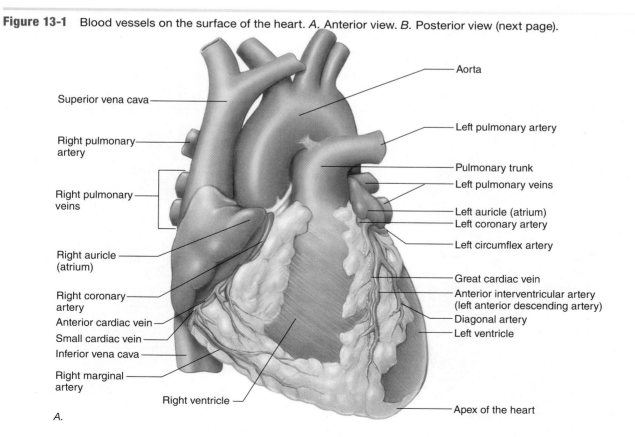

Superior vena cava

Right pulmonary artery

Right pulmonary veins

Right auricle (atrium)

Right coronary artery

Anterior cardiac vein

Small cardiac vein

Inferior vena cava

Right marginal artery

Right ventricle

A.

Aorta

Left pulmonary artery

Pulmonary trunk

Left pulmonary veins

Left auricle (atrium)

Left coronary artery

Left circumflex artery

Great cardiac vein

Anterior interventricular artery (left anterior descending artery)

Diagonal artery

Left ventricle

Apex of the heart

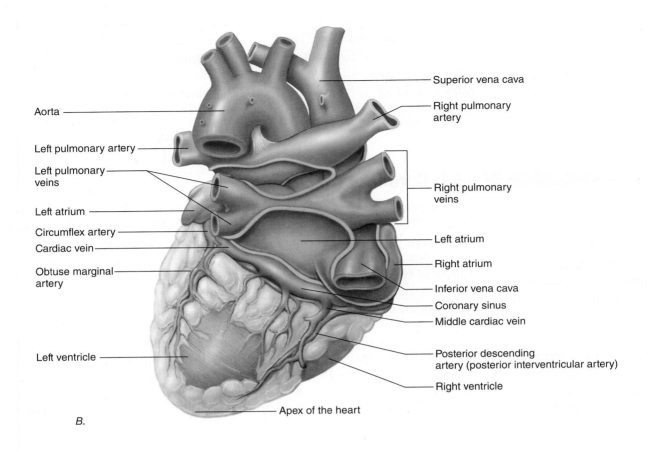

Aorta	Superior vena cava
	Right pulmonary artery
Left pulmonary artery	
Left pulmonary veins	
	Right pulmonary veins
Left atrium	
Circumflex artery	Left atrium
Cardiac vein	Right atrium
Obtuse marginal artery	Inferior vena cava
	Coronary sinus
	Middle cardiac vein
Left ventricle	Posterior descending artery (posterior interventricular artery)
	Right ventricle
B.	Apex of the heart

Figure 13-2 Blood vessels have three layers. *A.* The wall of an artery. *B.* The wall of a vein.

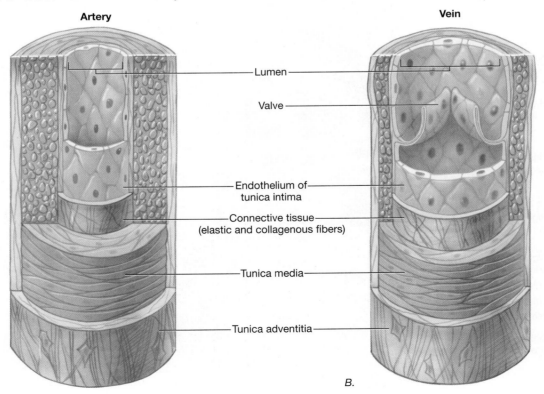

Artery   **Vein**

Lumen

Valve

Endothelium of tunica intima

Connective tissue (elastic and collagenous fibers)

Tunica media

Tunica adventitia

A.   *B.*

left anterior descending artery One of the primary branches of the left main coronary artery supplying blood to the anterior wall of the left ventricle.

left anterior descending artery (anterior interventricular artery), which supplies blood to both of the ventricles.

The coronary arteries, just like all arteries and veins, have three layers (Figure 13-2). The outermost layer of the artery is the tunica adventitia. This layer is comprised of tough fibrous connective tissue whose function is to keep the vessel open. The middle layer, the tunica media, is comprised of smooth muscle. Its job is to dilate and constrict in an effort to maintain normal blood pressure, thus maintaining homeostasis. When certain medications, such as nitroglycerine, are administered to the chest pain patient, they directly affect this layer of the artery. These medications are discussed later in this chapter.

The third and innermost layer is the tunica intima. This is the layer of the artery that comes in direct contact with the blood. It is a single-cell layer of endothelial cells that is normally very smooth, and this delicate layer is prone to disruption when atherosclerotic plaque is ruptured and peels away. When this happens chemicals are released into the blood stream, where they cause the platelets to stick together, and to the site of injury, forming a clot. The progressive growth of this clot reduces blood flow at the site of injury and causes ischemia distally to this site within the heart.

Checkpoint Question (LO 13.1)

1. Name the three layers of an artery.

_____

_____

13.2 Cardiac Symptoms

If normal blood flow through the coronary arteries is interrupted or diminished, a patient may experience symptoms of a heart attack. According to the National Institutes of Health's National Library of Medicine (MedlinePlus) estimates are that the average person waits three hours before seeking help for symptoms of a heart attack. The National Health and Nutrition Examination of 2006 indicates that there are over 10,200,000 people in the United States who suffer from angina. Based upon this, it is safe to say that, no matter where you work, patients will show up daily with chest pain and a variety of cardiac-related complaints.

Not all chest pain is cardiac in origin. Patients may experience chest pain due to inflammation of the costal cartilage or lungs, gastric or esophageal irritation, gallbladder, or dental pain, to name a few. The difficulty lies in knowing whether the patient's symptoms are related to a myocardial infarction (MI) or not. However, it is best *not* to discredit the patient with jaw pain as being a "dental problem" because, the one time that you do, your patient actually could be experiencing a heart attack.

angina An oppressive pain or pressure in the chest when the heart muscle does not receive enough oxygen due to partial or complete blockage of a coronary artery.

Chest pain or chest discomfort may present suddenly or gradually. It may stay in one location or may radiate or travel to other locations. It may be described as pressure or pain within the chest. The patient experiences chest pain or pressure when the heart muscle does not receive enough oxygen due to partial or complete blockage of a coronary artery. This discomfort or pain is referred to as **angina.**

To protect the patient, *consider all chest discomfort or pain as being cardiac in origin until proven otherwise.* It is better to consider discomfort or pain as a cardiac problem and be incorrect than to ignore chest pain or discomfort as a cardiac problem and have it turn out to be an untreated myocardial infarction or other serious cardiac condition. When chest pain is involved, always consider and treat the worse case scenario first.

Anginal symptoms are the heart's way of complaining that it is not receiving enough oxygen. The blockage of coronary arteries can cause ischemia, injury, and even death in the affected areas of the heart muscle. In addition to chest pain or pressure, patients may present with other complaints. The following is a list of complains that may occur due to blockage of the coronary arteries.

- Shortness of breath
- Sweating
- Chest pain
- Epigastric discomfort (bad indigestion)
- Neck pain
- Cough
- Back pain (between shoulder blades)
- Squeezing sensation
- Dizziness
- Pressure in the chest
- Nausea
- Fullness in the chest
- Tight band around the chest
- Palpitations
- Anxiety
- Sense of impending doom
- Jaw pain
- Arm pain (one or both arms)

It is not likely a patient would present with all the symptoms together, but any of these symptoms could indicate a possible cardiac problem. Frequently the patient describes the pain as "it feels like an elephant is sitting on my chest."

Unstable Angina

**unstable angina
(pre-infarction angina)**
A warning sign that the disease that has been causing angina has worsened. Signs and symptoms associated are less predictable, last longer, and are more painful than previously experienced.

Patients with a known cardiac condition or disease may experience angina. However, **unstable angina** is a signal to this patient that the angina that they have experienced in the past has changed or worsened. It is a warning sign that the cardiac disease has advanced and would likely indicate acute coronary syndrome (discussed later in this chapter). Unstable angina

TABLE 13-1   Signs of Unstable Angina—Chest Pain

Chest Pain	Example(s)
Change in severity and frequency	Pain is more frequent or severe; pain increases to three or more times a day.
Change in cause	Occurs with less and less exertion; occurs at rest or awakens the patient from sleep.
Change in duration	The symptoms last longer; often greater than 20 minutes.
Change in responsiveness to treatment	Pain is less responsive to nitroglycerin. The patient needs to take more nitroglycerin than previously for the same or less reduction of pain.

is a state between angina and myocardial infarction. Patients with unstable angina will experience symptoms at rest or with minimal exertion. Symptoms will become less predictable and will remain longer. Signs of unstable angina that may be confused with myocardial infarction are described in Table 13-1.

Checkpoint Question (LO 13.2)

1. Briefly describe why all chest pain is initially treated as cardiac in origin.

   _____

   _____

13.3 Atypical Patient Presentation

Every patient does not experience the same symptoms. It is important to know three groups of patients whose complaints and problems are often atypical (different). These include women, patients with diabetes, and the elderly.

Women

Chest pain is identified by doctors as the most important heart attack symptom in both women and men. However, women often present with different complaints. According to the Centers for Disease Control and Prevention, over 40% of women having a heart attack never experienced chest pain. This makes it very important to us as healthcare providers to be aware of other more subtle complaints that this large patient population may have. Cardiac symptoms are less predictable in women than men.

TABLE 13-2 Common Cardiac Symptoms in Women

Common Symptoms	Percentage of Occurrence*
Shortness of breath	58%
Weakness	55%
Unusual fatigue	43%
Cold sweat	39%
Dizziness	39%
Indigestion	39%

Percent of women who experience this symptom as a symptom of a cardiac event.

Women are more likely than men to experience some of the other common symptoms, particularly shortness of breath, nausea and/or vomiting, and back or jaw pain. Table 13-2 lists common cardiac symptoms and their occurrence in women.

Diabetes

atherosclerotic plaque Fatty deposits accumulated by elevated glucose levels.

Chronic diabetes or poorly managed diabetes with high blood glucose levels damages nerves and blood vessels. The elevated glucose level leads to an accumulation of fatty deposits called **atherosclerotic plaque.** The blood vessels can accommodate the presence of up to as much as 40% of this plaque. The vessels will expand and reshape or remodel themselves in an effort to maintain normal blood flow. Eventually, however, the vessel can no longer expand. The problem at this point is that the plaque continues to accumulate, further reducing blood flow to the heart muscle. The effect of the disease often leads to complications such as heart disease and stroke. Because of the damage to the blood vessels, a patient with diabetes is twice as likely to experience a heart attack or stroke. Heart attacks in people with diabetes are more serious and more likely to result in death.

Patient with diabetes have similar cardiac symptoms; however, the symptoms experienced by a patient with diabetes may be transient. The most common symptoms include:

- Chest pain or discomfort
- Pain or discomfort in arms, back, jaw, neck, or stomach
- Shortness of breath
- Sweating
- Nausea
- Light-headedness

neuropathy Common cause is chronic diabetes mellitus. May cause vascular and autonomic nervous system problems, with loss of ability to maintain blood pressure and loss or impaired sensation.

The problem for patients with diabetes is that their symptoms may be mild or absent due to a condition in which the heart rate stays at the same level during exercise, inactivity, stress, or sleep. Additionally, **neuropathy** (nerve damage) caused by diabetes may result in lack of pain during a heart attack.

Women have the additional benefit of protective hormones produced during their child-bearing years that help reduce the risk of cardiac problems. However, women with diabetes have an increased risk of heart disease because diabetes cancels out the benefits of these protective hormones.

Elderly

Various studies indicate that approximately 50% of elderly patients with an acute coronary syndrome reported atypical symptoms, including shortness of breath, nausea, profuse sweating, pain in the arms, and fainting. These symptoms are more likely to occur in patients with personal or family history of heart disease. Although classic symptoms of heart disease may be experienced by any patient regardless of age, gender, or medical history, elderly patients are likely to experience milder symptoms. As a result, they are more likely to delay medical treatment. The most common symptoms in elderly patients include:

- Shortness of breath
- Nausea
- Profuse sweating
- Pain in the arms
- Syncope
- Weakness or fatigue

Checkpoint Questions (LO 13.3)

1. Which of the following patient groups present atypically? Select a. or b.

   a. Children, African Americans, and men
   b. Patients with diabetes, women, and elderly

2. Why are these groups considered atypical?

   _____

   _____

   _____

13.4 Acute Coronary Syndrome

acute coronary syndrome (ACS) This is a broad term that refers to unstable angina, ST segment elevation MI (STEMI), and non-ST segment elevation MI (NSTEMI). ACS is usually associated with intracoronary plaque changes or thrombosis, where blood flow is suddenly stopped.

Once the 12-lead ECG is obtained or the cardiac monitor is attached to the patient with complaints, evidence may exist indicative of **acute coronary syndrome (ACS)**. According to the American Heart Association, ACS covers the spectrum of clinical conditions, ranging from unstable angina (discussed earlier in this chapter), to **ST segment elevation MI (STEMI)** or **non-ST segment elevation MI (NSTEMI)**. Compared to unstable angina, the discomfort associated with ACS will last more than just a few minutes.

ST Segment Elevation MI (STEMI)

According to the American College of Cardiology and the American Heart Association (ACC/AHA), between 75% and 80% of patients with MI will

ST segment elevation MI (STEMI) Classic MI with expected ST segment deviation and development of pathologic Q wave. Occurs 75%–80% of the time. Caused by complete occlusion of a coronary artery.

non-ST segment elevation MI (NSTEMI) A type of heart attack in which the classic signs and symptoms are not present. Caused by incomplete (partial) occlusion of a coronary artery. The patient often has vague complaints (e.g., fatigue), and inspection of the 12-lead ECG does not reflect the classic ST segment deviation or presence of pathologic Q wave. This type of patient requires further testing and assessment.

present with STEMI. STEMI refers to the classic MI, which occurs as a result of a complete occlusion of a coronary artery. Ischemia delays repolarization, and this has a direct effect on the ST segment. The changes to the ECG tracing include:

- ST segment depression or elevation
- T wave inversion
- Development of a pathologic Q wave

These changes are predictive of a patient experiencing an MI in the classic sense. However, not every patient has the classic presentation (Figure 13-3).

Non-ST Segment Elevation (NSTEMI)

The ACC/AHA also suggest that between 20% and 25% of MI patients will display non-ST segment elevation (NSTEMI). This clinical situation presents a challenge to the healthcare team because the "classic" signs and symptoms are not present. The healthcare team must be aware that patients without the classic signs and symptoms may present in the emergency department or clinic. NSTEMI often occurs because of an incomplete occlusion of a coronary artery. The patient is often asymptomatic but will frequently have vague symptoms of this "silent" MI. When the 12-lead ECG is examined, it will not display the classic MI morphologic changes. The doctor will order special blood tests to look for the presence of enzymes in the blood as a result of tissue death (infarction).

You might be thinking that the patient is not at risk for sudden death because of the "incomplete" occlusion, but you would be wrong. Sudden death is just as real and actually happens more often than with classic STEMI patients. The complaints of NSTEMI are not as clearly cardiac or the dramatic "Hollywood" MI complaints. Thus many of these patients die at home or on the job.

Checkpoint Question (LO 13.4)

1. List two changes in the cardiac complex that may indicate ischemia.

   a. _____

   b. _____

13.5 Heart Failure

Heart failure is when the heart muscle has sustained enough injury that it is unable to perform as an effective pump. This occurs when a lack of blood supply causes the tissue of the heart to die, making it unable to contract. Heart failure differs depending upon which side of the heart is affected. Recall from Chapter 2, that the left side of the heart receives the blood from the lungs and pumps the blood to the body. The right side of the heart receives the blood from the body and pumps the blood to the lungs. Since each side functions differently, failure is different based upon location of the heart muscle damage (Figure 13-4).

Figure 13-3 Anterolateral AMI. The isoelectric line has been identified with dark red lines. Note the ST segment elevation in V2 to V6 (V3 and V4 Anterior and V5 and V6 Lateral). Note: ST elevation in V2 provides evidence of a growing (extension) MI.

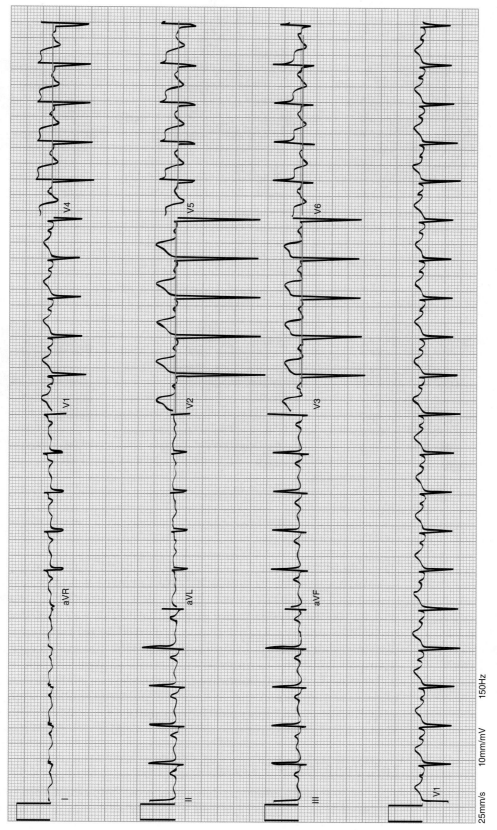

Figure 13-4   Effects of heart damage on function.

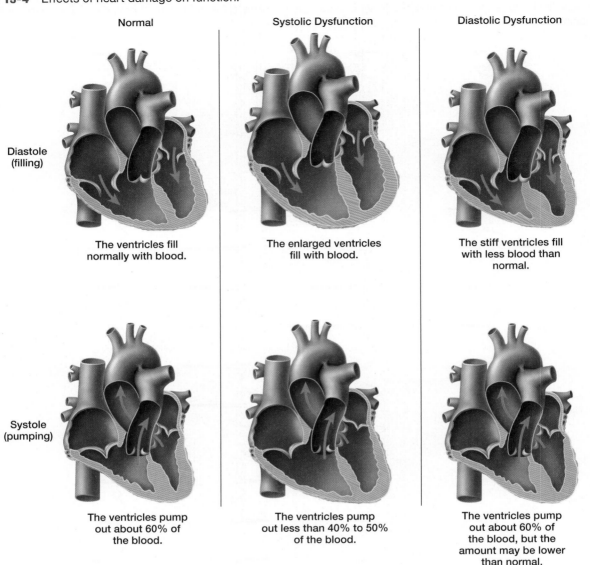

	Normal	Systolic Dysfunction	Diastolic Dysfunction

Diastole (filling)

The ventricles fill normally with blood.

The enlarged ventricles fill with blood.

The stiff ventricles fill with less blood than normal.

Systole (pumping)

The ventricles pump out about 60% of the blood.

The ventricles pump out less than 40% to 50% of the blood.

The ventricles pump out about 60% of the blood, but the amount may be lower than normal.

cardiogenic shock Inadequate flow of arterial blood, typically as a result of left heart failure.

The most common cause of pump failure is myocardial infarction. It is always important to remember that the heart is a pump. When the heart is damaged and doesn't work the way that it should, the tissues of the body will not be perfused (receive enough blood the way that they should) and sometimes not at all. This is often referred to as **cardiogenic shock.** Cardiogenic shock results in different effects on the systems of the body. For example, when the kidneys are not perfused well enough, urinary output is decreased. The elimination of waste from the body is very important to heart function. When the liver is not perfused well enough, special proteins important to blood clotting are reduced, increasing the patient's risk of bleeding in the event the patient is injured.

Left Ventricular Failure

The left ventricle plays perhaps the most important role of the heart in its job of providing oxygenated blood for systemic circulation. When the

pulmonary edema Abnormal collection of fluid within the pleural space (lungs) due to congestive heart failure (left venricle).

rales (crackles) caused by retained airway secretions. When caused by pulmonary edema, the sound may be described as inspiratory very short, soft, high-pitched lung sounds.

anorexia Decreased or loss of appetite.

pallor Pale skin.

left pump (ventricle) fails, blood will stall and back up in the lungs, often causing **pulmonary edema**. Respiratory assessment will often reveal noisy, "wet"-sounding lungs, referred to as **rales (crackles)**. Additional signs and symptoms of left heart failure include:

- Shortness of breath or trouble breathing
- Fatigue (tiredness)
- Tachycardia
- Confusion
- Shortness of breath
- **Anorexia** (lack of appetite)
- Decreased or absent urine production
- **Pallor** (pale skin)

Left heart failure always leads to right heart failure.

Right Ventricular Failure

Right ventricular failure has a different effect on the body. When the right ventricle fails, less blood is being pumped into the lungs. This in turn reduces the amount of blood reaching the left ventricle. The left heart can only pump out what it receives, and this reduction in cardiac output then affects blood pressure. Hypotension is one of the leading signs in right ventricular failure. Blood is not backing up in the lungs, so respiratory assessment will demonstrate clear "normal" breath sounds; however, it *is* still backing up on the venous side. This will frequently cause the patient's jugular veins to distend or "bulge." These three clinical signs are often referred to as the clinical triad (Figure 13-5). They don't always present together, but all three together represent an ominous sign. Signs and symptoms of right heart failure include:

- Hypotension
- Jugular vein distention

Figure 13-5 Clinical triad. These three symptoms are indicative of right-side heart failure and are considered ominous when presented together.

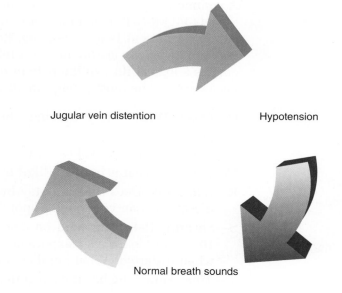

Jugular vein distention

Hypotension

Normal breath sounds

ascites Abnormal collection of serous fluid within the abdomen (peritoneal cavity). This may occur secondary to congestive heart failure.

- Clear lung sounds
- Swelling in the ankles, feet, legs, abdomen (pitting edema)
- **Ascites** (fluid collecting in the abdominal cavity)

Checkpoint Questions (LO 13.5)

1. True or False: Left ventricular failure leads to right ventricular failure.
2. Explain your answer.

_____

_____

13.6 Cardiac Patient Assessment and Immediate Treatment

Cardiac patients may present with a number of different physical complaints and duration of symptoms. It is important to approach all cardiac patients the same way. Two types of mnemonics (memory devices) can be used when assessing the patient: O-P-Q-R-S-T and S-A-M-P-L-E. The O-P-Q-R-S-T mnemonic device is used to evaluate pain, and the S-A-M-P-L-E mnemonic device gathers more information. No matter what method of questioning or evaluation is used, the information must be efficiently gathered, recorded, and/or reported to the physician or treating practitioner.

O-P-Q-R-S-T

A common approach is the use of the mnemonic (memory device) referred to as O-P-Q-R-S-T. This mnemonic will help you evaluate the pain or discomfort a patient is experiencing. Each letter of this memory device corresponds with a specific question related to the patient having pain. This creates a logical flow to the patient questioning and information gathering necessary for the most prompt medical care (Figure 13-6).

O—*Onset:* What were you doing when it started? Did it occur suddenly or gradually?

P—*Provoke:* What provokes (causes) the pain or makes it better or worse?

Q—*Quality:* What is the pain like? Is it sharp, dull, aching, etc.?

R—*Radiation:* Does the pain stay in one location or travel in a particular direction? Can you touch a spot that hurts the most?

S—*Severity:* Rate your pain on a scale of 0 to 10, with 0 = no pain and 10 = most pain ever experienced (Figure 13-7). What number was it when it started? What number is it now?

T—*Time:* How long has it been going on?

Figure 13-6 Patient pain assessment using a mnemonic (memory device): O-P-Q-R-S-T.

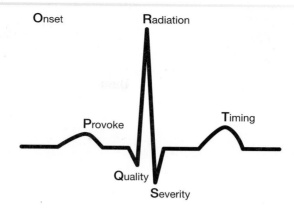

Figure 13-7 When evaluating the severity of pain that a patient is experiencing, a pain scale can be used. This is especially helpful for patients with language, educational, or other understanding barriers.

TCP Health Center

No Pain	Mild Pain	Moderate Pain	Severe Pain	Very Severe Pain	Worst Pain Imaginable
0 1	2 3	4 5	6 7	8 9	10
None	Annoying	Uncomfortable	Dreadful	Horrible	Agonizing

S-A-M-P-L-E

S-A-M-P-L-E is another mnemonic tool used when evaluating patients. O-P-Q-R-S-T is specific to the pain level, while the S-A-M-P-L-E memory tool includes additional information gathering (Figure 13-8).

S—*Signs and Symptoms:* Signs are actually things you can see, feel, or measure, such as pallor (pale skin), cyanosis (blue tint) to skin or other body parts such as lips or nail beds, or vital signs. Symptoms are patient complaints such as pain, tingling, or pressure. Note that the O-P-Q-R-S-T actually gathers information about pain, which is one of the most important symptoms to be evaluated so actually is part of the first step in the S-A-M-P-L-E mnemonic.

A—*Allergies:* Any known allergies are recorded and, for inpatients (patients admitted to a hospital), a wrist band identifying the allergy is placed on an arm. If there are no allergies, be sure to document this so it is known that the question has been asked.

M—*Medications:* All prescription, over-the-counter, and herbal medications should be recorded. Patients are encouraged to keep a list of their medications.

P—*Previous history:* Pertinent information related to the patient's cardiac health or previous cardiac events should be recorded.

L—*Last intake:* This would include food or liquids, when they were eaten, and how much.

E—*Events:* Anything that led up to the problem should be recorded.

Figure 13-8 Patient assessment using a mnemonic (memory device): S-A-M-P-L-E.

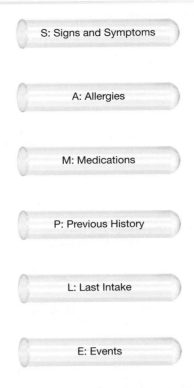

S: Signs and Symptoms

A: Allergies

M: Medications

P: Previous History

L: Last Intake

E: Events

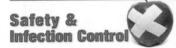

Safety & Infection Control

With a cardiac patient, you should gather and record information as quickly and clearly as possible to report to the physician or treating practitioner. It is not your responsibility to diagnose the patient. Remember that time is muscle—the patient's heart muscle!

Immediate Care

When providing care to chest pain patients, it is necessary that medical care be delivered immediately and effectively. Communication within the team creates success. This is a very busy time, so precise and complete communication is essential. Each member of the healthcare team typically will be assigned to perform very specific tasks.

Using the ACC/AHA guidelines, the following is a list of tasks to be performed within 10 minutes of the patient's arrival:

1. Assess pain level: quality, duration, location, radiation. Use the O-P-Q-R-S-T technique.
2. Check vital signs (see Appendix F), including pulse oximetry (Figure 13-9) which measures the oxygen saturation (SaO_2) of the blood.
   - Pulse and respiration reporting is more than just the number. It is important to report regularity and strength of the pulse, as well as regularity and respiratory effort. It will be important to report your observations to the doctor.

echocardiography Non-invasive diagnostic test that uses sound to study the heart and blood vessels; also known as an ultrasound.

Echocardiography. Sound waves are bounced off of structures within the patient. The sound waves create an image of the walls and chambers of the heart and the structures within it (Figure 13-11). This is an important tool in the assessment and diagnosis of cardiac patients. Many of these devices also have color Doppler, which

Figure 13-10 During a coronary angiography, radiopaque dye is injected into the patient to assist with visualizing the heart structures, and especially the coronary arteries.

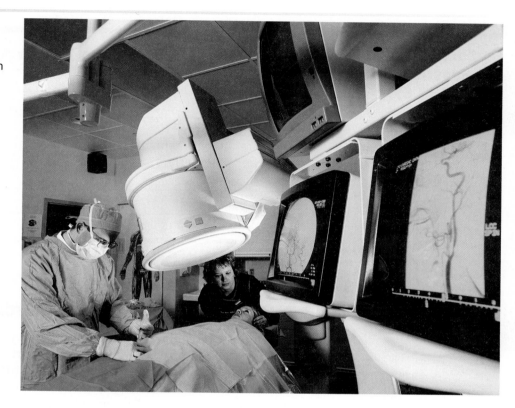

Figure 13-11 Echocardiography of the heart showing hypertrophy of the left ventricle. Echocardiography directs beams of ultrasonic waves through the chest wall, which are echoed by the heart tissues providing motion pictures of the heart.

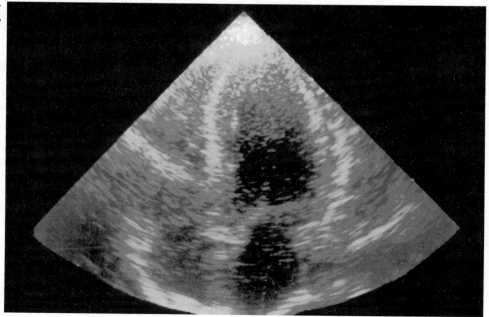

electrocardiogram (ECG)
A tracing of the heart's electrical activity recorded by an electrocardiograph.

is beneficial in observing blood flow and assessing function of the heart valves.

Electrocardiogram (ECG). Serial or repeated ECGs are performed at regular intervals over several hours to observe for subtle changes in the cardiac complexes.

Checkpoint Questions (LO 13.6)

1. List and describe the two common memory devices used in assessment of the cardiac patient.

   a. _____

   b. _____

2. Why are tools like this important in the care and management of the chest pain patient?

   _____

   _____

13-7 Further Treatment for the Cardiac Patient

Life-threatening irregular heartbeats, or dysrythmias, are the leading cause of death in the first few hours of a heart attack. Dysrythmias may be treated with medications or electrical cardioverson (defibrillation). In many instances it is necessary to perform other procedures. The following are common examples of interventional procedures. Not every patient is a good candidate for each procedure. Some are not strong enough, the occluded coronary vessel is not accessible enough, or there is not a facility with the capabilities to perform the intervention nearby.

Thrombolytic or Fibrinolytic Therapy (Clot Busters)

Thrombolytic or fibrinolytic therapy has been an important addition to the world of emergency cardiovascular care. Known as clot busters, these medications are used to prevent or break down clots that cause blocked coronary vessels. In order to understand this type of therapy, you must first understand how clots are formed. The three main components of a blood clot are platelets, thrombin, and fibrin. During thrombus formation, circulating prothrombin is activated to the active clotting factor, thrombin, by activated platelets. Fibrinogen is activated to fibrin by the newly activated thrombin. Fibrin is then formed into the fibrin matrix. This cascade of events all takes place while platelets are being adhered and aggregated.

thrombolytic agent
Medications administered intravenously that posses the ability to lyse or dissolve a clot.

fibrinolytic agent Medications administered to break down the fibrin in a blood clot essentially dissolving it. Ie. One type is recombinant Tissue Plasminogen Activator (rTPA).

Thrombolytic agents work by converting plasminogen to the natural fibrinolytic agent, plasmin. Plasmin lyses clots by breaking down the fibrinogen and fibrin contained in a clot. **Fibrinolytic agents** work by breaking down the fibrin in the clot, causing lysis (destruction) of the clot. The small remaining fragments of this clot are metabolized by the liver and kidneys and eliminated from the body.

These agents are especially beneficial in regions of the country where an interventional cath lab or cardiovascular operating room is not immediately available. The sooner the symptomatic cardiac patient receives this drug, the better the chances of survival. It is often referred to as door-to-drug or door-to-needle time. Thrombolytic or fibrinolytics can be given in the pre-hospital setting to further reduce the time to treatment. The goal is a door-to-drug or door-to-needle time of less than 30 minutes. Every effort must be made to expedite the intervention. The medicine is given through an IV.

Thrombolytic or fibrinolytic therapy is not appropriate in cases of:

- Brain bleeding (intracranial hemorrhage)
- Stroke within the past three months (or possibly longer)
- Head trauma within the past three months
- Bleeding disorders
- Bleeding ulcers
- Pregnancy
- Uncontrolled high blood pressure
- Recent trauma or surgery

Thrombolytics will dissolve formed clots anywhere in the body, so it is important to realize the systemic (entire body) impact. The patient is at risk for hemorrhage from other locations of recent injury or even at the IV puncture site itself.

Angioplasty and Stents

Angioplasty, also called **percutaneous transluminal coronary angioplasty (PTCI)** or **percutaneous coronary intervention (PCI)**, is a procedure very commonly used to open the arteries for some types of myocardial infarctions. It should be performed within 90 minutes (plus or minus 30 minutes) of arriving at the hospital and no later than 12 hours after a heart attack. With improvements within the healthcare system, some hospitals are breaking the 60 minute mark today.

Angioplasty is a procedure performed to open narrowed or blocked blood vessels that supply blood to the heart. A small catheter with a balloon is inserted into a peripheral artery and threaded with the aid of radiopaque dye and flouroscopy. Once the catheter is placed at the proper location, the balloon is inflated, causing the intravascular plaque to be compressed against the vessel walls. This procedure is effective in reestablishing blood flow to the ischemic myocardium. Angioplasty by itself has a chance of closing so, as discussed below, typically a stent is also used. As a matter of fact, according to Heartsite.com, in 30% to 60% of cases, the build-up of material can be large enough to cause the blockage to return to its original (or worse) severity. This occurs over a 6-week to 6-month duration of time and is known as **restenosis**.

A coronary artery **stent** is a small, metal mesh tube that opens up inside a coronary artery (Figure 13-12). The stent appears as a matrix of criss-crossed metal forming a small tube. Stents look similiar to Chinese handcuffs. A stent is often placed after angioplasty to help prevent reocclusion of the coronary artery. Some stents have medication within them (drug-eluting stent) that helps to prevent the artery from closing again.

angioplasty Surgical repair of blood vessels.

percutaneous transluminal coronary angioplasty (PTCI) Similar to PCI, but now it is specific to a coronary vessel. A catheter with a balloon is inserted, placed at the location of the obstructed coronary artery, and inflated. The intent is to outwardly compress the plaque and re-establish blood flow to the region of tissue distal to the occlusion.

percutaneous coronary intervention (PCI) Another name for angioplasty. This minimally invasive procedure is performed with a sheath and catheter to inject dye for flouroscopic examination to determine the specific location of a narrowed or occluded artery. Once this portion of the procedure is performed, a catheter with a balloon is inserted, and the balloon is placed at the location of the obstruction and inflated. The intent is to outwardly compress the plaque and re-establish blood flow to the region of tissue distal to the occlusion.

restenosis When a blood vessel that has been treated with angioplasty returns to a blocked state or becomes reoccluded.

stent A small, metal mesh tube that opens up inside a coronary artery to keep it patent.

Figure 13-12 Coronary angioplasty with stent.

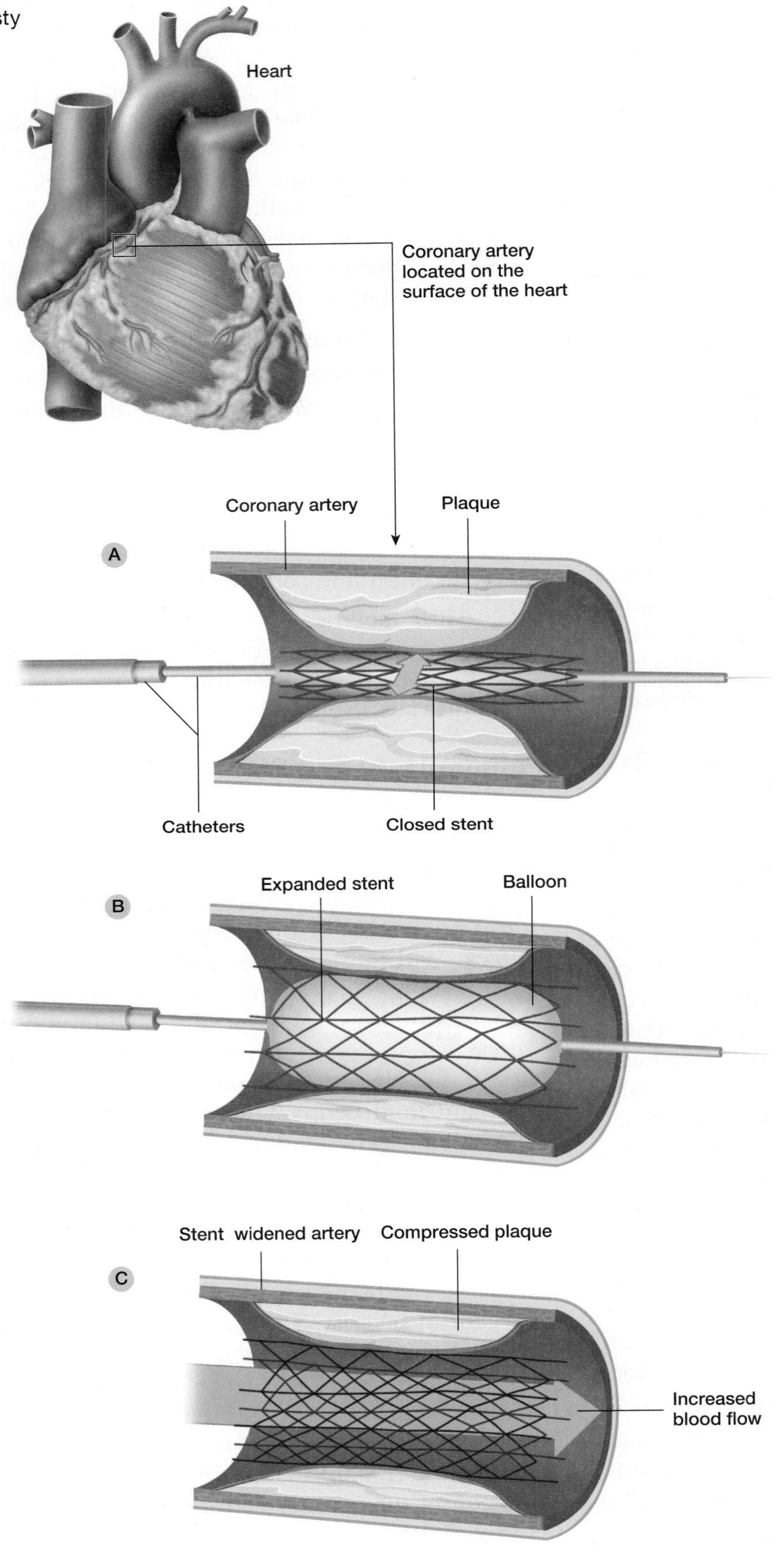

Heart

Coronary artery located on the surface of the heart

A

Coronary artery

Plaque

Catheters

Closed stent

B

Expanded stent

Balloon

C

Stent widened artery Compressed plaque

Increased blood flow

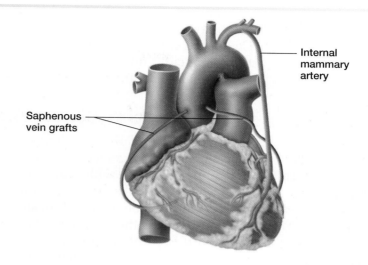

Figure 13-13 Placement of vessels for coronary artery bypass graft (CABG).

Internal mammary artery

Saphenous vein grafts

Coronary Artery Bypass Graft Surgery (CABG)

Coronary angiography is performed for diagnostic purposes. When this test is performed, sometimes it reveals extensive coronary artery disease or disease in the left main coronary artery. Disease of the left main coronary artery is a very dangerous circumstance requiring immediate intervention. Occlusion of the proximal left main coronary artery leads to cardiogenic shock and sudden death and is often referred to as the "**widow maker.**" Occlusion of this vessel will lead to death of the septum and the anterior and lateral wall of the left ventricle, with subsequent left pump failure and death.

Coronary artery bypass graft (CABG) surgery is performed while the patient is under anesthesia and placed on a heart–lung machine. The doctor will either graft the internal mammary artery directly to the heart just past the occlusion to reestablish blood flow, or the doctor will obtain grafts from the greater saphenous vein in the leg. Typically the doctor will connect the vein graft to the ascending aorta and attach it to a point on the heart just distal to an occluded vessel. Whichever vessel is used, the intent is to reestablish blood flow to ischemic regions of the heart due to blood vessel disease (Figure 13-13).

Coumadin Clinic

Coumadin clinics provide an essential service to patients taking the oral anticoagulant Coumadin. Patients are prescribed this drug due to either a heart rhythm disturbance such as atrial fibrillation or a problem with **hypercoagulopathy**. In either case, the drug is used to reduce the clot formation in the blood.

The Coumadin works by decreasing the activity of vitamin K. So while taking Coumadin the patient needs to keep his or her vitamin K blood level consistent. A sudden increase in vitamin K will decrease the effect of Coumadin. Once this therapy is initiated, the patient is placed on a specific diet that restricts foods that will affect the clotting of the blood. Patients must limit the intake of foods that are high or moderately high in vitamin K, such as spinach, kale, broccoli, turnips, romaine lettuce, and collard greens.

widow maker Proximal occlusion of the left main coronary artery leads to potential for anterior, lateral, and septal wall MI. It has been long-associated with cardiogenic shock and death.

coronary artery bypass graft (CABG) surgery Surgical intervention performed by taking a grafted or transplanted blood vessel and attaching it to the heart at a point beyond an occluded coronary artery to reestablish blood flow.

hypercoagulopathy An increased ability of the blood to form clots.

Patients are also required to take their Coumadin at the same time each day and have their bleeding times checked on a regular basis at a Coumadin clinic. This helps ensure the dose of Coumadin remains within the therapeutic range. These patients are carefully monitored to prevent embolic and bleeding events.

Enhanced External Counter Pulsation Therapy (EECP)

enhanced external counter pulsation (EECP) Treatment for chronic angina patients who do not have other options due to health status. This procedure is performed five days a week for several weeks, with the intent of developing collateral blood vessels—essentially creating a "natural" bypass around narrowed or blocked arteries.

External counter pulsation therapy is performed on patients with recurrent angina or, more recently, on heart failure patients who are typically not strong enough to withstand major surgery such as heart catheterization or CABG. **Enhanced external counter pulsation (EECP)** is a safe, noninvasive, well-tolerated, and clinically effective outpatient physical therapy modality. During the treatment, the patient lies on a comfortable treatment table with large blood pressure-like cuffs wrapped around their legs and buttocks (Figure 13-14). They are designed to systematically inflate and deflate in coordination with the contraction and relaxation phases of the

Figure 13-14 Enhanced external counter pulsation (EECP®) therapy.

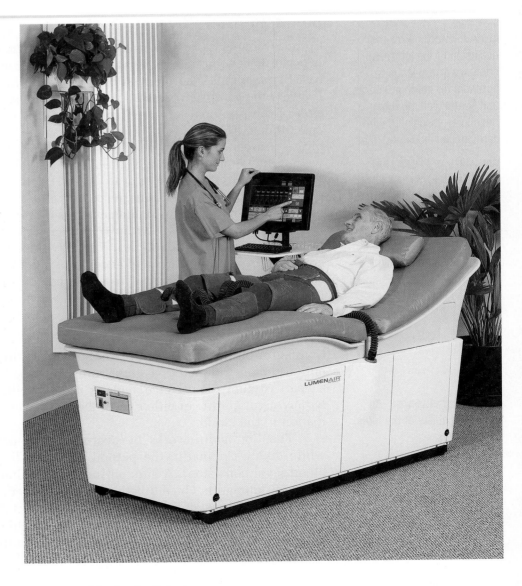

collateral blood vessels
Side-by-side, as in small vessels providing additional blood flow to a region of tissue.

heart. The idea behind it is to increase the intravascular pressure in an effort to promote the growth of new **collateral blood vessels** and in essence create a "natural" bypass to bridge areas of the heart where occlusions or narrowing of blood vessels have occurred. Each EECP treatment generally lasts one hour per day and is performed five days per week for a total of seven weeks.

Checkpoint Question (LO 13.7)

1. What is the difference between coronary artery bypass graft surgery and enhanced external counter pulsation therapy?

_____

_____

Chapter Summary

Learning Outcomes	Summary	Pages
13.1 Identify the major coronary arteries, and describe the structure of arteries.	The coronary arteries are responsible for supplying oxygen and nutrients to the heart muscle. The main coronary artery and specific branch supply blood to the different regions of the heart. Knowing the vessels and anatomic structures in the heart within the affected area is beneficial to risk assessment of the patient experiencing an acute coronary syndrome.	309–311
13.2 Describe typical cardiac symptoms and unstable angina.	Not all chest pain is cardiac in origin; however, all chest discomfort or pain is considered cardiac until proven otherwise. Chest pain may present gradually or quickly, stay in one location or radiate to other locations. Anginal symptoms are the heart's way of telling us it is not receiving enough oxygen. Unstable angina is a signal to a patient that the angina they have has changed or gotten worse. Signs of unstable angina may be confused with an MI.	311–313
13.3 Summarize atypical patient types and presentation.	Not every patient with MI presents with the same complaints. Women, patients with diabetes, and the elderly are three groups who present atypically.	313–315
13.4 Compare ST segment elevation and non-ST segment elevation.	Acute coronary syndrome is a broad term that refers to patients presenting with unstable angina, ST segment elevation MI (STEMI), or non-ST segment elevation MI (NSTEMI). STEMI refers to the classic MI, it occurs 75%–80% of the time. NSTEMI patients don't present with the classic signs and symptoms, it occurs 20%–25% of the time. NSTEMI patients may be asymptomatic so the healthcare team must be alert to this type of patient.	315–316

(Continued)

Learning Outcomes	Summary	Pages
13.5 Explain heart failure.	Heart failure occurs when the heart muscle has sustained enough injury that it is unable to function as an effective pump. The most common cause of heart failure is MI. Left and right ventricular failure have different effects on the body.	316–320
13.6 Identify assessment and immediate treatment for the cardiac patient.	O-P-Q-R-S-T and S-A-M-P-L-E are common mnemonics, or memory tools, used to ensure a consistent approach to information gathering when interviewing cardiac patients. When providing care to the cardiac patient, it is necessary that medical care be delivered immediately and effectively. Communication within the team creates success.	320–326
13.7 Discuss continued treatment for the cardiac patient.	Additional tests are often used to evaluate the heart and its function. Interventional procedures may be performed for patients in certain circumstances and may include fibrinolytic therapy, angioplasty with stenting of vessels, and CABG surgery. There are other types of treatment prescribed for cardiac patients, such as Coumadin therapy and EECP, depending upon the specific diagnosis or patient's health state. When working with a cardiac patient, if there is a chance the patient will be having an invasive procedure, ensure the consent is signed before the patient receives narcotics.	326–331

Chapter Review

True / False

Read each statement and determine if it is true or false. Circle the T or F. For false (F) statements, correct them to "make them true" on the lines provided.

T F **1.** All chest pain is cardiac in origin. (LO 13.2)

_____

T F **2.** Angina is the heart's way of complaining it needs more oxygen. (LO 13.2)

_____

T F **3.** All acute myocardial infarctions present with ST segment elevation. (LO 13.4)

_____

T F **4.** The "A" in S-A-M-P-L-E refers to ascites. (LO 13.6)

_____

T F **5.** Patients must sign a consent for procedures before receiving narcotics. (LO 13.5)

_____

T F **6.** Fibrinolytic agents may be used on any patient. (LO 13.7)

_____

T F **7.** Beta blockers decrease heart rate and blood pressure. (LO 13.6)

_____

T F **8.** The circumflex artery supplies blood to the right atrium and ventricle. (LO 13.1)

_____

Multiple Choice

9. What is the name of the innermost layer of an artery? (LO 13.1)
   a. Tunica adventitia
   b. Tunica media
   c. Tunica os
   d. Tunica intima

10. Which major coronary artery and vessel supplies blood to both ventricles? (LO 13.1)
   a. Circumflex artery
   b. Left anterior descending
   c. Right descending
   d. Right main and marginal artery

11. Which of the following complaints may be cardiac in origin? (LO 13.2)
    a. Dental pain
    b. Nausea
    c. Indigestion
    d. All responses are correct

12. Symptoms of unstable angina include which of the following? (LO 13.2)
    a. Chest pain that lasts greater than 20 minutes
    b. More frequent or severe chest pain
    c. Occurs with less exertion
    d. All responses are correct

13. Which three groups of patients often present with atypical symptoms of MI? (LO 13.3)
    a. Women, infants, and children
    b. Women, elderly, and patients with diabetes
    c. Men, women, and children with diabetes
    d. All responses are correct

14. Due to damage to blood vessels, patients with diabetes are _____ as likely as a nondiabetic individual to experience a stroke or heart attack. (LO 13.3)
    a. 10 times
    b. 5 times
    c. twice
    d. not

15. Which of the following are included when referring to acute coronary syndrome? (LO 13.3)
    a. STEMI, NSTEMI, and unstable angina
    b. STEMI, NSTEMI, and stable angina
    c. STEMI, NSTEMI, and diabetes
    d. STEMI, NSTEMI, and CVA

16. What percentage of patients may present with STEMI? (LO 13.4)
    a. 20%–25%
    b. 40%–45%
    c. 75%–80%
    d. 100%

17. What percentage of patients may present with NSTEMI? (LO 13.4)
    a. 20%–25%
    b. 40%–45%
    c. 75%–80%
    d. 100%

18. Heart failure is simply defined as _____. (LO 13.5)
    a. pulmonary edema
    b. hyperlipidemia
    c. pulmonary failure
    d. pump failure

19. Which type of heart failure causes fluid to back up in the lungs, causing pulmonary edema? (LO 13.5)
    a. Right atrial
    b. Right ventricular
    c. Left atrial
    d. Left ventricular

20. Mnemonic devices are commonly used in medicine to _____. (LO 13.6)
    a. create a complex tool for specialists only
    b. decrease communication and efficiency of patient care
    c. increase the amount of time before the patient receives care
    d. increase efficiency and present a more logical flow to patient care

21. What does the "S" in S-A-M-P-L-E refer to? (LO 13.6)
    a. Signs and symptoms
    b. Signs of distress
    c. Pain scale
    d. All responses are incorrect

22. In emergency cardiovascular care "Time is _____." (LO 13.6)
    a. relative
    b. money
    c. muscle
    d. not important

23. Nitroglycerin causes blood vessels to _____ and blood pressure to _____. (LO 13.6)
    a. constrict, increase
    b. relax, increase
    c. constrict, decrease
    d. relax, decrease

24. Which procedure allows visualization of the coronary arteries and placement of a stent? (LO 13.7)
    a. Coronary artery bypass
    b. Echocardiography
    c. Cardiac catheterization
    d. Enhanced external counter pulsation

25. Coumadin is used to _____. (LO 13.7)
    a. increase heart rate
    b. increase clot formation in blood
    c. decrease heart rate
    d. decrease clot formation in blood

Fill in the Blank

26. List at least five things that must be done when caring for a cardiac patient within the first 10 minutes of their arrival. (LO 13.6)

    _____   _____

    _____   _____

    _____   _____

27. List five blood tests that the doctor might order when caring for a chest pain patient. (LO 13.6)

    _____   _____

    _____   _____

    _____

28. Occlusion of the proximal left main coronary artery is often referred to as the _____ _____. (LO 13.7)

29. Name two vessels that are commonly used in CABG surgery. (LO 13.7)

_____   _____

Critical Thinking Application *What Should You Do?*

30. A 68-year-old male is complaining of substernal chest pressure. The pressure is radiating to his left shoulder. This patient has no history of heart disease, diabetes, hypertension (HTN), or stroke. His father died from a heart attack at the age of 62. This patient is moderately anxious. He is not obese, and his vital signs are within normal limits except for a blood pressure (BP) of 90/48. (LO 13-2, 13-6)

  a. Is this patient at risk?
  b. Why would this patient be anxious?
  c. What are the tasks that must be performed within the first 10 minutes of arrival?
  d. Why are these tasks performed within the first 10 minutes?
  e. What do you think this patient is experiencing?

Get Connected *Internet Activity*

Visit the McGraw-Hill Higher Education Online Learning Center at **www.mhhe.com/boothecg3e** to review additional Internet resources about the following topics.

- Angina
- ACC/AHA 2007 Guidelines for the Management of Patients with Unstable Angina/Non–ST-Elevation myocardial infarction
- Heart failure animation
- Diagnosis and treatment of chest pain and acute coronary syndrome (ACS)
- Sample chest pain algorithm
- Typical vs. atypical presentation

 ## Using the Student CD

Now that you have completed the material in the chapter text, return to the student CD and complete any chapter activities you have not yet done. Practice your terminology with the "Key Term Concentration" game. Review the chapter material with the "Spin the Wheel" and "ECG Challenge" games. Take the final chapter test, and complete the troubleshooting question; email or print your results to document your proficiency for this chapter.

Basic 12-Lead ECG Interpretation

14

Chapter Outline

- The Views of a Standard 12-Lead ECG and Major Vessels (p. 337)
- Ischemia, Injury, and Infarction (p. 342)
- Electrical Axis (p. 346)
- Bundle Branch Block (p. 348)
- Left Ventricular Hypertrophy (p. 350)

Learning Outcomes

14.1 Discuss the anatomic views seen on a 12-lead ECG and the coronary artery that commonly supplies that region of tissue.

14.2 Identify common morphologic changes associated with ischemia, injury, and infarction.

14.3 Define axis deviation, and list the steps utilized to determine the presence of axis deviation.

14.4 Define bundle branch block (BBB), identify what makes BBB unique, differentiate left from right BBB, and list the steps to determine the presence of BBB.

14.5 Describe left ventricular hypertrophy (LVH), and list the steps to determine the presence of LVH.

Key Terms

anatomically contiguous lead
axis deviation
hypertrophy
myocardial infarction

myocardial injury
myocardial ischemia
pathologic Q wave
physiologic Q wave

14.1 The Views of a Standard 12-Lead ECG and Major Vessels

In Chapter 3, we discussed how the 12-lead ECG produces 12 different tracings of the heart. Now it is time to explain what a standard 12-lead is specifically looking at. . .essentially what each lead sees.

Consider each lead as being a photograph, like taking a picture of a car. If you stand in front of the car and take the picture, it is the front view of the car. If you stand behind the same car and take a picture, it's still the car but simply from a different angle.

A standard 12-lead ECG focuses directly on the left ventricle but considers the heart from slightly different angles (Table 14-1 and Figure 14-1). Each lead is looking for problems or damage to vessels and heart muscle tissue in specific areas.

Consider Figures 14-2 to 14-7. Each figure identifies the area on the heart involved and the lead tracing affected by the involvement.

TABLE 14-1   Standard 12-Lead Views

Leads	Portion of Heart Viewed	Main Coronary Artery and Branch
II, III, aVF	Inferior wall of left ventricle	Right coronary – Marginal branch
V1 & V2	Septal wall	Left coronary – Septal branch
V3 & V4	Anterior wall of left ventricle	Left coronary – Left anterior descending
I, aVL, V5 & V6	Lateral wall of left ventricle	Left coronary – Left circumflex

Checkpoint Question (LO 14.1)

1. Why do you think a doctor may order a right-side or posterior 12-lead ECG?

_____

_____

Figure 14-1   Typically, a 12-Lead ECG focuses on the left ventricle but considers the heart from slightly different angles.

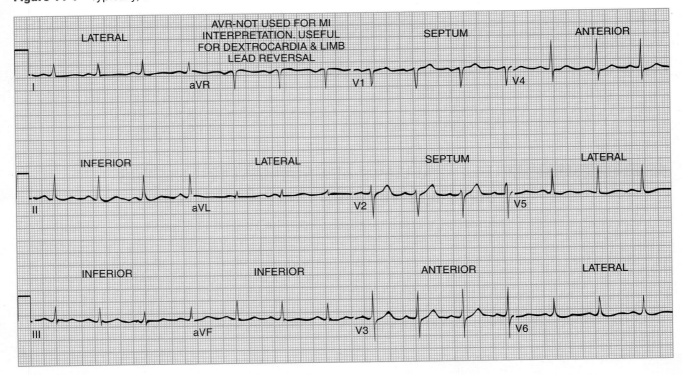

Figure 14-2 Localization of myocardial injury and infarction. *A.* Anterior View *B.* Posterior View.

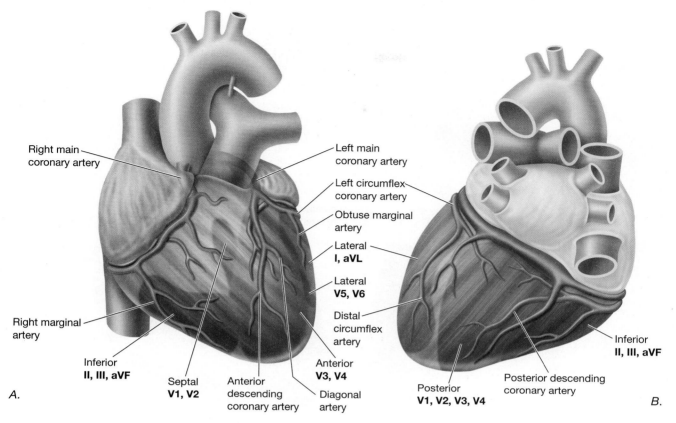

Right main coronary artery

Left main coronary artery

Left circumflex coronary artery

Obtuse marginal artery

Lateral
I, aVL

Lateral
V5, V6

Distal circumflex artery

Anterior
V3, V4

Right marginal artery

Inferior
II, III, aVF

Septal
V1, V2

Anterior descending coronary artery

Diagonal artery

Posterior
V1, V2, V3, V4

Posterior descending coronary artery

Inferior
II, III, aVF

A.

B.

Figure 14-3 Inferior infarction. *A.* Anterior View *B.* Posterior View.

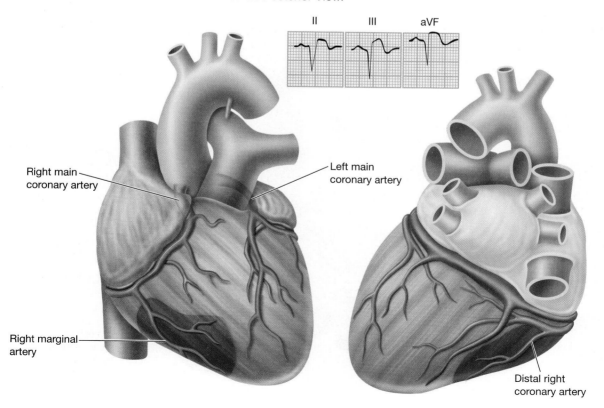

II   III   aVF

Right main coronary artery

Left main coronary artery

Right marginal artery

Distal right coronary artery

A.

B.

Figure 14-4 Lateral infarction. *A.* Anterior View *B.* Posterior View.

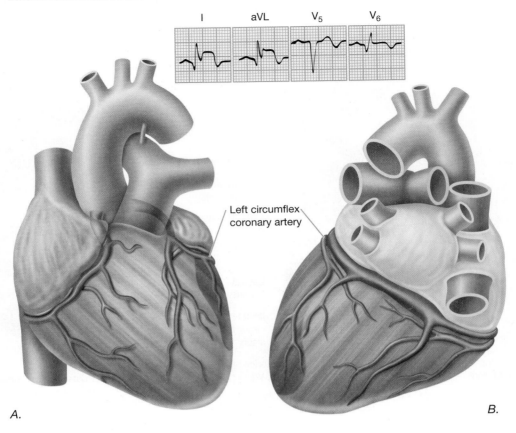

A.

B.

Left circumflex coronary artery

Figure 14-5 Septal infarction.

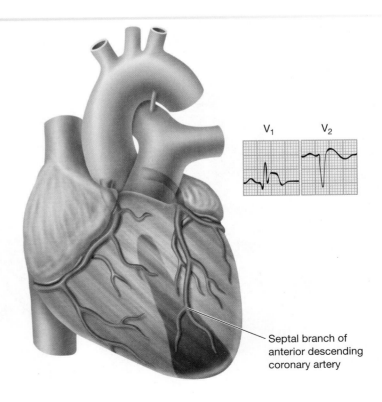

Septal branch of anterior descending coronary artery

Figure 14-6   Anterior infarction.

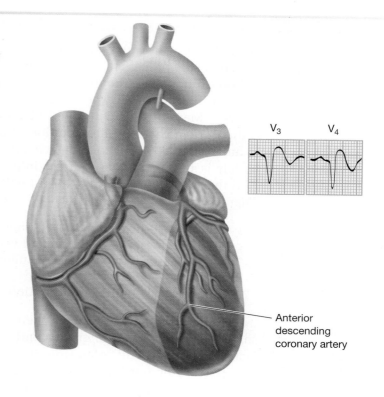

Anterior descending coronary artery

Figure 14-7   Posterior infarction. A posterior wall infarction may result from occlusion of the posterior descending artery which is formed by the right main coronary artery in 90% of the population. Much less frequently, occlusion of the distal portion of the left circumflex artery (10% of the population) may also cause a posterior wall MI.

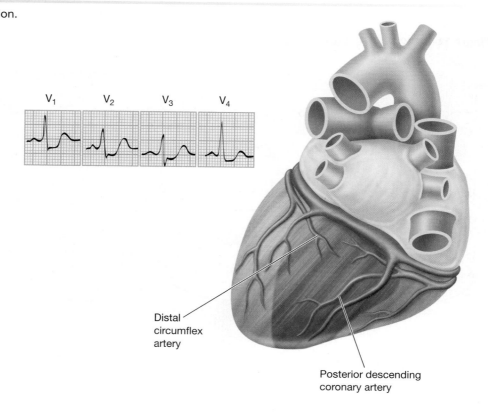

Distal circumflex artery

Posterior descending coronary artery

14.2 Ischemia, Injury, and Infarction

When learning how to interpret a rhythm strip, you were taught a very specific five-step process that is to be followed each and every time, regardless of how complicated the dysrhythmia may be. In this chapter you will still use the five steps you were taught but simply add two more steps to the process. Many people consider 12-lead interpretation to be so much more difficult than rhythm interpretation. Presented here are the basics for you to build your skill and competence quickly.

It is important that you get into the habit of analyzing the 12-lead ECG the same way each time. Begin with the five-step process. Recall from Chapter 5:

Step 1: Determine the ECG rhythm or regularity
Step 2: Determine the atrial and ventricular rate
Step 3: Identify the P wave configuration
Step 4: Measure the PR interval
Step 5: Measure the QRS duration and analyze the configuration

Follow the first five steps, then view leads in groups looking at the same part of the heart in groups and reading from left to right. Focus on ischemia, injury, and infarction; these often cause morphologic changes to a portion or portions of the cardiac complexes. Ischemia and injury often cause a delay in repolarization. This delay is represented by either ST segment depression or elevation (Figure 14-8). Recall from Chapter 4 that the ST segment is normally in line with the isoelectric line or baseline.

Figure 14-8 12-lead ECG with ST deviation.

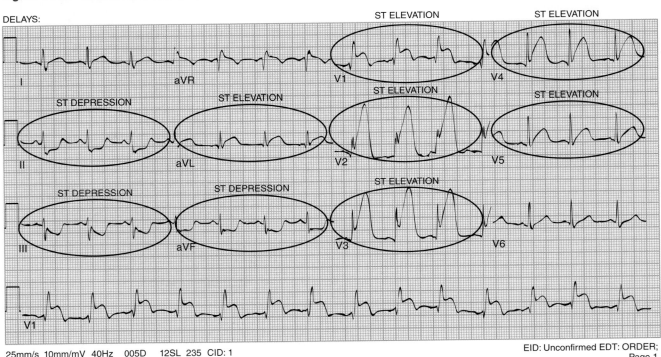

25mm/s 10mm/mV 40Hz 005D 12SL 235 CID: 1

EID: Unconfirmed EDT: ORDER;
Page 1

myocardial ischemia A reduction or interruption in blood flow and oxygen to the myocardium, possibly for a short period of time.

anatomically contiguous lead Two or more leads looking at the same part of the heart, or numerically consecutive chest leads.

Think of ischemia, injury, and infarction as a dangerous continuum of worsening cardiac conditions when blood flow to the myocardium is decreased or interrupted for even a few minutes. ST segment depression is often indicative of **myocardial ischemia**. The depression of the ST segment must be 1 mm or more. When seen in two or more anatomically continuous leads, ST segment depression of 1 mm or more is indicative of myocardial ischemia. An **anatomically contiguous lead** is defined as two or more leads "looking" at the same part of the heart, or numerically consecutive chest leads. For example, leads II and III look at the inferior wall of the left ventricle, and V3 and V4 are numerically consecutive chest leads that look at the anterior wall of the left ventricle. Examples of anatomically contiguous leads include:

- II, III, aVF
- I, aVL
- V1, V2, V3, V4, V5, V6 (Figure 14-9)

When analyzing the ST segment, it is important to compare the PR segment, ST segment, and TP segments. This will provide you with the segment prior to and after the ST segment. This step is critical for the purpose of analysis. By taking a straight edge or cardiac ruler and lining up the segments, it will assist in identifying any deviation of the ST segment from the isoelectric line.

Another indicator of ischemia is T wave inversion. T waves are normally a positively deflected waveform. In some cases of ischemia, the T wave will become negatively deflected. T wave inversion may be seen by itself as shown in Figure 14-10. Most often T wave inversion is seen with concurrent ST segment elevation (Figure 14-11).

myocardial injury Reduction or interruption of blood flow persists for a few minutes; the affected myocardium will transition from myocardial ischemia to a worsened state.

Myocardial ischemia occurs when there is a reduction or interruption in blood flow and oxygen to the myocardium. This may be for just a short period. If this reduction or interruption of blood flow persists for more than a few minutes, the affected myocardium will transition from myocardial ischemia to a more worsened state referred to as **myocardial injury**. ST segment elevation is morphologic evidence of acute injury pattern. ST segment elevation of 1 mm or more that is seen in two or more anatomically

Figure 14-9 Anatomically contiguous leads.

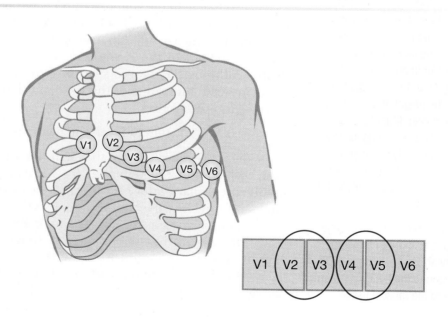

Figure 14-10 T wave inversion.

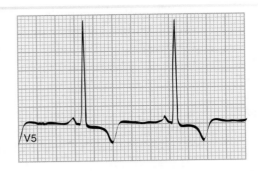

Figure 14-11 T wave inversion with ST elevation.

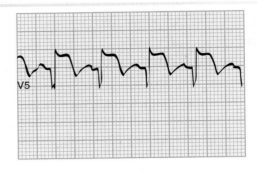

contiguous leads is indicative of myocardial injury. ST segment elevation may be accompanied by T wave inversion.

When ST segment elevation is seen on a 12-lead ECG, it is often referred to either as myocardial injury, acute injury pattern, or acute MI (AMI). *When you see ST elevation, it means the problem is happening right now, and the tissue is* not *dead yet!* It is in that state between ischemic and dead. . . "stunned" would be a good way to describe it. Unless immediate and effective intervention is established, the tissue soon will begin to die.

Evidence of tissue death (infarction) is often seen as a change in the width and/or depth of the Q wave. A normal or **physiologic Q wave** (Figure 14-12*A*) is defined as one in which the width measures less than 0.04 second and the depth measures less than one-third of the height of the R wave in that lead.

The change in the shape of the Q wave as a result of tissue death (infarction) is called a pathologic Q wave. A **pathologic Q wave** (Figure 14-12*B*) is defined as measuring 0.04 second and/or greater than or equal to one-third the height of the R wave in that lead tracing. This indicates tissue death. Pathologic Q waves seen in two or more anatomically contiguous leads indicate that some of the tissue in that part of the heart is now dead (**myocardial infarction**).

(infarcted = tissue necrosis = tissue death)

There are many factors that will determine how dangerous the infarction will be and the potential for recovery. This will depend upon the involved coronary artery or arteries, location and extent of the infarction, vital structures involved, and time, just to name a few.

When viewing a 12-lead ECG look for the changes (ST depression, ST elevation, T wave inversion, and Pathologic Q wave. just described. However, it is most important to know that these changes must be seen in at least two or more anatomically contiguous leads in order to consider the changes as being ischemia, injury, or infarction.

physiologic Q wave Also known as a normal Q wave, it will measure less than 0.04 second in duration and less than 1/3 the height of the R wave in that lead.

pathologic Q wave ECG evidence of myocardial infarction. A pathologic Q wave must measure 0.04 second or wider in duration and/or be greater than or equal to 1/3 the height of the R wave in that lead. Must be seen in two or more contiguous leads to be clinically meaningful. Absence of Q waves does not eliminate the possibility of MI.

myocardial infarction (MI) (heart attack) A blockage of one or more of the coronary arteries causing lack of oxygen to the heart and damage to the muscle tissue.

Figure 14-12 Q Waves. *A.* Physiologic Q wave. *B.* Pathologic Q wave.

A.

Physiologic Q wave

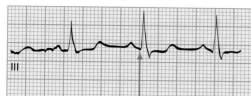

III

B.

Pathologic Q wave

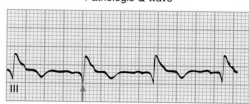

III

Not all patients will present with the classic morphologic changes discussed in this chapter. Some patients will not present with any changes at all. This presents the healthcare professional with a situation where other testing will be necessary. Recall from Chapter 13 these tests may include blood tests to look for specific markers (enzymes) that are only present when heart muscle death occurs, echocardiography, and/or coronary angiography.

Safety & Infection Control

ST Segment Elevation

Not every instance of ST segment elevation is indicative of myocardial injury. Time, experience, and further training will help you will learn what those instances are. The bottom line is the safety of the patient. ST segment elevation of any kind must *always* be reported.

Checkpoint Questions (LO 14.2)

1. Consider wandering baseline. Why is it important to eliminate this type of artifact from a 12-lead tracing?

   _____

   _____

2. Define myocardial ischemia.

   _____

   _____

3. What morphologic change provides evidence of myocardial injury?

   _____

   _____

4. Describe anatomically contiguous leads.

   _____

   _____

5. What is a pathologic Q wave.

   _____

   _____

14.3 Electrical Axis

axis deviation Orientation of the heart within the chest.

hypertrophy Abnormal thickening of the ventricular wall due to chronic pressure overload; is often caused by hypertension.

Electrical **axis deviation** essentially refers to the changes that occur on the 12-lead ECG as a result of the position of the heart within the patient's chest. When the heart is not in its normal location, the deflection of the QRS complex will change due to being displaced within the chest. If you would imagine a circle divided into four large equal quadrants superimposed over a person's chest, the patient's heart would be located normally in the direction of the left lower quadrant (Figure 14-13).

Different things may cause the heart to become displaced from its normal location. Displacement of the heart is often seen in conditions such as pregnancy, birth defects, and left ventricular hypertrophy. During pregnancy, the large third-trimester fetus temporarily displaces the heart toward the upper left quadrant. In the case of pregnancy, once the baby is delivered, the heart typically returns to the normal location. With congenital defects, the location of the heart within the chest may also be displaced.

Left ventricular hypertrophy is different. **Hypertrophy,** an abnormal thickening of the ventricular wall due to chronic pressure overload, is often caused by hypertension. The effort the heart must exert in order to maintain normal cardiac output is increased due to increased peripheral vascular resistance. This is the same process that would occur if you went to the gym every day and lifted weights: over time, your muscles would become thicker. As the wall of the ventricle thickens, the heart may become displaced toward the upper left quadrant. This increased muscle thickness also translates to more electrical activity (think QRS complex); the more electrical activity, the larger the QRS complex.

Axis deviation may be either left or right. Left axis deviation is the most common. Other types of deviation are less common but do occur. Table 14-2 provides examples.

Axis deviation changes the direction of ventricular depolarization. A simple way to determine the presence of axis deviation is to refer to leads

Figure 14-13 Axis determination-quadrants.

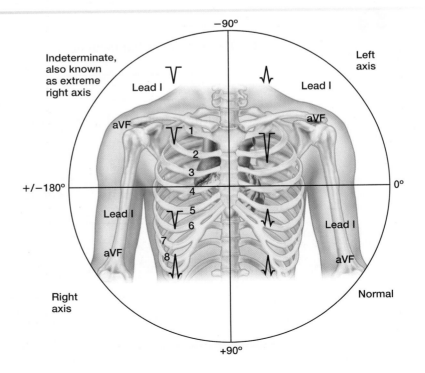

TABLE 14-2 **Causes of Axis Deviation**

Deviation	Possible Cause
Left axis deviation (most common)	Left ventricular hypertrophy Pregnancy Obesity Emphysema Hyperkalemia
Right axis deviation (Right axis deviation is considered normal in children and tall, thin adults.)	Right ventricular hypertrophy Anterolateral wall MI
Extreme right axis deviation (referred to as indeterminate, NW territory or No Man's Land)	Situs transversus or dextrocardia (The heart is on the right side of the chest.) Pacemaker rhythms COPD patients Hyperkalemia (Extreme right axis deviation may also indicate lead reversal.)

Figure 14-14 Axis deviation.

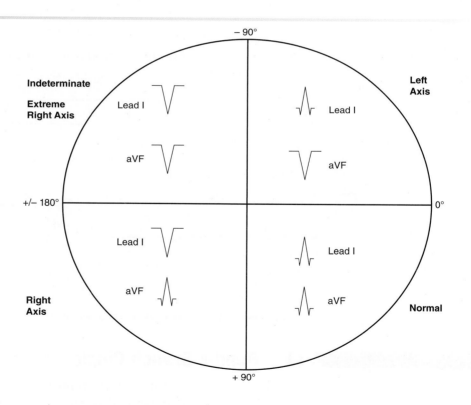

I and aVF. When "normal," both of these leads will have a predominantly positive QRS complex. If either or both of these leads have a prominently negative ventricular depolarization, the electrical axis is something other than "normal," Focus on the QRS complex when referring to leads I and aVF. Review Figure 14-14 and use these steps.

> **Step One:** If lead I is positive (up) and aVF is also positive (up), the axis is said to be "normal."
> **Step Two:** If lead I is positive (up) and aVF is negative (down), the patient has left axis deviation.
> **Step Three:** If lead I is negative (down) and aVF is positive (up), the patient has right axis deviation.
> **Step Four:** If lead I is negative (down) and aVF is also negative (down), the patient has extreme right axis deviation (also referred to as indeterminate).

Checkpoint Questions (LO 14.3)

1. What are the two leads we refer to when determining the presence of axis deviation?

   _____

   _____

2. When determining the electrical axis, on which portion of the cardiac complex should attention be focused?

   _____

   _____

3. Use the two views below from the 12-lead ECG tracing to determine the electrical axis.

   _____

   _____

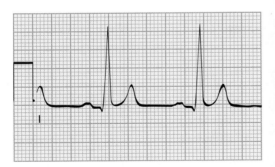
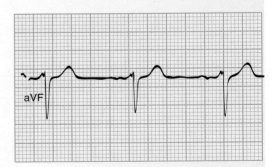

14.4 Bundle Branch Block

As was discussed in Chapter 10, bundle branch blocks occur when one or both of the ventricular pathways are damaged or delayed due to cardiac disease, drugs, or other conditions. When an area of one of the bundle branches is damaged, electrical current will not be able to travel through that tissue to reach the myocardial tissue in its usual fashion. Current will travel down the good bundle and will activate the myocardial tissue in that corresponding ventricle only. The other ventricle must then receive the impulse as current travels from one cell to the next until the entire myocardial contraction occurs. It is similar to the knocking down of a line of dominoes, where each domino represents a cardiac cell. The cell will not contract until the next cell delivers the energy. Current traveling via the abnormal pathways will take longer to achieve the full ventricular contraction. This longer time frame is similar to driving a car to a specific destination and having to find an alternate route or detour when the road is closed. This is what happens to the current traveling through the heart's conduction pathway when it has a blocked bundle branch. The increased length of time is reflected in a wider than normal QRS duration (0.12 second or greater). Remember that the QRS duration is a measurement of just how long it takes for current to travel through ventricular myocardial tissue.

Characteristics of the right and left bundle branch block will be similar over monitoring leads I, II, and III. Specific characteristics of the right or left bundle branch will be present when monitoring with leads V1 to V6. Although bundle branch block (BBB) is seen in the precordial leads, to distinguish RBBB from LBBB, lead VI is referenced (Figure 14-15). If the QRS is positively deflected, it is an RBBB. RBBB often has a classic RSR pattern in V1 and is often referred to as "bunny ears" or "bunny branch block." If the QRS is negative or a QS complex, it is an LBBB.

When analyzing V1 to determine the presence of bundle branch block you must look for the following:

1. Evidence of atrial activity (P wave). Remember the problem is within the ventricles, so we must see a P wave to tell us that the electrical activity was initiated above the ventricles.
2. QRS complex that measures 0.12 second or more in duration.

The question now becomes," which direction is the QRS going and how do you determine this?" Starting at the J point of the QRS, move backward into the ventricular depolarization. If it is going down (negative), it is a left bundle branch block (Figure 14-16A). If it is going up (positive), it is a right bundle branch block (Figure 14-16B).

Figure 14-15 Bundle branch blocks. *A.* RBBB. Note that the QRS is positively deflected. *B.* LBBB. Note that the QRS is either negative or a QS complex is present.

A.

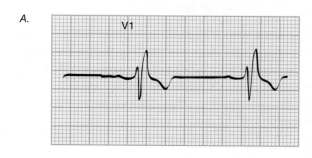

B.

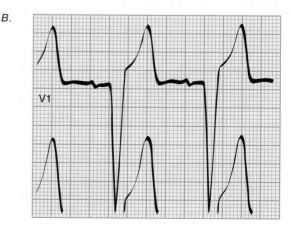

Figure 14-16 Bundle branch blocks. *A.* Left bundle branch block (LBBB). *B.* Right bundle branch block.

A.

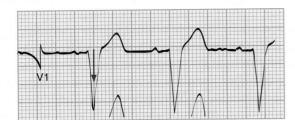

B.

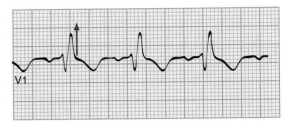

Checkpoint Questions (LO 14.4)

1. Review the following tracings, identify the type of BBB, and then explain how you determined your answers.

a. _____

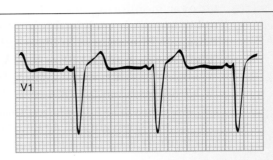

b. _____

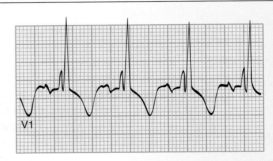

14.5 Left Ventricular Hypertrophy (LVH)

Left ventricular hypertrophy is an abnormal thickening of the ventricular wall due to pumping against increased vascular resistance over a period of time. As the wall thickens, the depth and height of the ventricular depolarization will increase. More muscle equals more electricity, which is shown as greater amplitude of the QRS complex. This means taller and deeper ventricular depolarization waves will be seen.

When determining the presence of left ventricular hypertrophy, you will follow a few simple steps (Figure 14-17).

1. Refer to V1 and V2. Measure and select the deeper of the two views. Measure from the isoelectric line down to the tip of the deepest QS complex, count the millimeters, and write this number down.

2. Refer to V5 and V6. Measure and select the taller of the two views. Measure from the isoelectric line to the tip of the tallest R wave, then count the number of millimeters and write it down.

3. Add the two numbers together. If it adds up to 35 or more millimeters, clinically you would suspect left ventricular hypertrophy.

Figure 14-17   Assessing for the presence of left ventricular hypertrophy.

A.

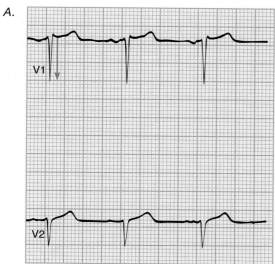

Step 1: Analyze V1 and V2. Measure from the isoelectric line down to the tip of the deepest QS complex. The image to the left measures 12 mm. Write down that number.

12 mm

B.

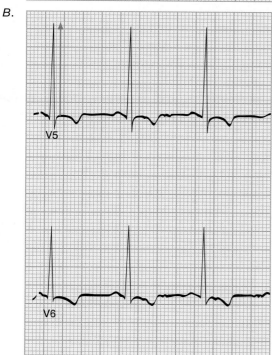

Step 2: Analyze V5 and V6. Measure from the isoelectric line up to the tip of the tallest R wave. The image to the left measures 24 mm. Write down that number.

24 mm

Step 3: Combine the deepest QS complex measurement with the tallest R wave measurement. If the numbers measure 35 mm or greater when combined, clinically you must suspect left ventricular hypertrophy.

12 + 24 = 36 mm

1. Review the following tracing. Do you suspect left ventricular hypertrophy? Explain how you determined your answer.

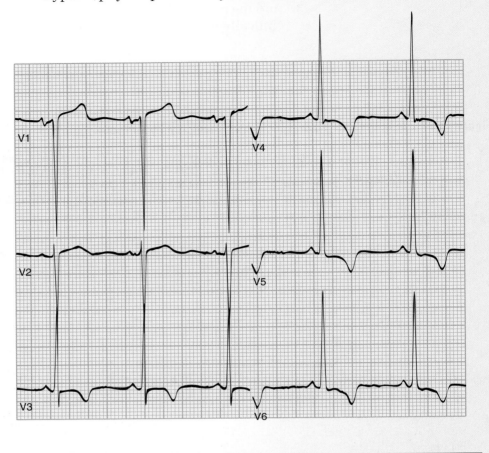

_____

_____

Chapter Summary

Learning Outcomes	Summary	Page
14.1 Discuss the anatomic views seen on a 12-lead ECG and the coronary artery that commonly supplies that region of tissue.	Leads II, III, aVF view the inferior wall of left ventricle. Leads V1 and V2 view the lateral wall of left ventricle.	337–341
14.2 Identify common morphologic changes associated with ischemia, injury, and infarction.	Think of ischemia, injury, and infarction as a dangerous continuum of worsening cardiac condition when blood flow to the myocardium is decreased or interrupted for even a few minutes. ST segment depression of 1 mm or more seen in two or more anatomically contiguous leads is indicative of myocardial ischemia. ST segment elevation of 1 mm or more seen in two or more anatomically contiguous leads is indicative of myocardial injury. The change in the shape of the Q wave as a result of tissue death is called a pathologic Q wave. Pathologic Q waves seen in two or more anatomically contiguous leads indicate that some of the tissue in that part of the heart is now dead (myocardial infarction).	342–345
14.3 Define axis deviation, and list the steps utilized to determine the presence of axis deviation.	Electrical deviation causes morphologic changes within the 12-lead ECG as a result of the position of the heart within the patient's chest. When the heart is not in its normal location the deflection of the QRS complex will change due to being displaced within the chest.	346–348
14.4 Define bundle branch block (BBB), identify what makes BBB unique, differentiate left from right BBB, and list the steps to determine the presence of BBB.	Bundle branch blocks occur when one or both of the ventricular pathways are damaged or delayed due to cardiac disease, drugs, or other conditions. The electrical current will not be able to travel through that tissue to reach the myocardial tissue in its usual fashion. The increased length of time is reflected in a wider than normal QRS duration (0.12 second or greater). Refer to lead V1 to differentiate between right and left BBB. • LBBB presents with a P wave and a QS complex measuring 0.12 second or more. • RBBB presents with a P wave and has an R wave that often has two points, or "bunny ears." It also measures 0.12 seconds or more in duration.	348–350
14.5 Describe left ventricular hypertrophy (LVH), and list the steps to determine the presence of LVH.	Left ventricular hypertrophy is an abnormal thickening of the ventricular wall due to pumping against increased vascular resistance over a period of time. As the wall thickens, the depth and height of the ventricular depolarization will increase. More muscle equals more electricity and thereby greater amplitude of the QRS complex. This means taller and deeper ventricular depolarizations will be seen.	350–352

Chapter Review

Matching

_____ **1.** axis deviation (LO 14.3)

_____ **2.** contiguous leads (LO 14.3)

_____ **3.** hypertrophy (LO 14.5)

_____ **4.** myocardial infarction (LO 14.2)

_____ **5.** myocardial injury (LO 14.2)

_____ **6.** myocardial ischemia (LO 14.2)

_____ **7.** pathologic Q wave (LO 14.3)

_____ **8.** physiologic Q wave (LO 14.3)

_____ **9.** right marginal branch (LO 14.1)

a. abnormal thickening

b. reduction or interruption in blood flow and oxygen to the myocardium

c. measuring 0.04 second and/or greater than or equal to one-third the height of the R wave

d. supplies blood to both surfaces of the right ventricle

e. tissue death to the heart muscle

f. measures less than 0.04 second, and the depth measures less than one-third of the height of the R wave

g. ST segment elevation of 1 mm or more seen in two or more anatomically contiguous leads

h. ECG changes due to position of heart

i. looks at the same part of the heart or numerically consecutive leads

Multiple Choice

10. Which leads look at the lateral wall of the left ventricle? (LO 14.1)
   a. II, III, and aVF
   b. V1 and V2
   c. V3 and V4
   d. I, aVL, V5, and V6

11. Which leads look at the septal wall of the left ventricle? (LO 14.1)
   a. II, III, and aVF
   b. V1 and V2
   c. V3 and V4
   d. I, aVL, V5, and V6

12. Which leads look at the inferior wall of the left ventricle? (LO 14.1)
   a. II, III, and aVF
   b. V1 and V2
   c. V3 and V4
   d. I, aVL, V5, and V6

13. Which leads look at the anterior wall of the left ventricle? (LO 14.1)
    a. II, III, and aVF
    b. V1 and V2
    c. V3 and V4
    d. I, aVL, V5, and V6

14. Which major coronary artery and vessel supply the inferior wall of the left ventricle? (LO 14.1)
    a. Left main and circumflex artery
    b. Left main and left anterior descending
    c. Left main and septal
    d. Right main and right acute marginal branch

15. Which major coronary artery and vessel supply the septal wall of the left ventricle? (LO 14.1)
    a. Left main and circumflex artery
    b. Left main and left anterior descending
    c. Left main and septal
    d. Right main and right acute marginal branch

16. Which major coronary artery and vessel supply the lateral wall of the left ventricle? (LO 14.1)
    a. Left main and circumflex artery
    b. Left main and left anterior descending
    c. Right main and septal
    d. Right main and right acute marginal branch

17. Which major coronary artery and vessel supply the anterior wall of the left ventricle? (LO 14.1)
    a. Left main and circumflex artery
    b. Left main and left anterior descending
    c. Right main and septal
    d. Right main and right acute marginal branch

18. Signs of ischemia may include (LO 14.2)
    a. ST segment elevation.
    b. ST segment depression only.
    c. ST segment depression and T wave inversion.
    d. pathologic Q wave.

19. Signs of injury may include (LO 14.2)
    a. ST segment elevation.
    b. ST segment depression only.
    c. ST segment depression and T wave inversion.
    d. pathologic Q wave.

20. Which of the following is the moslt line sign of an infarction? (LO 14.2)
    a. ST segment elevation.
    b. ST segment depression only.
    c. ST segment depression and T wave inversion.
    d. pathologic Q wave.

21. What are the two views referred to when determining electrical axis? (LO 14.3)
    a. V1 and V2
    b. V3 and V4
    c. I and aVF
    d. III and aVR

22. Which direction is the QRS complex in normal axis point for lead I and aVF? (LO 14.3)
    a. Down, down
    b. Up, down
    c. Down, up
    d. Up, up

23. Which direction is the QRS complex in right axis point lead I and aVF? (LO 14.3)
    a. Down, down
    b. Up, down
    c. Down, up
    d. Up, up

24. Which direction is the QRS complex in extreme axis point lead I and aVF? (LO 14.3)
    a. Down, down
    b. Up, down
    c. Down, up
    d. Up, up

25. Which direction is the QRS complex in left axis point lead I and aVF? (LO 14.3)
    a. Down, down
    b. Up, down
    c. Down, up
    d. Up, up

26. Which leads are referred to when analyzing a 12-lead ECG for the presence of left ventricular hypertrophy? (LO 14.5)
    a. V2, V3 and V5, V6
    b. I, aVL and II, III
    c. V1, V2 and V5, V6
    d. 1, aVL and aVR, V4

27. When totaled, how many millimeters is the minimum necessary to clinically suspect hypertrophy? (LO 14.5)
    a. 3
    b. 5
    c. 35
    d. 350

28. Which of the following most accurately describes the difference between LBBB and RBBB when viewing lead V1? (LO 14.4)
    a. The QRS complex is less than 0.12 second for RBBB and greater than 0.12 seconds for LBBB.
    b. The QRS is positive for LBBB and negative for RBBB.
    c. The QRS is negative for LBBB and positive for RBBB.
    d. The QRS complex is greater than 0.12 second for RBBB and less than 0.12 seconds for LBBB.

Fill in the Blank

29. What are the two criteria for determining the presence of bundle branch block? (LO 14.4) _____ _____

30. List two major causes of ischemia within the heart. (LO 14.2) _____ _____

31. Left BBB is a _____ deflection. (LO 14.4)

32. Right BBB is a _____ deflection. (LO 14.4)

33. The view referred to when differentiating left from right BBB is _____. (LO 14.4)

34. BBB changes the _____ of the QRS complex, and hypertrophy changes the _____ of the QRS complex. (LO 14.4 and 14.5)

35. Define anatomically contiguous. (LO 14.2) _____

_____

Critical Thinking Application *Rhythm Identification*

36. Identify the location of the ischemia on this 12-lead ECG, and explain your answer. (LO 14.2)

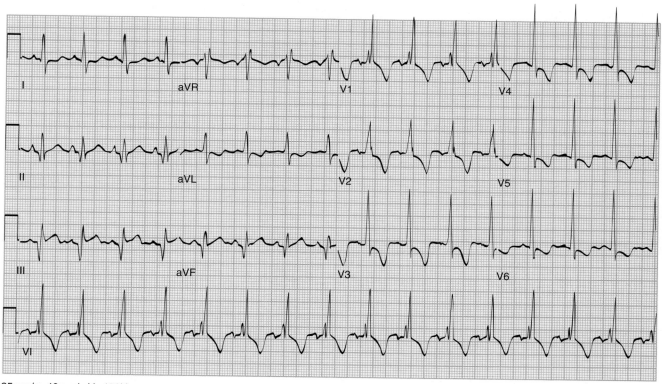

25mm/s 10mm/mV 150Hz

_____

_____

37. Identify the location of the infarction on this 12-lead ECG, and explain your answer. (LO 14.2)

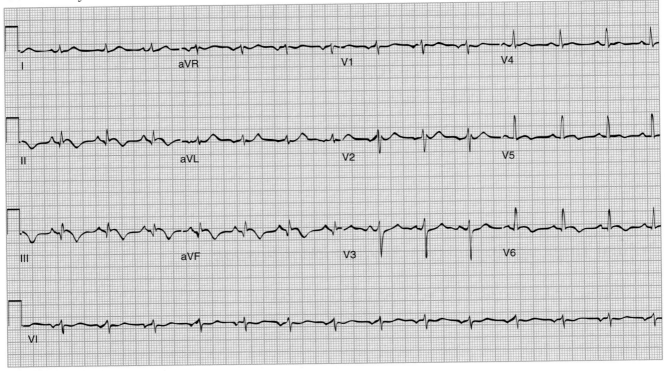

25mm/s 10mm/mV 150Hz

38. Identify the location of the AMI on this 12-lead ECG, and explain your answer. (LO 14.2)

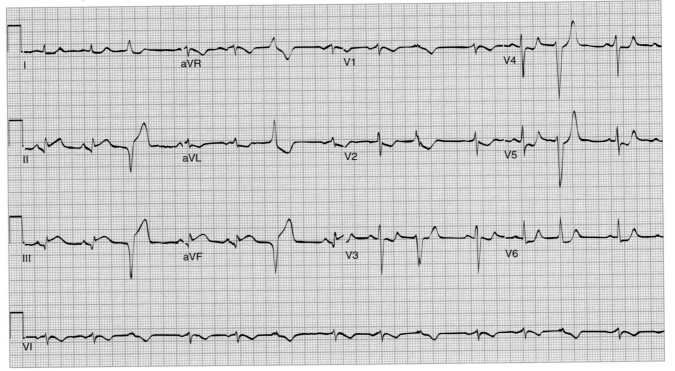

25mm/s 10mm/mV 150Hz

39. Identify the location of the AMI on this 12-lead ECG, and explain your answer. (LO 14.2)

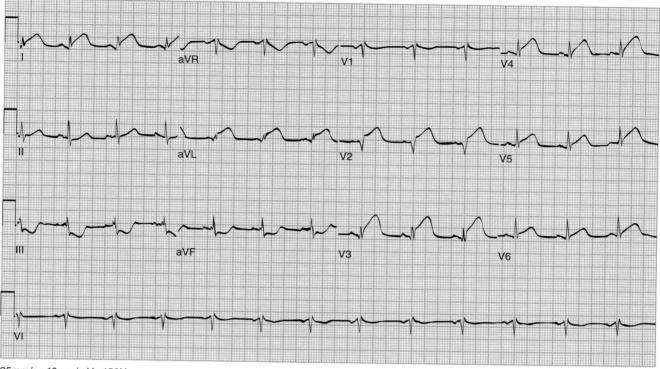

25mm/s   10mm/mV   150Hz

40. Identify the electrical axis, and explain your answer. (LO 14.3)

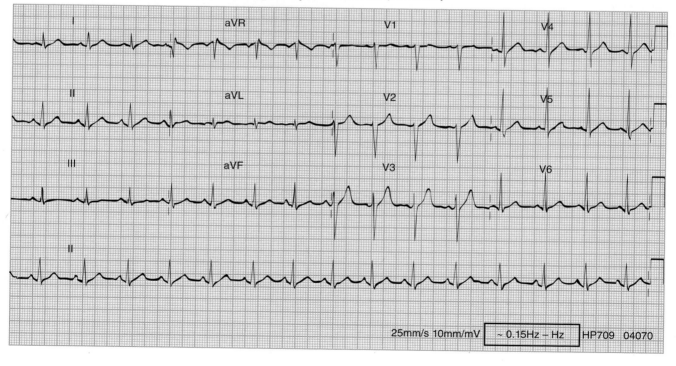

25mm/s 10mm/mV   ~ 0.15Hz – Hz   HP709   04070

41. Identify the electrical axis, and explain your answer. (LO 14.3)

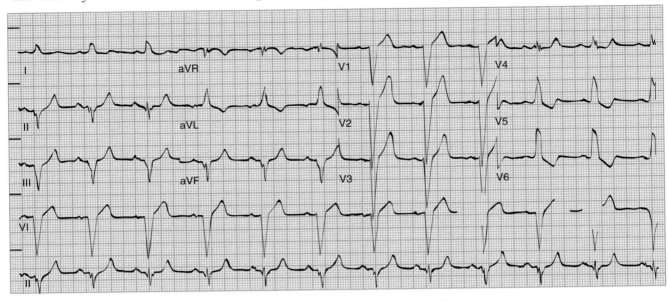

42. Identify the electrical axis, and explain your answer. (LO 14.3)

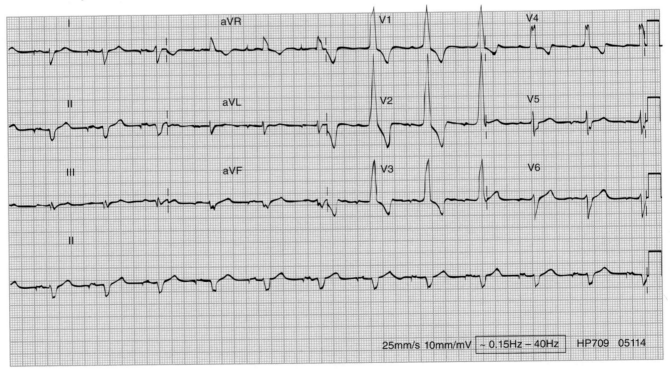

25mm/s 10mm/mV ~ 0.15Hz – 40Hz HP709 05114

43. Identify the bundle branch block, and explain your answer in the space provided. (LO 14.4)

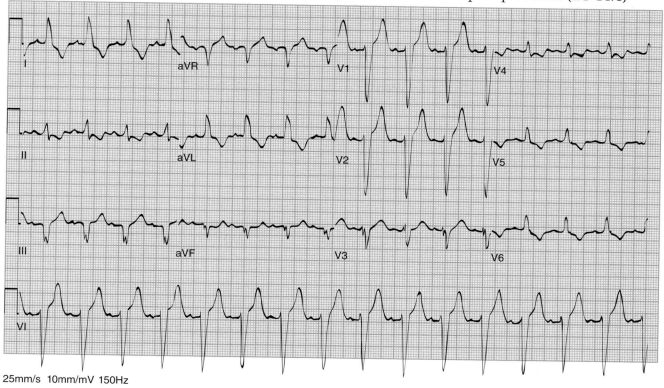

25mm/s 10mm/mV 150Hz

44. Identify the bundle branch block, and explain your answer in the space provided. (LO 14.4)

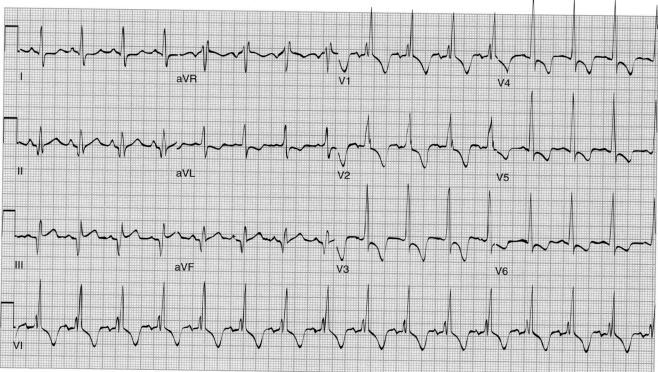

25mm/s 10mm/mV 150Hz

45. Review the figure, and determine if left ventricular hypertrophy is present. Explain your answer. (LO 14.5)

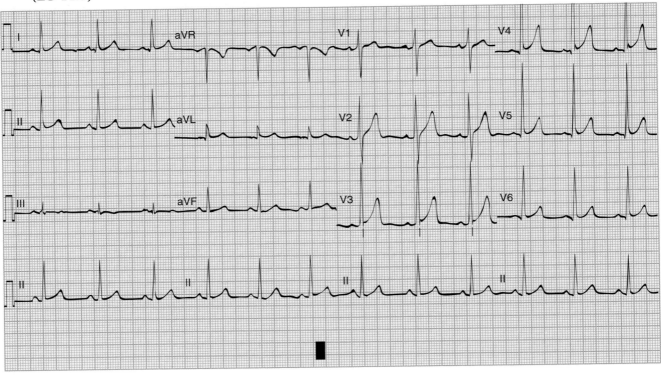

Get Connected *Internet Activity*

Visit the McGraw-Hill Higher Education Online Learning Center *Electrocardiography for Healthcare Professionals* Web site at **www.mhhe.com/boothecg3e** to complete the following activity.

1. Use the following Web sites or search for another Internet resource and create a detailed chart, bulletin board, brochure, report, or presentation about a topic introduced in this chapter.

   American Heart Association [http://www.americanheart.org/presenter.jhtml?identifier=251]

   Home Page of Barbara Ritter, EdD,FNP-BC,CS,CEN,PHN [http://nps.freeservers.com/ekg.htm]

   ECG Learning Center [http://library.med.utah.edu/kw/ecg/tests/index.html]

Using the Student CD

Now that you have completed the material in the chapter text, return to the student CD and complete any chapter activities you have not yet done. Practice your terminology with the "Key Term Concentration" game. Review the chapter material with the "Spin the Wheel" and "ECG Challenge" games. Take the final chapter test, and complete the troubleshooting question; email or print your results to document your proficiency for this chapter.

Cardiovascular Medications

Beta Blockers

Drugs in this class include:

- Atenol**ol** (Tenormin®)
- Metoprol**ol** (Toprol XL®, Lopressor®)
- Propranol**ol** (Inderal®)
- Sotal**ol** (Betapace®, Sotalex®)
- Labetol**ol** (Normodyne®, Trandate®)
- Carvedil**ol** (Coreg®)

Note: The majority of drugs in this class end in *ol.*

Beta blockers are used to treat angina pectoris (chest pain caused by lack of blood/oxygen to the heart muscle), hypertension (high blood pressure), various heart rhythm disturbances such as atrial fibrillation, and PVCs.

Cardiac Glycoside

Drugs in this class include:

- Digoxin (Lanoxin®, Digitek®)

Digitalis, the most common and well-known of the cardiac glycosides, is extracted from the foxglove plant. It has been used for over 100 years to treat atrial fibrillation and congestive heart failure. Digitalis increases the force of the heart's contractions and slows the heart rate. This medication is especially helpful in treating patients with congestive heart failure (CHF). Digoxin is specifically a medication with a host of side effects (i.e., visual disturbances, various cardiac dysrhythmias, and even depression of the ST segment, also known as the digitalis effect).

Calcium Channel Blockers

Drugs in this class include:

- Amlodipine (Norvasc®)
- Diltiazem (Cardizem®)
- Verapamil (Calan®, Isoptin®)
- Nifedipine (Adalat®, Procardia®)

Calcium channel blockers are used to treat a variety of cardiac conditions including hypertension, angina pectoris, and certain types of rapid heart beat conditions such as Afib and Paroxysmal SVT. They are also used to treat coronary artery spasms and after a heart attack for patients who cannot tolerate beta blockers.

ACE Inhibitors

Drugs in this class include:

- Enalapril (Vasotec®)
- Lisinopril (Prinivil®, Zestril®)
- Captopril (Capoten®)
- Benazepril (Lotensin®)

Note: The majority of drugs in this class end in *il.*

The angiotensin-converting enzyme (ACE) inhibitors are named because they work by inhibiting (blocking) the conversion of angiotensin I to angiotensin II in the lungs. Angiotensin II is a potent hormone that constricts arterioles and raises blood pressure. As a result, ACE inhibitors lower the blood pressure. ACE inhibitors are also used in the treatment of patients with congestive heart failure. They work by lowering the overall resistance in the vascular beds, making it easier for the heart to pump the blood.

Antiarrhythmic Medications

There are many different classes of antiarrhythmic medications because the electrical conduction system of the heart is so complex. Each antiarrhythmic-class medication affects the speed or way that electricity flows through the heart. Beta blockers, calcium channel blockers and digitalis are antiarrhythmics. Two other classes of antiarrhythmic medications include sodium channel blockers and postassium channel blockers. Example medications that are used for treatment of arrhythmias, especially during cardiac care, include atropine, epinephrine, isuprel, and lidocaine.

Anticoagulants (Blood Thinners)

Drugs in this class include:

- Warfarin (Coumadin®)
- Heparin
- Enoxaparin (Lovenox®)

This group of drugs is extremely useful in the treatment of blood clot conditions. These medications are administered by a number of different methods, including orally or by injection. These medications all work to stop blood from clotting, or to prevent clots from forming or enlarging. They *do not* lyse (break up or destroy) existing clots.

- Oral Medications

Coumadin (warfarin) is the most commonly prescribed oral "blood thinner." It is prescribed in the treatment of heart valve conditions (including patients with artificial valves and for valve prolapse when blood is not flowing in the proper direction). It is also prescribed for other medical conditions in which blood clotting is a problem and embolization is a risk.

- Intravenous or Subcutaneous Medications

Heparin and Lovenox are very potent intravenous blood thinners. This type of thinner is generally used in an inpatient setting to quickly stop the development of an ongoing blood clot as seen in serious unstable angina, certain strokes, and acute pulmonary embolism. They have no effect on blood platelets.

Warfarin (as previously noted) is primarily used in the treatment of atrial fibrillation and in patients who have artificial metallic heart valves. Warfarin use significantly reduces the risk of embolism development in patients with atrial fibrillation.

Antiplatelet Agents

Drugs in this class include:

- Aspirin (Bayer®)
- Clopidogrel (Plavix®)
- Ticlopidine (Ticlid®)

Antiplatelet medications decrease platelet aggregation (clumping) and inhibit thrombus (clot) formation. They are effective in the arterial circulation where anticoagulants (blood thinners) have little effect.

These medications may be used by patients with any of the following:

- Coronary artery disease
- Heart attack
- Angina (chest pain)
- Stroke and transient ischemic attacks (TIAs)
- Peripheral artery disease
- Angioplasty and stent placement
- Heart bypass surgery
- Atrial fibrillation, to prevent the formation of blood clots

Aspirin is a very potent antiplatelet that has been found to lower the risk of heart attacks and to improve the prognosis with a heart attack. Data have also shown a reduced stroke risk in patients who take prophylactic aspirin. It is a first-line drug administered to "chest pain" patients presenting for emergency care of acute coronary syndromes. Aspirin is routinely prescribed to men over 40 years and postmenopausal women to reduce their risk of clot formation.

Plavix (clopidogrel) keeps platelets in the blood from sticking together and forming clots. These clots are the direct cause of cardiovascular incidents such as heart attacks and strokes. Plavix is useful in angioplasty/coronary stent implantation to prevent postprocedure closure of the treated artery.

Fibrinolytics

Also known as "clot busters," these medications are most commonly used in an inpatient setting where they rapidly dissolve clots wherever they are located; for example, inside a heart artery (causing a heart attack) or inside a brain artery (causing a stroke). The clot is lysed quickly once the clot buster is administered. These drugs can also be used to treat large pulmonary embolisms and clots that are causing obstruction of a prosthetic (metallic) valve.

Because of the way clot busters work, they can increase the risk of bleeding elsewhere in the body (IV site, intracranial, etc.) when administered. Unfortunately, the category of people with the greatest need of these medications are also at the greatest risk for complications as a result of this medication.

Diuretics

Diuretics act by removing salt and water from the body through the action of the kidneys (elimination). Diuretics are used primarily in the treatment of congestive heart failure (CHF) and are often used in the treatment of hypertension (high blood pressure). *Caution must be observed when treating patients with diuretics* as salt and water are not the only elements removed by the action of medications in this class. Other essential electrolytes may be eliminated as well (e.g., potassium, calcium, magnesium, etc.), which may contribute to the development of cardiac dysrhythmias.

Cholesterol-Lowering Agents (Statins)

Drugs in this class include:

- Atorvastatin (Lipitor®)
- Pravastatin (Pravachol®)
- Rosuvastatin (Crestor®)
- Simvastatin (Zocor®)

Cholesterol-lowering medications work to lower the LDL (low-density lipoprotein or "bad") cholesterol in the blood. Some of these drugs also raise the HDL (high-density lipoprotein or "good") cholesterol. This class of drugs has been shown to reduce the incidence of heart attack and death in patients with high cholesterol and coronary artery disease. Some statins may reverse atherosclerotic plaque within blood vessels, thereby reducing the potential for sudden cardiac death and potentially reducing the need for surgical intervention. There are always drawbacks: This category of medications is also potentially hepatotoxic, and high doses of statins may in some cases destroy the liver.

Nitrates

Drugs in this class include:

- Nitroglycerin (Nitor-Dur®, Nitrolingual®, Nitrostat®)
- Isosorbide dinitrate (Dilatrate-SR®, Isordil®)
- Isosorbide mononitrate (ISMO®)

Nitrates are the most commonly prescribed vasodilators, or medications that widen the blood vessels. They are frequently used for relief of ischemic chest pain in patients with coronary vascular disease and angina (chest pain). They work by relaxing smooth muscles, most notably the muscles of the heart and blood vessels. As a result, pressure on blood vessel walls is reduced, which allows more blood to circulate with less effort by the heart. Nitrates affect veins as well as arteries, but their vasodilatory effect is more pronounced on veins. Nitrates prevent and relieve angina by relieving vasoconstriction and restoring blood flow and oxygen to ischemic heart muscle.

Nitrates can be administered intravenously, sublingually (via metered spray or tablet), transdermally (ointments or skin patches), and orally.

Safety note: Don't ever handle nitrates with your bare hands!

Extra Precautions for Patients Taking Nitrates

- If a patient is already taking any medication to treat hypertension and/or **erectile dysfunction** (e.g., Viagra, Cialis, Levitra) the addition of nitrates can be dangerous. When taken in combination, these can increase the effects of nitrates on blood pressure, causing profound irreversible hypotension, cardiac arrest, and even death.

Inotropic Agents (Also Known as Cardiotonics)

Drugs in this class include:

- Adenosine (Adenocard®)
- Dobutamine (Dobutrex®)

Inotropes or inotropic agents affect the heart's contractile force. These medications strengthen the pumping action of the heart and, as a result, reduce cardiac workload (myocardial oxygen demand). They are commonly used to treat patients with heart failure or tachydysrhythmias. Cardiac glycosides such as digitalis are also considered inotropic agents.

Chemical Stress Testing Agents

There are two categories of chemical stress testing agents. The cardioactive agents have an effect on the heart and the imaging agents allow the heart to be visualized during the test.

Cardioactive Drugs

- Dobutamine (Dobutrex®)—increase cardiac output and heart rate, coronary artery vasodilation
- Adenosine (Adenocard®)—coronary artery vasodilation
- Persantine (Dipyridamole®)—coronary artery vasodilation
- Regadenoson (Lexiscan®)—coronary vasodilation

Imaging Agents

- Cardiolite®
- Thallium®
- Myoview®

Standard and Isolation Precautions

Key Components to Standard Precautions

Handwashing (or using an antiseptic handrub)

- After touching blood, body fluids, secretions, excretions, and contaminated items
- Immediately after removing gloves
- Between patient contacts

Gloves

- For contact with blood, body fluids, secretions, and contaminated items
- For contact with mucous membranes and nonintact skin

Masks, Goggles, Face Masks

- Protect mucous membranes of eyes, nose, and mouth when contact with blood and body fluids is likely

Gowns

- Protect skin from blood or body fluid contact
- Prevent soiling of clothing during procedures that may involve contact with blood or body fluids

Linen

- Handle soiled linen to prevent touching skin or mucous membranes
- Do not prerinse soiled linens in patient care areas

Patient Care Equipment

- Handle soiled equipment in a manner to prevent contact with skin or mucous membranes and to prevent contamination of clothing or the environment
- Clean reusable equipment prior to reuse

Environmental cleaning

- Routinely care for, clean, and disinfect equipment and furnishings in patient care areas

Sharps

- Avoid recapping used needles
- Avoid removing used needles from disposable syringes
- Avoid bending, breaking, or manipulating used needles by hand
- Place used sharps in puncture-resistant containers

Patient Resuscitation

- Use mouthpieces, resuscitation bags, or other ventilation devices to avoid mouth-to-mouth resuscitation

Patient Placement

- Place patients who contaminate the environment or cannot maintain appropriate hygiene in private rooms

Hand Hygiene Practices and Procedures

Recommended Practices

- Wash hands at the beginning of the work day. Wash your hands with soap and water whenever they are visibly contaminated with blood or other body fluids.
- If hands are not visibly contaminated, an alcohol-based hand rub can be used.
- Wash hands at the end of the work day before leaving the facility.

Indications for Hand Hygiene

- Before putting on and after removing gloves
- Between patient contacts; between different procedures on same patient
- After touching blood, body fluids, secretions, excretions, and contaminated objects
- After handling specimen containers or tubes
- After restroom visits, eating, combing hair, handling money, and any other time your hands get contaminated
- Before inserting any invasive device
- After having contact with a patient's skin
- After having contact with wound dressings (bandages)
- After having contact with inanimate objects near a patient
- Before eating, applying cosmetics, or contact lens manipulation

Basic Steps for Handwashing

- Remove all rings and jewelry.
- Turn on water, and adjust temperature to warm.*
- Wet hands liberally without leaning your body against sink area.
- Apply soap, and work up a good lather.
- Use circular motions while applying friction, being sure to interlace fingers to clean between them for 2 minutes at the start of your work day, 15–30 seconds in between patients, and 1–2 minutes when hands are really soiled.

- Rinse each hand, allowing water to run from wrist toward fingertips, keeping fingers pointing downward. Contamination under fingernails should be removed with a tool designed for that purpose, such as an orange stick.
- Repeat above steps if hands are very soiled.
- Dry hands thoroughly by patting with paper towels; discard paper towels into waste receptacle.
- Turn off water with a clean, dry paper towel, if indicated.*
- Clean area using dry paper towels only if indicated.*

Advantages of Alcohol-Based Hand Rubs (Foam or Gels)

- Kill bacteria and viruses more effectively and more quickly than hand-washing with soap and water.
- Less damaging to the skin than soap and water, resulting in less skin irritation.
- Requires less time than handwashing.
- Dispensers can be placed in more accessible areas.

Basic Steps for Alcohol-Based Hand Rubs

- Make sure there is no visible dirt or contamination.
- Apply ½ to 1 teaspoon of alcohol cleanser, either foam or gel, to one hand. Check the manufacturer's directions for proper amount.
- Rub your hands together vigorously, making sure all surfaces are covered.
- Continue rubbing until your hands are dry.

* Many facilities have sensors that turn water on automatically when the hands are lowered to the faucet. Other facilities have a knee or foot device that is used to turn the water on.

TABLE B-1 Personal Protective Equipment (PPE) Practices

Type	When Used	Rules for Use
Gloves	For hand contact with blood, mucous membranes, and other potentially infectious materials or when nonintact skin is anticipated, when performing vascular access procedures, or when handling contaminated items or surfaces	• Does not replace handwashing • Perform hand hygiene before applying and after removing gloves • When removing gloves, do not touch the outside (contaminated) area of the gloves • Keep gloved hands away from the face • Avoid touching or adjusting other PPE • Remove if torn, and perform hand hygiene before putting on new gloves • Limit surfaces and items touched • Extend gloves over isolation gown cuffs

(Continued)

Gown	During procedures and patient care activities when contact of clothing/ exposed skin with blood/body fluids, secretions, or excretions is anticipated	• To put on gown
		  — Opening is in the back
		  — Secure at neck and waist
		• To remove gown
		  — Unfasten ties
		  — Peel gown away from neck and shoulder—do not touch outside
		  — Turn contaminated outside toward the inside
		  — Fold or roll into a bundle
		  — Discard

Mask	During patient care activities likely to generate splashes or sprays of blood, body fluids, secretions, or excretions	• Must fully cover nose and mouth
		• Respirator masks such as N95, N99, and N100 must be used for airborne precautions
		• To put on mask
		  — Place over nose, mouth, and chin
		  — Fit flexible nosepiece over nose bridge
		  — Secure on head with ties or elastic
		  — Adjust to fit
		• To remove mask
		  — Untie the bottom tie, then untie the top tie
		  — Remove from face—do not touch the outside
		  — Discard

Eye protection	During patient care activities likely to generate splashes or sprays of blood, body fluids, secretions, or excretions	• Goggles should fit snugly over and around the eyes
		• Personal glasses are not an acceptable substitute
		• Can use a face shield that protects face, nose, mouth, and eyes
		• Face shield should cover forehead, extend below chin, and wrap around side of face
		• Position goggles over eyes and secure to the head using the earpieces or headband
		• Position face shield over face and secure on brow with headband
		• Remove goggles or face shield
		  — Grasp ear or head pieces with ungloved hands
		  — Lift away from face—do not touch outside
		  — Place in designated receptacle for reprocessing or disposal

Isolation (Transmission-Based) Precautions*

There are three categories of Transmission-Based Precautions:

1. Contact Precautions
2. Droplet Precautions
3. Airborne Precautions

Transmission-Based Precautions are used when the route(s) of transmission is (are) not completely interrupted using Standard Precautions alone. For some diseases that have multiple routes of transmission (e.g., severe acute respiratory syndrome, SARS), more than one Transmission-Based Precautions category may be used. When used either singly or in combination, they are always used in addition to Standard Precautions.

Contact Precautions

Contact Precautions are intended to prevent transmission of infectious agents, including important microorganisms, which are spread by direct or indirect contact with the patient or the patient's environment. Certain infections require the use of Contact Precautions, including patients infected or colonized with multidrug-resistant organisms. Contact Precautions also apply where the presence of excessive wound drainage, fecal incontinence, or other discharges from the body suggest an increased potential for extensive environmental contamination and risk of transmission. A single-patient room is preferred for patients who require Contact Precautions. When a single-patient room is not available, consultation with infection control personnel is recommended to assess the various risks associated with other patient placement options (e.g., cohorting, keeping the patient with an existing roommate). In multipatient rooms, at least 3 feet of spatial separation between beds is advised to reduce the opportunities for inadvertent sharing of items between the infected/colonized patient and other patients. Healthcare personnel caring for patients on Contact Precautions wear a gown and gloves for all interactions that may involve contact with the patient or potentially contaminated areas in the patient's environment. Donning PPE upon room entry and discarding before exiting the patient room is done to contain pathogens, especially those that have been implicated in transmission through environmental contamination, such as vancomycin-resistant enterococci, *Clostridium difficile,* noroviruses, and other intestinal tract pathogens.

Droplet Precautions

Droplet Precautions are intended to prevent transmission of pathogens that are spread through close respiratory or mucous membrane contact with respiratory secretions. Because these pathogens do not remain infectious over long distances in a healthcare facility, special air handling and ventilation are not required to prevent droplet transmission. Infectious agents for which Droplet Precautions are indicated include pertussis, influenza virus, adenovirus, rhinovirus, *Neisseria meningitides*, and group A streptococcus (for the first 24 hours of antimicrobial therapy). A single-patient room is preferred for patients who require Droplet Precautions. When a single-patient room is not available, consultation with infection control personnel is recommended to assess the various risks associated with other patient placement options (e.g., cohorting, keeping the patient with an existing roommate). Spatial separation of at least 3 feet and drawing the curtain between patient beds is especially important for patients in multi-bed rooms with infections transmitted by the droplet route. Healthcare personnel wear a mask (a respirator is not necessary) for close contact with infectious patients; the mask is generally donned upon room entry. Patients on Droplet Precautions who must be transported outside of the room should wear a mask if tolerated and follow respiratory hygiene/cough etiquette.

Airborne Precautions

Airborne Precautions prevent transmission of infectious agents that remain infectious over long distances when suspended in the air (e.g., rubeola virus [measles], varicella virus [chickenpox], *M. tuberculosis*, and possibly SARS-CoV). The preferred placement for patients who require Airborne Precautions is in an airborne infection isolation room (AIIR). An AIIR is a single-patient room that is equipped with special air handling and ventilation capacity that meet the American Institute of Architects/Facility Guidelines Institute (AIA/FGI) standards for AIIRs. Some states require the availability of such rooms in hospitals, emergency departments, and nursing homes that care for patients with *Mycobacterium tuberculosis*. A respiratory protection program that includes education about use of respirators, fit-testing, and user seal checks is required in any facility with AIIRs. In settings where Airborne Precautions cannot be implemented due to limited engineering resources (e.g., physician offices), masking the patient, placing the patient in a private room (e.g., office examination room) with the door closed, and providing N95 or higher level respirators or masks if respirators are not available for healthcare personnel will reduce the likelihood of airborne transmission until the patient is either transferred to a facility with an AIIR or returned to the home environment, as deemed medically appropriate. Healthcare personnel caring for patients on Airborne Precautions wear a mask or respirator mask that is donned prior to room entry. Whenever possible, nonimmune healthcare workers should not care for patients with vaccine-preventable airborne diseases (e.g., measles, chickenpox, and smallpox).

Applications of Transmission-Based Precautions

Diagnosis of many infections requires laboratory confirmation. Since laboratory tests, especially those that depend on culture techniques, often require two or more days for completion, Transmission-Based Precautions must be implemented while test results are pending based on the clinical presentation and likely pathogens. Use of appropriate Transmission-Based Precautions at the time a patient develops symptoms or signs of transmissible infection, or arrives at a healthcare facility for care, reduces transmission opportunities.

Discontinuation of Transmission-Based Precautions

Transmission-Based Precautions remain in effect for limited periods of time (i.e., while the risk for transmission of the infectious agent persists or for the duration of the illness. For some diseases (e.g., pharyngeal or cutaneous diphtheria, respiratory syncytial virus, RSV), Transmission-Based Precautions remain in effect until culture or antigen-detection test results document eradication of the pathogen and, for RSV, symptomatic disease is resolved. For other diseases (e.g., *M. tuberculosis*), state laws/regulations and healthcare facility policies may dictate the duration of precautions. In immunocompromised patients, viral shedding can persist for prolonged periods of time (many weeks to months) and transmission to others may occur during that time; therefore, the duration of contact and/or droplet precautions may be prolonged for many weeks.

Application of Transmission-Based Precautions in Ambulatory and Home Care Settings

Although Transmission-Based Precautions generally apply in all healthcare settings, exceptions exist. For example, in home care, AIIRs are not available. Furthermore, family members already exposed to diseases such as varicella and tuberculosis would not use masks or respiratory protection, but visiting phlebotomists or other healthcare workers would need to use such protection. Similarly, management of patients colonized or infected with multidrug-resistant organisms may necessitate Contact Precautions in acute-care hospitals and in some long-term care facilities when there is continued transmission, but the risk of transmission in ambulatory care and home care has not been defined. Consistent use of Standard Precautions may suffice in these settings, but more information is needed.

Adapted from Centers for Disease Control Guidelines for Isolation Precautions 2007 (www.cdc.gov).

Medical Abbreviations, Acronyms, and Symbols

The following are common medical abbreviations, acronyms, and symbols. Always check the facility where you are employed for the acceptable medical abbreviations, acronyms, and symbols used. Avoid using abbreviations and symbols designated as Do Not Use by The Joint Commission (TJC) or Error-Prone as designated by the Institute for Safe Medication Practices.

Medical Abbreviation	Term
Numbers	
1°	First degree
2°	Second degree
2de	Two-dimensional echocardiography
3°	Third degree
A	
a k amputation	Above the knee amputation
A&OX3	Alert and oriented to person, place, and date
a&w	Alive and well
a-line	Arterial line
a-p	Anterior and posterior
a-p&lat	Anteroposterior and lateral
a-v	Atrioventricular
a/n or abnl	Abnormal
a/o	Alert and oriented

(Continued)

Medical Abbreviation	Term
AAA	Abdominal aortic aneurysm
ABG	Arterial blood gas
AC	Before eating or meal
ACLS	Advanced cardiac life support
ad lib	Ad libitim (as desired)
ADAT	Advance diet as tolerated
AEA	Above elbow amputation
AF	Atrial fibrillation
Afl or a flutter	Atrial flutter
Agit	Agitation
AHHD	Arteriosclerotic hypertensive heart disease
AICD	Automatic implanted cardiac defibrillator
AIDS	Acquired immunodeficiency syndrome
AIMI	Anteroinferior myocardial infarction
AIVR	Accelerated idioventricular rhythm
AKA	Above the knee amputation
Amb	Ambulate
AODM	Adult-onset diabetes mellitus
Appt	Appointment
Apw	Aortopulmonary window
ARDS	Acute respiratory distress syndrome
ARF	Acute renal failure
AS	Aortic stenosis
ASAP	As soon as possible
ASCVD or ASCVHD	Atherosclerotic cardiovascular disease
ASD	Atrial septal defect
ASHD	Atherosclerotic heart disease
ASHVD	Atherosclerotic hypertensive vascular disease
ASMI	Anteroseptal myocardial infaction

ASVD	Arteriorsclerotic vascular disease
ASVHD	Arteriosclerotic vascular heart disease
AVS	Arteriovenous shunt
AV	Atrioventricular
AWMI	Anterior wall myocardial infarction
B	
BBB	Bundle branch block
BID	Twice a day
bil	Bilateral
BKA	Below the knee amputation
BP or b/p	Blood pressure
BPM or bpm	Beats per minute
BRP	Bathroom privileges
BS	Bowel or breath sounds
BW	Body weight
Bx	Biopsy
C	
c̄	With
C&S	Culture and sensitivity
CA	Cancer
CABG	Coronary artery bypass graft
CAD	Coronary artery disease
CAT	Computerized axial tomography
CBC	Complete blood count
CBG	Capillary blood gas
CC	Chief complaint
CCU	Cardiac care unit
CF	Cystic fibrosis
CHB	Complete heart block
CHF	Congestive heart failure

(Continued)

Medical Abbreviation	Term
CI	Cardiac index
CNS	Central nervous system
CO	Cardiac output
c/o	Complaining of
COLD	Chronic obstructive lung disease
COPD	Chronic obstructive pulmonary disease
CP	Chest pain
CPAP	Continuous positive airway pressure
CPK	Creatine phosphokinase
CPK-mb	Creatine phosphokinase myocardial band
CPR	Cardiopulmonary resuscitation
CRF	Chronic renal failure
CT	Computerized tomography
CVA	Cerebrovascular accident
CVC	Central venous catheter
CVHD	Cardiovascular heart disease
CVP	Central venous pressure
CXR	Chest x-ray
D	
DAT	Diet as tolerated
DDx	Differential diagnosis
D5W	5% dextrose in water
DI	Diabetes insipidus
DIC	Disseminated intravascular coagulopathy
DIG	Digoxin
DJD	Degenerative joint disease
DKA	Diabetic ketoacidosis

DM	Diabetes mellitus
DNR	Do not resuscitate
DOA	Dead on arrival
d/s	Discharge summary
DOB	Date of birth
DOD	Date of discharge
DOE	Dyspnea on exertion
DTR	Deep tendon reflexes
DVT	Deep venous thrombosis
DX or Dx	Diagnosis
E	
EBL	Estimated blood loss
ECG or EKG	Electrocardiogram
ET	Endotracheal
ETT	Endotracheal tube
ETOH	Ethanol
Eval	Evaluation
F	
FBS	Fasting blood sugar
FEV	Forced expiratory volume
FTT	Failure to thrive
FU	Follow-up
FUO	Fever of unknown origin
fekg	Fetal electrocardiogram
fem pop, fem-pop, or fem/pop	Femoral popliteal
Fx	Fracture

(Continued)

Medical Abbreviation	Term
G	
GI	Gastrointestinal
Gr	Grain; 1 grain = 60 to 65 mg
GSW	Gun shot wound
gt or gtt	Drops
GTT	Glucose tolerance test
GU	Genitourinary
GXT	Graded exercise tolerance (stress test)
H	
HA	Headache
HAV	Hepatitis A virus
HBP	High blood pressure
HCT	Hematocrit
HDL	High density lipoprotein
HEENT	Head, eyes, ears, nose, throat
Hep A	Hepatitis A
Hep B	Hepatitis B
Hep lock or hep-lock	Heparin lock
Hgb	Hemoglobin
H/H	Hemoglobin/hematocrit
HIV	Human immunodeficiency virus
HO	History of
HOB	Head of bed
HOH	Hard of hearing
HPI	History of present illness
HR	Heart rate
HSV	Herpes simplex virus
HTN	Hypertension
Hx	History

I	
I&D	Incision and drainage
IASD	Interatrial septal defect
I&O	Intake and output
ICS	Intercostal space
ICU	Intensive care unit
IPPB	Intermittent positive pressure breathing
ID	Infectious disease or identification
IDDM	Insulin-dependent diabetes mellitus
IHSS	Idiopathic hypertropic subaortic stenosis
IM	Intramuscular
IMCU	Intermediate medical care unit
IMV	Intermittent mandatory ventilation
INF	Intravenous nutritional fluid
IPPB	Intermittent positive pressure breathing
IRBBB	Incomplete right bundle branch block
IRDM	Insulin-resistant diabetes mellitus
ITP	Idiopathic thrombocytopenic purpura
IV	Intravenous
IVC	Inferior vena cava
IVP	Intravenous pyelogram
IWMI	Inferior wall myocardial infarction
J	
JODM	Juvenile-onset diabetes mellitus
JVD	Jugular venous distention
K	
KOR	Keep open rate
KVO	Keep vein open

(Continued)

Medical Abbreviation	Term
L	
L	Left
LAD	Left axis deviation or left anterior descending
LAE	Left atrial enlargement
LAHB	Left anterior hemiblock
LAP	Left atrial pressure
LBBB	Left bundle branch block
LLL	Left lower lobe
LMP	Last menstrual period
LOC	Loss of consciousness or level of consciousness
LP	Lumbar puncture
LPN	Licensed practical nurse
LUL	Left upper lobe
LUQ	Left upper quadrant
LV	Left ventricle
LVAD	Left ventricular assist device
LVEDP	Left ventricular end diastolic pressure
LVF	Left ventricular failure
LVH	Left ventricular hypertrophy
LWMI	Lateral wall myocardial infarction
M	
MAP	Mean arterial pressure
MAST	Medical antishock trousers
MI	Myocardial infarction or mitral insufficiency
mL	Milliliter
mm	Millimeter
MLE	Midline episiotomy

MRI	Magnetic resonance imaging
MRSA	Methicillin-resistant *Staphylococcus aureus*
msec	Millisecond
MSSA	Methicillin-sensitive *Staphylococcus aureus*
MVA	Motor vehicle accident
N	
n&v, n + v, or n/v	Nausea and vomiting
n/a	Not applicable
NAD	No active disease
NAS	No added salt
NCV	Nerve conduction velocity
NED	No evidence of recurrent disease
NG	Nasogastric
NGT	Nasogastric tube
NIDDM	Non-insulin-dependent diabetes mellitus
NKA	No known allergies
NKDA	No known drug allergies
NMR	Nuclear magnetic resonance
NPO	Nothing by mouth
NRM	No regular medication
NSAID	Non-steroidal anti-inflammatory drugs
NSR	Normal sinus rhythm
NT	Nasotracheal
NTG	Nitroglycerine
O	
OD	Overdose
OOB	Out of bed
OR	Operating room

(Continued)

Medical Abbreviation	Term
P	
P	Para
PA	Posteroanterior
PAC	Premature atrial contraction
PaO_2	Peripheral arterial oxygen content
PAP	Pulmonary artery pressure
PAT	Paroxysmal atrial tachycardia
PC	After eating
PCWP	Pulmonary capillary wedge pressure
PDA	Patent ductus arteriosus
PDR	*Physicians' Desk Reference*
PE	Pulmonary embolus, or physical exam, or pleural effusion
PEEP	Positive end expiratory pressure
PFT	Pulmonary function tests
PI	Pulmonic insufficiency disease
PMH	Previous medical history
PMI	Point of maximal impulse
PND	Paroxysmal nocturnal dyspnea
Pneumo	Pneumothorax
PO	By mouth
POD	Post-op day
PP	Postprandial
PR	By rectum
PRBC	Packed red blood cells
Pre-op or preop	Preoperative
PRN	As needed
PS	Pulmonic stenosis
PSVT	Paroxysmal supraventricular tachycardia
PT	Prothrombin time or physical therapy

Pt	Patient
PTCA	Percutaneous transluminal coronary angioplasty
PTT	Partial thromboplastin time
PUD	Peptic ulcer disease
PVC	Premature ventricular contraction
PVD	Peripheral vascular disease
PVI	Peripheral vascular insufficiency
PVT	Paroxysmal ventricular tachycardia
PEMI	Posterior wall myocardial infarction
PWP	Pulmonary wedge pressure
Q	
q	Every
qh	Every hour
q4h, q6h, . . .	Every 4 hours, every 6 hours, etc.
qid	Four times a day
QNS	Quantity not sufficient
R	
R	Right
RA	Rheumatoid arthritis or right atrium
RAD	Right atrial axis deviation
RAE	Right atrial enlargement
RAP	Right atrial pressure
RBBB	Right bundle branch block
RBC	Red blood cell
RDA	Recommended daily allowance
RLL	Right lower lobe
RML	Right middle lobe
R/O	Rule out
ROM	Range of motion

(Continued)

Medical Abbreviation	Term
ROS	Review of systems
RRR	Regular rate and rhythm
RT	Respiratory or radiation therapy
r/t	Related to
RTC	Return to clinic
RUL	Right upper lobe
RV	Residual volume
RVH	Right ventricular hypertrophy
Rx	Treatment
Rxn	Reaction
S	
s̄	Without
s̄s̄	One-half
s/s	Signs and symptoms
SA	Sinoatrial
SBE	Subacute bacterial endocarditis
SEM	Systolic ejection murmur
SG	Swan-Ganz
SGA	Small for gestational age
SICU	Surgical intensive care unit
sig	Write on label
SIMV	Synchronous intermittent mandatory ventilation
sl	Sublingual
SOAP	Subjective, objective, assessment, plan
SOB	Shortness of breath
SR	Sinus rhythm
Subcut	Subcutaneous
ST	Sinus tachycardia
stat	Immediate

SVT	Supraventricular tachycardia
Synch	Synchronized
Syst	Systolic
Sx	Symptoms
T	
TB	Tuberculosis
TIA	Transient ischemic attack
tid	Three times a day
TKO	To keep open
TLC	Total lung capacity
TNTC	Too numerous to count
TO	Telephone order
TPN	Total parenteral nutrition
TV	Tidal volume
tw	Twice a week
TX	Treatment, transplant
U	
ud	As directed
UGI	Upper gastrointestinal
URI	Upper respiratory infection
US	Ultrasound
V	
V1	Chest lead I
V2	Chest lead II
V3	Chest lead III
V4	Chest lead IV
V5	Chest lead V

(Continued)

Medical Abbreviation	Term
V6	Chest lead VI
VC	Vital capacity
VO	Verbal or voice order
V/Q	Ventilation-perfusion
VS	Vital signs
VSS	Vital signs stable
VT	Ventricular tachycardia
VF or vfib	Ventricular fibrillation
W	
WD	Well developed
WF	White female
WM	White male
WN	Well nourished
WNL	Within normal limits
WPW	Wolff-Parkinson-White
X	
XRT	X-ray therapy
Y	
yo	Years old

The Joint Commission has determined that the following abbreviations should not be used and are prone to errors. Although you may need to recognize these abbreviations, they should not be used in healthcare practice to avoid errors.

Abbreviation	Potential Problem	Preferred Term
U (for unit)	Mistaken as zero, four, or cc	Write "unit"
IU (for international unit)	Mistaken as IV (intravenous) or 10 (ten)	Write "international unit"
Q.D., QD, qd, q.d., Q.O.D., QOD, q.o.d, qod (Latin abbreviation for once daily and every other day)	Mistaken for each other. The period after the Q can be mistaken for an "I" and the "O" can be mistaken for "I"	Write "daily" and "every other day"
Trailing zero (X.0 mg), Lack of leading zero (.X mg)	Decimal point is missed	Never write a zero by itself after a decimal point (X mg), and always use a zero before a decimal point (0.X mg)
MS MSO_4 $MgSO_4$	Confused for one another; can mean morphine sulfate or magnesium sulfate	Write "morphine sulfate" or "magnesium sulfate"

Other Abbreviations, Acronyms, and Symbols to Avoid

μg (for microgram)	Mistaken for mg (milligrams) resulting in one thousand-fold dosing overdose	Write "mcg"
c.c. (for cubic centimeter)	Mistaken for U (units) when poorly written	Write "mL" for milliliters
> (greater than) < (less than)	Misinterpreted as the number "7" or the letter "L"; confused for one another	Write "greater than" and "less than"
Abbreviations for drug names	Misinterpreted due to similar abbreviations for multiple drugs	Write drug names in full
Apothecary units	Unfamiliar to many practitioners Confused with metric units	Use metric units
@	Mistaken for the number "2" (two)	Write "at"
H.S. (for half-strength or Latin abbreviation for bedtime)	Mistaken for either half-strength or hour of sleep (at bedtime) q.H.S. mistaken for every hour. All can result in a dosing error	Write out "half-strength" or "at bedtime"
T.I.W. (for three times a week)	Mistaken for three times a day or twice weekly, resulting in an overdose	Write "3 times weekly" or "three times weekly"
S.C. or S.Q. (for subcutaneous)	Mistaken as SL for sublingual, or "5 every"	Write Subcut, or "subcutaneously"
D/C (for discharge)	Interpreted as discontinue whatever medications follow (typically discharge meds)	Write "discharge"
A.S., A.D., A.U. (Latin abbreviation for left, right, or both ears) O.S., O.D., O.U. (Latin abbreviation for left, right, or both eyes)	Mistaken for each other (e.g., AS for OS, AD for OD, AU for OU, etc.)	Write: "left ear," "right ear" or "both ears;" "left eye," "right eye," or "both eyes

Appendix D

Correlation of Textbook Learning Outcomes to Certification Standards

National Healthcareer Association (NHA) EKG Technician Correlation Chart

Areas of Competencies	Learning Outcomes
I. Describe the Cardiovascular System	2.2, 2.3, 2.5, 13.1
a. Locate the heart and surrounding structures.	2.2
b. Diagram and label the parts of the heart and list the functions of each labeled part.	2.2, 13.1
c. Trace the flow of blood through the cardiopulmonary system.	2.3
d. Identify and describe the electrical conduction system.	2.5
II. Identify Legal and Ethical Responsibilities	1.5, 3.4, 3.5, 4.2, 4.9, 5.3, 7.6, 11.4, 12.4, 13.6
a. Recognize and practice legal and ethical responsibilities as they relate to an EKG aide.	1.5, 3.5, 4.2, 5.3, 7.6, 11.4, 12.4, 13.6
b. Maintain a safe and efficient work environment.	1.5, 3.5, 4.2, 5.3
c. Maintain EKG equipment so it will be safe and accurate.	1.5, 3.4, 4.9
III. Demonstrate Knowledge of, Apply, and Use Medical Instrumentation Modalities	3.1, 3.3, 3.5, 4.4, 4.6, 4.7, 4.10, 4.12, 5.2–5.6, 6.7
a. Calibrate and standardize the cardiograph instrument.	3.3, 3.5, 4.6
b. Identify three types of lead systems.	3.1
c. State Einthoven's triangle.	3.1
d. Demonstrate proper lead placement including lead placement for patients with special needs.	3.1, 4.4, 4.10, 4.12
e. Identify artifacts and mechanical problems.	4.7
f. Perform a 12-lead EKG.	4.6
g. Recognize normal sinus rhythm.	5.2, 5.3
h. Report any rhythm that is not normal sinus rhythm.	5.4, 5.5–5.7
i. Recognize a cardiac emergency as seen on the EKG.	5.7
j. Use documentation skills to identify electrocardiographs.	5.4, 5.5–5.7
IV. Perform Patient Care Techniques in the Healthcare Facility	1.4, 1.5, 4.1, 4.5, 6.4–6.6, 11.1, 11.4, 11.5, 12.4, 12.5, 13.6
a. Describe the physical and mental preparation of the patient for EKG testing.	1.5, 4.1, 11.4, 12.4, 12.5
b. Identify patient and verify the requisition order.	1.5, 4.1, 11.4
c. Prepare patient for EKG testing.	1.5, 4.1, 11.4, 12.4, 12.5

Areas of Competencies	Learning Outcomes
d. Measure and record patient's vital signs and recognize and report abnormalities.	1.4, 6.4–6.6, 11.1, 13.6
e. State precautions required when performing an EKG.	1.5, 4.5, 11.5
f. Demonstrate understanding of the chain of infection.	1.5, 4.5
V. Recognize Normal and Abnormal Monitoring and Testing Results	3.6, 5.2–5.7, 6.1–6.6, 7.1–7.6, 8.1–8.5, 9.1–9.8, 10.1–10.4, 14.1–14.5
a. Measure waves, segments, complexes, rates, and intervals.	3.6, 5.2–5.7, 6.2–6.6, 7.2–7.6, 8.2–8.5, 9.2–9.8, 10.2–10.4, 14.2, 14.4, 14.5
b. Identify electrical axis.	14.3
c. List purposes for pacemakers and indications for insertion.	10.1
d. Recognize normal and deviations from normal sinus rhythms.	5.3–5.7
e. Recognize normal and deviations from normal atrial rhythms.	6.1–6.6
f. Recognize normal and deviations from normal atrioventicular rhythms.	7.1–7.6
g. Recognize normal and deviations from normal ventricular rhythms.	9.1–9.8
h. Recognize normal and deviations from normal types of heart blocks.	8.1–8.4
i. Recognize normal and deviations from normal pacemaker rhythms.	5.3, 10.1, 10.3
j. Recognize normal and deviations from normal types of myocardial ischemia and infarction.	14.2
k. Recognize normal and deviations from normal 12-lead EKG results.	14.1–14.5
l. Recognize and describe AV block.	8.1–8.4, 14.4
VI. Describe Cardiovascular Drugs, Their Actions, Use, and Adverse Effects	5.2, 11.3, 11.4, 13.5, 13.6, Appendix A
a. Describe mechanisms by which cardiovascular drugs work.	13.6, Appendix A
b. List common cardiovascular drugs.	11.4, 13.6, Appendix A
c. Identify and respond to cardiac emergency.	13.5, 13.6, Appendix A
d. State actions and adverse effects of commonly used cardiovascular drugs.	5.2, 11.3, 11.4, Appendix A
e. Differentiate between normal and abnormal EKG changes due to drugs.	11.3, 13.6, Appendix A
f. State reasons for pharmacological stress testing.	11.3, Appendix A
VII. Demonstrate Knowledge of Other Cardiovascular Diagnostic Modalities	11.1–11.3, 11.7, 12.1–12.3, 13.3, 13.4, 13.6, 13.7, 14.2–14.5
a. Describe the Holter monitoring and scanning exercise treatment.	12
b. Describe other modalities of cardiovascular diagnosis and interpretation.	11, 13, 14

Cardiovascular Credentialing International (CCI) Certified Cardiographic Technician Correlation

A. Basic Cardiovascular Anatomy and Physiology	Learning Outcomes
I. Heart	2.2
a. Size	2.2
b. Location	2.2
c. Layers	2.2
1. Pericardium	2.2
2. Epicardium	2.2
3. Myocardium	2.2
4. Endocardium	2.2
d. Chambers	2.2
1. Atrial	2.2
2. Ventricular	2.2
e. Valves	2.2
1. Semilunar	2.2
2. Atrioventricular	2.2
II. Heart and Coronary Circulation	2.3, 13.1
a. Blood flow	2.3, 13.1
1. Through the heart	2.2
2. Systemic through the body	2.2
3. Coronary Arterial	2.3, 2.6, 13.2, 14.2–14.5
a. Myocardial wall distribution	2.3
b. Ischemic changes	2.6, 13.2, 14.2
c. Patterns of injury	14.2–14.5
d. Infarction types	14.2
4. Right and left oxygen saturations	2.2
b. Arteries (major)	2.2, 2.3
1. Systemic	2.2
2. Coronary	2.2, 2.3
c. Veins	2.2, 2.3
1. Major systemic	2.2
2. Coronary	2.2, 2.3
d. Capillaries	2.3
e. Arterioles	2.3
f. Venules	2.3
III. Physiology	2.2–2.6, 5.2, Appendix A
a. Cardiac valve function	2.2
b. Pressures	2.5, Appendix F
1. Determination of mean pressure	2.5, Appendix F
2. Blood pressure	2.5, Appendix F
a. Measurement	2.5, Appendix F
b. Pulse pressure determination	2.5, Appendix F
3. Aortic pulse pressure	2.5, Appendix F
4. Pressure difference in the right and left heart	2.4
c. Cardiac output (relationship to)	2.3, Appendix F
1. Heart rate	2.3, Appendix F
2. Stroke volume	2.3, Appendix F

A. Basic Cardiovascular Anatomy and Physiology	Learning Outcomes
d. Control Mechanisms	2.3, Appendix A
1. Blood pressure	2.3, Appendix F
2. Cardiac output	12.3, Appendix F
3. Peripheral resistance	Appendix A, Appendix F
4. Baroreceptors/chemoreceptors	Appendix F
5. Compliance	Appendix F
6. Preload	Appendix F
7. Afterload	Appendix E
8. Contractility	2.5
e. Cardiac Cycle	2.2–2.6, 5.2, 5.3
1. Relationship to the EKG	2.5, 5.2
2. Relationship to heart sounds	2.4
3. Relationship to valve opening and closure	2.2, 2.3
f. Normal values	2.6, 5.3
1. Measurement sites of heart rate	2.5, 5.2
2. Blood pressure	2.5
IV. Conduction System	2.5
a. Nodes	2.5
b. Pathway	2.5
c. Blood supply	2.3, 2.5
d. Heart rate	2.5
1. Factors affecting heart rate	2.5
2. Blood pressure	2.5, Appendix F
V. Anatomical Terms	Appendix E
a. Definition and position of:	Appendix E
1. Anterior –ventral	Appendix E
2. Posterior –dorsal	Appendix E
3. Superior	Appendix E
4. Inferior	Appendix E
5. Medial	Appendix E
6. Lateral	Appendix E
7. External	Appendix E
8. Internal	Appendix E
9. Superficial	Appendix E
10. Distal	Appendix E
11. Sagittal	Appendix E
12. Peripheral	Appendix E
13. Visceral	Appendix E
14. Parietal	Appendix E
15. Transverse or horizontal	Appendix E
16. Proximal	Appendix E

B. ECG Techniques and Recognition	Learning Outcomes
I. Define, identify, measure, explain and analyze:	3.3, 3.6, 5.2, 11.2, 13.4, 14.2
a. Waveforms	3.3, 3.6
1. P, Q, R, S, and T waves	3.6
2. Baseline values	3.3, 3.6
3. Normal sinus rhythm	5.3
b. ECG Measurement	3.6, 5.2, 11.2, 13.4, 14.2

(Continued)

B. ECG Techniques and Recognition	Learning Outcomes
1. Time	3.6
2. Heart rate	3.6
3. Voltage	3.6, 5.2
4. Axis/hexaxial system	3.3
5. Intervals	3.6, 5.2
6. Segments	5.2
7. Complexes	3.6, 5.2
8. Normal and abnormal ST segment	5.2, 11.2, 13.4, 14.2
II. ECG Leads	3.1
a. Bipolar leads	3.1
b. Umpolar leads	3.1
c. Precordial leads	3.1
d. Einthoven's triangle and law	3.1
III. ECG, Holter, and Stress Testing Instrumentation	1.6, 3.2, 3.3, 4.6, 4.7, 4.10, 4.12, 11.4, 12.6, 12.7
a. ECG calibration methods	3.3
b. Single channel	3.2
c. Three channel	3.2, 4.12
d. Troubleshooting	1.6, 4.7, 11.4
e. Paper speed	3.3, 4.10, 12.6, 12.7
IV. Recognition of Recording Errors	3.2–3.4, 4.4, 4.6, 4.12
a. Incorrect standardization	4.6
b. Incorrect paper speed	4.6
c. Lead reversals	3.3, 4.12
d. Incorrect lead placement	3.4, 4.4
V. Recognition of Recording Artifacts	4.7
a. Electrical interference	4.7
b. Somatic tremor	4.7
c. Wandering baseline	4.7
d. Other causes	4.7
VI. Patient and Electrical Safety Hazards of Electrical Apparatus	4.5
a. Common hazards (broken cords, plugs, and sockets)	4.5
b. Subtle hazards (current leakage)	4.5
c. Ground connectors	4.5
d. Pacemaker hazards	4.5
e. Electrical shock	4.5
VII. Distinguish, Interpret, and Describe:	5, 6, 7, 8, 9, 10 (entire chapters)
a. Recognition of Cardiac Arrhythmias	5, 6, 7, 8, 9, 10
1. Sinus arrhythmias	5.3–5.7
2. Sinus bradycardia	5.4
3. Sinus tachycardia	5.5
4. Atrial arrhythmias/PSVT	6 (entire chapter)
5. Ventricular arrhythmias	9 (entire chapter)
6. AV disassociation/aberration	7 (entire chapter)
7. SA Blocks/sinus pause	5.7
8. Bundle branch block	10.6–10.8
9. Heart blocks	8 (entire chapter)
a. First degree block	8.2

b. Second degree block	8.3, 8.4
i. Type I	8.3
ii. Type II	8.4
10. Third degree block	8.5
11. Cardiac pacemakers	2.5, 10.3
12. Wolff-Parkinson White	
13. ST segment and T wave alterations	5.2, 11.2, 13.4, 14.2
14. Ambulatory electrocardiography artifacts	12.1
b. Recognition and Interpretation of Normal and Abnormal 12-lead Electrocardiogram	14 (entire chapter)
15. Myocardial infarction	14.2
a. Injury	14.2
b. Ischemia	14.2

C. Basic Cardiovascular Electrophysiology	**Learning Outcomes**
Define, Identify, and Explain:	2, 3, 4
I. Basic Electrophysiology	2.4–2.6, 9.2
a. Cardiac cycle	2.4
b. Electrical conduction system	2.5
c. Refractory	9.2
d. Transmembrane potential	2.6
1. Polarization	2.6
2. Depolarization	2.6
3. Repolarization	2.6
e. Action potential	2.6
1. Phase 0	
2. Phase 1	
3. Phase 2	
4. Phase 3	
5. Phase 4	

D. Stress Test Techniques, Indications, and Contraindications	**Learning Outcomes**
I. Stress Testing	11 (entire chapter)
a. Indications	11.2, 11.3
b. Contraindications	11.3
c. Protocols	11.7
1. Bruce	11.7
2. Modified Bruce	11.7
3. Naughton	11.7
d. Prep techniques	11.4
e. Test interpretation	11.8
f. Calculation	11.7
1. Double product	11.7
2. METs	11.7
g. Bicycle procedures	11.6
h. Thallium/Muga stress test	11.3
II. Interpretation of the Exercise ECG	11.8
III. Ergometers	11.6
a. Arms	11.6
b. Leg	11.6
c. Treadmill	11.6

(Continued)

IV. Pharmacologic	11.3, Appendix A
a. Dipyridamole	11.3, Appendix A
b. Dobutamine	11.3, Appendix A
c. Thallium	11.3, Appendix A
d. Cardiolyte	11.3, Appendix A
E. Holter Monitoring	**Learning Outcomes**
I. Concepts of Holter Monitoring	12 (entire chapter)
a. Indications	12.1
b. Contraindications	12–2
c. Preparation techniques	12.5
d. Lead placement	12.6
e. Interpretation	12.1, 12.7
1. Recognition of artifact	12.1
2. Advanced ECO interpretation	12.3
F. Cardiac Medications	**Learning Outcomes**
I. Categories	1.4, 2.6, 5.2, 11.4, 13.6, Appendix A
a. Antihypertensives	Appendix A
b. Nitrates	Appendix A
c. Calcium Channel Blockers	Appendix A
d. Beta Blockers	11.4, 13.6, Appendix A
e. Cardiac Olycosides	Appendix A
f. Antiarrhythmics	1.4, 2.6, 5.2
II. Indications	11.2–11.4, 13.6, Appendix A
a. Effect on heart rate	11.2, Appendix A
b. Effect on blood pressure	11.4, 13.6
c. Correlation to arrhythmias	11.2
d. Routes of administration	11.3
e. Emergency cardiac medications	13.6, Appendix A
1. Epinephrine	Appendix A
2. Atropine	Appendix A
3. Verapamil	Appendix A
4. Lidocaine	Appendix A
5. Oxygen	13.6
6. Isuprel	Appendix A

CCI Certified Rhythm Analysis Technician (CRAT) Content Outline

	CRAT Duties and Tasks	Required Knowledge	Learning Outcomes
A	Complying with Governing Regulations	5%	
A.1	Obtain/maintain prescriptions/orders	Communication skills; Documentation protocol; Federal guidelines (e.g., Medicare, HIPAA)	1.5, 4.1, 11.4, 13.6
A.2	Maintain HIPAA compliance		1.5
A.3	Obtain patient demographics		1.5, 4.1, 13.6
A.4	Verify patient identification		1.5, 3.3, 4.2, 11.4
B	Interacting with Patients and Others	10%	
B.1	Familiarize patients regarding services	Adhesive sensitivity; Chain of command; Communicate discrepancies; Communicate with appropriate departments; Customer service; Documentation protocol; Electrodes; Emergency protocols; Function of monitor; How to protect the monitor from water damage; How to respond to discrepancies; Identification of paced rhythms; Medical terminology; Monitor types (e.g., Holter, Event, Transtelephonic, Ambulatory Cardiac Telemetry); Notification criteria; Symptoms as they relate to arrhythmias; Types of monitor malfunctions; Use of patient diary	1.5, 4.2, 4.10, 11.3, 11.4, 12.4
B.2	Educate patients on when to call for help		11.3, 11.5
B.3	Educate patients on electrical hazards, broken wires		3.4, 4.5, 11.5, 12.4
B.4	Obtain patient symptoms, activities, location		4.1, 11.4
B.5	Service cardiac patients (customer service)		4.11, 4.13, 13.6, 13.7
B.6	Communicate with ordering physician or physician's office		4.1, 11.5, 11.6
B.7	Communicate with patients' family members		1.5, 1.6, 4.10
B.8	Communicate with other offices (scheduling, order verification, etc.)		4.1, 4.8, 12.7
B.9	Seek advice regarding findings		4.8, 11.8
B.10	Conduct interdepartmental interactions		4.8, 12.7
C	Identify Normal ECG Components and Cardiac Anatomy	19%	
C.1	Identify P-wave	Basic understanding of heart anatomy and physiology; ECG interpretation; Identification of paced rhythms; Lead placements; Waveform intervals	3.5, 5.2
C.2	Identify and measure the PR interval		3.5, 5.2
C.3	Identify and measure a QRS complex		3.5, 5.2
C.4	Identify T-wave		3.5, 5.2
C.5	Identify the standards for ECG recording		3.1, 4.4–4.13
C.6	Calculate the atrial rate		5.2
C.7	Calculate the ventricular rate		5.2
C.8	Identify the relationship of the atrial and ventricular rates		5.2
C.9	Evaluate P-P and R-R interval regularity		5.2

(Continued)

	CRAT Duties and Tasks	Required Knowledge	Learning Outcomes
C.10	Identify the chambers of the heart		2.2
C.11	Identify the valves of the heart		2.2
C.12	Identify the conduction system of the heart		2.5
D	Determine Patient's Cardiac Rhythm	55%	
D.1	Identify sinus rhythm	Appropriate leads for application; Basic math; Correct pacemaker TTM application; Correct event/ Holter monitor application; ECG interpretation; Electrode placement; Identification of paced rhythms; Lead placements; Symptoms as they relate to arrhythmias; Waveform intervals	5.3–5.7
D.1.a	Identify normal sinus rhythm		5.3
D.1.b	Identify sinus arrhythmia		5.6
D.1.c	Identify sinus tachycardia		5.5
D.1.d	Identify sinus bradycardia		5.4
D.1.e	Identify sinus arrest		5.7
D.2	Identify atrial rhythm		6.1
D.2.a	Identify wandering atrial pacemaker		6.3
D.2.b	Identify rhythms with premature atrial ectopy (PAC, Couplets, Triplets, Runs, Multifocal)		6.2
D.2.c	Identify atrial tachycardia		6.4
D.2.d	Identify supraventricular tachycardia		7.6
D.2.e	Identify atrial fibrillation (general characteristics)		6.6
D.2.e.1	Identify atrial fibrillation with a slow ventricular response		6.6
D.2.e.2	Identify atrial fibrillation with a rapid ventricular response		6.6
D.2.f	Identify atrial flutter		6.5
D.2.f.1	Identify atrial flutter with a ratio of ventricular response		6.5
D.2.f.2	Identify atrial flutter with a variable ventricular response		6.5
D.3	Identify junctional rhythm		7.1
D.3.a	Identify rhythms with premature junctional ectopy		7.2
D.3.b	Identify junctional escape rhythms		7.3
D.3.c	Identify accelerated junctional rhythms		7.4
D.3.d	Identify junctional tachycardia		7.5
D.4	Recognize ventricular rhythms		9.1
D.4.a	Identify rhythm with premature ventricular ectopy (PVCs, Couplets, Triplets)		9.2

	CRAT Duties and Tasks	Required Knowledge	Learning Outcomes
D.4.b	Identify idioventricular rhythms (agonal, escape, and accelerated)		9.4
D.4.c	Identify ventricular tachycardia		9.6
D.4.d	Identify ventricular fibrillation		9.7
D.4.e	Identify ventricular standstill		9.7, 9.8
D.5	Recognize asystole		9.8
D.6	Recognize conduction defects		7.6, 8.1, 9.1
D.6.a	Identify first degree AV block		8.2
D.6.b	Identify second degree type one AV block		8.3
D.6.c	Identify second degree type two AV block		8.4
D.6.d	Identify third degree AV block		8.5
D.6.d.1	Identify third degree AV block with a junctional escape rhythm (narrow QRS)		8.5
D.6.d.2	Identify third degree AV block with a ventricular escape rhythm (wide QRS)		8.5
D.6.e	Identify presence of intraventricular conduction delay (Bundle Branch Block)		14.4
D.7	Determine paced events		10.3–10.6
D.7.a	Identify paced atrial rhythm		10.1
D.7.b	Identify paced ventricular rhythm		10.1
D.7.c	Identify AV sequential (atrioventricular) paced rhythm		10.1
D.7.d	Identify P-wave synchronous, ventricular paced rhythm		13.5
D.7.e	Identify loss of pacing capture		10.3
D.7.f	Identify loss of sensing		10.3
D.7.g	Identify failure to pace		10.3
E	Troubleshoot ECG	6%	
E.1	Recognize artifact on ECG tracings	Causes of interference; ECG interpretation; Electrode placement; Electromagnetic interference; Identification of paced rhythms; Lead placements; Monitor troubleshooting; Types of monitor malfunctions	3.3, 4.7
E.1.a	Recognize artifact on ECG tracings from wandering baseline		4.7
E.1.b	Recognize artifact on ECG tracings from somatic tremor, patient movement		4.7
E.1.c	Recognize artifact on ECG tracings from EMI/60 cycle interference		4.7

(Continued)

	CRAT Duties and Tasks	Required Knowledge	Learning Outcomes
E.2	Identify inappropriate electrocardiograph paper speed		3.3
E.3	Identify inappropriate gain of the ECG signal		3.3
E.4	Identify causes of artifact		3.3, 4.7
E.5	Identify lead reversals		3.3, 4.12
F	Compile ECG Results	5%	
F.1	Insert preliminary findings	Appropriate rhythm strips; Documentation protocol; Identification of paced rhythms; Medical terminology	4.8, 11.6, 12.7
F.2	Compare test results to past tests		3.2, 4.7
F.3	Respond if notification criteria are met (Dispatch EMS if needed)		6.4, 6.6, 7.3–7.5, 8.2, 8.4, 9.2–9.6, 10.3, 10.4, 11.5, 13.6, 13.7, 14.2
F.4	Correlate findings with patient symptoms or risk		4.7, 5.3
F.5	Create patient report		4.8, 11.6, 12.7
	Totals		**100%**

ECG Technician Certification Exam Content Outline National Center for Competency Testing ®

Approximate % of Exam	Content Categories	Learning Outcomes
32%	Medical Terminology	
	• Foundations	Appendix C, Glossary
	• Abbreviations	Appendix C
	• Cardiac and circulatory terms	2 (entire chapter)
26%	Anatomy and Physiology	
	• Structures (primarily cardiac and circulatory)	2.2, 2.5, 4.3, 13.1
	• Functions (primarily circulation and electrical conduction)	2.1, 2.3–2.5
24%	Rhythm	
	• Basic ECG concepts	3.1–3.4
	• Electrical heart functions (cardiac cycle)	2.4
	• Electrocardiography, including lead placement, safety, QC	3.5, 3.6, 4 (entire chapter)
18%	Basic Interpretations	
	• Scope of practice	1.4, 5.1, 7.6, 12.4
	• ECG strip analysis (P, Q, R, S, T wave interpretations)	3.6, 5.1, 5.2
	• Recognition of normal sinus rhythm, sinus bradycardia, and tachycardia	5.3–5.5
	• Troubleshooting; recognizing artifact, tracing problems	1.6, 4.7, 11.4, 12.3
	• Basic interpretation of common arrhythmias and blocks	5, 6, 7, 8, 9, 10 (entire chapters)
	• Recognize myocardial infarction	14.2
100%	Total	

Appendix E

Anatomical Terms

Anatomical terms are used to describe the location of body parts and various body regions. In order to correctly use these terms, it is assumed that the body is in the anatomical position. See Figures E-1 and E-2 and Table E-1.

Figure E-1   Directional terms provide mapping instructions for locating organs and body parts.

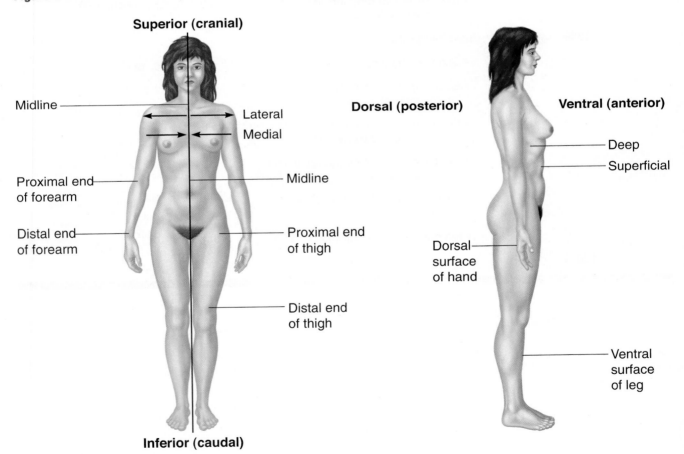

Figure E-2 Spatial terms are based on imaginary cuts or planes through the body.

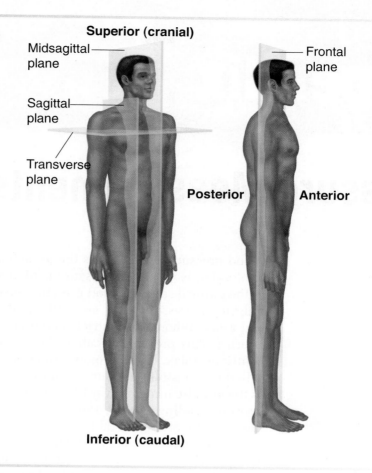

Superior (cranial)

Midsagittal plane

Sagittal plane

Transverse plane

Frontal plane

Posterior   Anterior

Inferior (caudal)

TABLE E-1   Anatomical Terms

Term	Definition
Anterior (ventral)	Toward the front of the body
Posterior (dorsal)	Toward the back of the body
Superior	Above or closer to the head
Inferior	Below or closer to the feet
Medial	Closer to the midline of the body
Lateral	Farther away from the midline of the body
External	Outward or moving toward the exterior of a hollow form
Internal	Inward the movement towards the middle of a hollow form
Superficial	Close to the surface
Distal	Farther away from a point of attachment or from the center of the body
Sagittal	Divides into a left and right side
Peripheral	Near the surface or outside
Visceral	Near the inside
Parietal	Near the side or top
Transverse or horizontal	Divides into superior (top) and inferior (bottom)
Proximal	Closer to a point of attachment or from the center of the body

Appendix F

Pressure Measurements

Blood pressure is defined as the force that blood exerts on the inner walls of blood vessels. Blood pressure is highest in arteries and lowest in veins. In the clinical setting, blood pressure refers to the pressure in arteries. Arterial blood pressure rises and falls as the ventricles of the heart contract and relax. When the ventricles contract, blood pressure is greatest in the arteries. This pressure is called the systolic pressure or systole. When the ventricles relax, blood pressure in arteries is at its lowest. This pressure is called the diastolic pressure or diastole. Blood pressure is usually reported as the systolic number over the diastolic number. For example, in the blood pressure reading 120/80, 120 denotes the systolic pressure and 80 refers to the diastolic pressure (Table F-1).

You can feel the surge of blood through arteries when you take a pulse. The pulse is created as the artery expands when pressure increases and then subsequently relaxes as blood pressure decreases. Common places to feel a pulse are the carotid and radial arteries (Table F-1). Many factors affect blood pressure, the most common being cardiac output, blood volume, vasoconstriction, and blood viscosity (thickness). Cardiac output is the total amount of blood pumped out of the heart in one minute. As cardiac output increases and decreases, blood pressure increases and decreases. When a person loses a large amount of blood, his blood pressure significantly decreases. If blood pressure falls too low, vasoconstriction, which is the tightening of blood vessel walls, helps to raise blood pressure. In contrast, if blood pressure is too high, vasodilation, which is the widening of blood vessels, decreases the blood pressure. Under certain circumstances,

TABLE F-1   Normal Range Values for Blood Pressure and Pulse

Vital Sign	Age				
	0–1 years	1–6 years	6–11 years	11–16 years	Adult
Pulse (beats per minute)	80–160	75–130	75–115	55–110	60–100
Blood Pressure (mm Hg)					
Systolic	74–100	80–112	80–120	88–120	<120
Diastolic	50–70	50–80	50–80	58–80	<80

such as dehydration, blood becomes more viscous, or thicker, than normal. This also decreases blood pressure.

Blood pressure is controlled to a large extent by the amount of blood pumped out of the heart. The amount of blood entering the heart should be equal to the amount of blood pumped out of the heart. The heart has a way to ensure that this happens. When blood enters the left ventricle, the wall of the ventricle is stretched. The more the wall is stretched, the harder it will contract and the more blood it will pump out. This is referred to as *Starling's Law*. If only a small amount of blood enters the left ventricle, it will not be stretched very much and therefore will not contract very forcefully. In this case, not much blood is pumped out of the heart.

Baroreceptors also help regulate blood pressure. Baroreceptors measure blood pressure and are located in the aorta and carotid arteries. If pressure increases in these blood vessels, this information is sent to the cardiac center in the medulla oblongata. The cardiac center then knows to decrease the heart rate, which lowers blood pressure. If pressure gets too low in the aorta, baroreceptors pick up this information and relay it to the cardiac center. The cardiac center then increases the heart rate to raise blood pressure.

In addition to blood pressure and pulse the pulse pressure (aortic pulse pressure) and the mean arterial pressure may be measured. The pulse pressure is the difference between the systolic and diastolic pressure. To calculate use this formula.

$$PP = (diastolic + systolic) \text{ divided by } 2$$

The mean arterial pressure (MAP) is the average arterial pressure during a single cardiac cycle. It reflects the hemodynamic perfusion pressure of the vital organs. The simple way to calculate the patients MAP is to use the following formula:

$$MAP = [(2 \times diastolic) + systolic] \text{ divided by } 3$$

Measuring and Recording Vital Signs Electronically

When you measure and record vital signs electronically, follow the step-by-step guide in the following sections.

1. Gather needed equipment include electronic vital sign machine and method of documenting results.
2. Introduce yourself to the client.
3. Identify the client using two forms of identifcation including name, birthdate and/or medical record number from the identification bracelet or client's chart.
4. Explain the procedure. Since clients may not know what an electronic vital signs machine is, let them know the purpose and exactly what you are doing.
5. Provide for client privacy if needed.
6. Wash your hands.
7. Ask the client to rest in a sitting or lying position. The client's arm should be close to the level of the heart and relaxed. The palm should be up. Raise the sleeve above the level of the pulse site.
8. Remind the client that the cuff will become tight. Normally, more pressure is applied with automatic cuffs.
9. Choose the appropriate-sized cuff.

10. Position the extremity so that it is slightly flexed, relaxed, and at the level of the heart. Apply the cuff . Apply the finger probe if available.

11. Push the power button on the face of the machine. The machine usually performs a self-test when it is first turned on. Check the manufacturer's directions for the machine you are using.

12. Press the start button. The cuff will begin to inflate.

13. Since the machine is very sensitive to any movement, the client should be reminded to stay very still. If there is too much movement, the cuff will usually begin inflating again. If this occurs, press the stop button, remove the cuff, and allow the extremity to rest 1 to 2 minutes before attempting to measure the blood pressure again.

14. When the blood pressure has been taken, the systolic and diastolic blood pressure will appear in boxes on the machine screen.

15. The pulse rate is recorded as well and will be displayed in the screen. If a finger probe is the level of oxygen in the blood will be recorded as well.

16. The machine automatically releases the air from the bladder. Remove the cuff, note the results, and turn the power off.

17. Record the blood pressure, pulse, and other measurements correctly.

18. Return the machine to the proper area and plug it into an outlet or place it on the charging base.

19. Wash your hands.

20. Report to your supervisor any findings that are a significant change from a previous result or outside the normal range. A change of 30 mm Hg or more in either the systolic or the diastolic reading should be reported.

Glossary

A

AC (alternating current) interference   Unwanted markings on the ECG caused by other electrical current sources.

action potential   The change in the electrical potential of the heart muscle when it is stimulated; depolarization followed by repolarization.

acute coronary syndrome (ACS)   This is a broad term that refers to unstable angina, ST segment elevation MI (STEMI), and non-ST segment elevation MI (NSTEMI). ACS is usually associated with intracoronary plaque changes or thrombosis, where blood flow is suddenly stopped.

advanced cardiac life support (ACLS):   A set of clinical interventions for the urgent treatment of cardiac arrest and other life threatening medical emergencies, as well as the knowledge and skills to deploy those interventions.

ambulate   To walk; ambulating is walking.

anatomically contiguous lead   Two or more leads looking at the same part of the heart, or numerically consecutive chest leads.

angina   An oppressive pain or pressure in the chest when the heart muscle does not receive enough oxygen due to partial or complete blockage of a coronary artery.

angiogram   An invasive procedure during which x-rays are taken of a blood vessel after injection of a radiopaque substance.

angioplasty   Surgical repair of blood vessels.

angle of Louis   A ridge about an inch or so below the suprasternal notch where the main part of the sternum and the top of the sternum, known as the manubrium, are attached.

anorexia   Decreased or loss of appetite.

anterior axillary line   An imaginary vertical line starting at the front axilla that extends down the left side of the chest.

anti-arrhythmic   Type of medication given to prevent cardiac rhythm abnormalities.

aorta   The largest artery of the body; transports blood from the left ventricle of the heart to the entire body.

aortic semilunar valve   Valve located in the aorta that prevents the backflow of blood into the left ventricle.

apnea   The absence of breathing.

arrhythmia   Abnormal heartbeats.

arteriosclerosis   An abnormal thickening and hardening of the arterial walls with resulting loss of elasticity.

artifact   Unwanted marks on the ECG tracing caused by activity other than the heart's electrical activity.

ascites   Abnormal collection of serous fluid within the abdomen (peritoneal cavity). This may occur secondary to congestive heart failure.

asystole   When no rhythm or electrical current is traveling through the cardiac conduction system.

atherosclerotic plaque   Fatty deposits accumulated by elevated glucose levels.

atrial kick   When blood is ejected into the ventricles by the atria immediately prior to ventricular systole.

atrioventricular (AV)   Related to the atria and ventricles of the heart.

atrioventricular (AV) node   Delays the electrical impulse to allow the atria to complete their contraction.

atrioventricular delay   The measurement from the atrial spike to the ventricular spike, or from the beginning of the P wave to the ventricular spike on a pacemaker tracing.

atrium (pl. atria)   Top two chambers of the heart.

augmented   Normally small ECG lead tracings that are increased in size by the ECG machine in order to be interpreted.

auscultation   Listening to the body sounds, such as heart, lung, and stomach, using a stethoscope.

automatic external defibrillator (AED)   A lightweight, portable device that recognizes abnormal rhythm and determines if the rhythm is considered a "shockable rhythm."

automaticity   The ability of the heart to initiate an electrical impulse without being stimulated by another or independent source.

autonomic nervous system (ANS)   A system that is in charge of the body's automatic functions, such as the heart rate.

AV   Atrioventricular; related to the atria and ventricles.

axis deviation   Orientation of the heart within the chest.

B

beta blockers   Drugs used to treat hypertension.

bigeminy   Pattern in which every other complex is a premature beat.

biphasic The waveform that has two phases; an equally positive (upward) and negative (downward) deflection on the ECG tracing.

bipolar A type of ECG lead that measures the flow of electrical current in two directions at the same time.

blocked or nonconducted impulse Impulse occurs too soon after the preceding impulse, causing a period when no other impulses can occur in the ventricles.

body mechanics Using movements that maintain proper posture and avoid muscle and bone injuries.

bolus A concentrated amount of medication or fluid to be administered over a prescribed period of time.

bradycardia A slow heart rate, usually less than 60 beats per minute.

bundle branch block Impulse is delayed or blocked within the bundle branches of the normal conduction pathway.

bundle branches Left and right branches of the bundle of His that conduct impulses down either side of the interventricular septum to the left and right ventricles.

bundle of His (atrioventricular or AV bundle) Located next to the AV node; provides the transfer of the electrical impulse from the atria to the ventricles.

C

capture The ability of the heart muscle to respond to electrical stimulation and depolarize the myocardial tissue.

Cardiac Care Units (CCU) A specialized patient care location for patients with cardiovascular disorders that require cardiac monitoring.

cardiac cycle The contraction and relaxation of the heart.

cardiac enzymes (cardiac markers or cardiac bio-markers) Chemicals found in the blood stream that are indicators of myocardial cell death (infarction). Common examples include troponin, CK-MB, and myoglobin.

Examples of Test and Peak Serum Level

Blood Test	Benefit	Peak Level in Blood
Troponin	Most specific	12 hours
CK-MB	Good test if there is not any skeletal muscle damage	10–24 hours
Myoglobin	Not specific to the heart, but useful in nontrauma related cardiac patients due to early presence in blood stream	2 hours

cardiac output Observation guidelines used to assess the blood supply to the vital organs of the body to maintain normal function.

cardiogenic shock Inadequate flow of arterial blood, typically as a result of left heart failure.

cardiologist A physician who specializes in the study of the heart.

cardiopulmonary resuscitation (CPR) To provide ventilations (breaths) and chest compressions (blood circulation) for a person who shows no signs of breathing or having a heartbeat.

cardiovascular Related to the heart and blood vessels (veins and arteries).

cardiovascular disease (CVD) Narrowing of the arteries surrounding the heart, causing a reduction in the blood flow to the heart.

cardioversion The use of electricity to change an abnormally fast or cardiac dysrhythmia to a normal rhythm.

Cerebrovascular accident (CVA) A stroke. Caused by a hemorrhage in the brain or more often by a clot lodged in cerebral artery.

chemical stress test An invasive type of exercise electrocardiography in which thallium or another a radiopaque substance (one that is visible with an x-ray machine), is injected into the body to permit viewing the vessels around the heart. Other medications may also be injected if the patient is unable to exercise. These medications cause the heart rate to increase or the coronary blood vessels to dilate.

circumflex artery One of the primary branches of the left main coronary artery, which winds around, supplying blood to the lateral wall of the left ventricle.

Code Blue Typically means that a patient is unresponsive and needs assistance immediately.

collateral blood vessels Side-by-side, as in small vessels providing additional blood flow to a region of tissue.

complexes Atrial or ventricular contractions as they appear on the ECG; complete ECG waveforms.

conductivity The ability of the heart cells to receive and transmit an electrical impulse.

congestive heart failure (CHF) Failure of the heart to pump an adequate amount of blood to the body tissue.

contractility The ability of the heart muscle cells to shorten in response to an electrical stimulus.

coronary circulation The circulation of blood to and from the heart muscle.

contiguous leads Referring to similar views of the heart (e.g., II, III, and aVF inferior leads, or numerically consecutive chest leads).

coronary angiography A radiopaque dye is injected into the patient to assist with visualizing the heart structures and especially the coronary arteries.

coronary artery bypass graft (CABG) surgery Surgical intervention performed by taking a grafted or transplanted blood vessel and attaching it to the heart at a point beyond an occluded coronary artery to reestablish blood flow.

crash cart   A cart or tray used during emergencies containing medication/equipment at site of medical/surgical emergency for life support

coupling   Two PVCs that occur back to back.

D

defibrillator   A machine that produces and sends an electrical shock to the heart, which is intended to correct the electrical pattern of the heart.

deoxygenated blood   Blood that has little or minimal oxygen (oxygen-poor blood).

depolarization   The electrical activation of the cells of the heart that initiates contraction of the heart muscle.

dextrocardia   When the heart is on the opposite or right side of the chest.

diabetes mellitus (DM)   A condition characterized by a lack of production of insulin, resulting in elevated glucose (sugar) in the blood stream.

diastole   The phase of the cardiac cycle when the heart is expanding and refilling; also known as the relaxation phase.

direct contact   A mode of transmission of infection that occurs from one person to another.

dissociative   To remove from association as with atrioventricular (AV) dissociation or a condition in which the atria and ventricles do not activate in a synchronous fashion but beat independent of each other.

dysrhythmia   Irregularity or lost of rhythm of the heartbeat.

E

echocardiography   Noninvasive diagnostic testing that uses sound to study the heart and blood vessels; also known as an ultrasound.

ectopic pulse   Electrical impulse(s) that come from outside of the normal pacemaker site or electrical conduction pathway.

eICU   Electronic Intensive Care Unit; an off-site unit of the hospital that monitors patients remotely through wired or wireless connections.

Einthoven triangle   A triangle formed by three of the limb electrodes—the left arm, the right arm, and the left leg; it is used to determine the first six leads of the 12-lead ECG.

electrocardiogram (ECG)   A tracing of the heart's electrical activity recorded by an electrocardiograph.

electrocardiograph   An instrument used to record the electrical activity of the heart.

electrocardiology   The study of the heart's electrical activity.

electrodes   Small sensors placed on the skin to detect the electrical activity from the heart.

electronic pacemaker   A device that delivers a small, measured amount of electrical energy to cause myocardial depolarization. Most artificial pacemakers are electronic.

emphysema   Decreased respiratory function usually caused by smoking, chronic bronchitis, or old age.

enhanced external counter pulsation therapy (EECP)   Treatment for chronic angina patients who do not have other options due to health status. This procedure is performed five days a week for several weeks, with the intent of developing collateral blood vessels—essentially creating a "natural" bypass around narrowed or blocked arteries.

ER   Emergency room; patient care location that provides urgent care.

escape rhythm   A rhythm that occurs when the SA node fails to initiate the electrical activity and one of the backup pacemaker sites takes over.

excitability   The ability of the heart muscle cells to respond to an impulse or stimulus.

F

failure to pace   Pacemaker does not send electrical impulse to myocardium.

failure to sense   The pacemaker does not recognize or sense the patient's own inherent heartbeats. Also known as malsensing.

false positive   When a diagnostic test indicates that disease is present but, in reality, the test result is negative and no disease is present.

fibrinolytic agent   Medications administered to break down the fibrin in a blood clot, essentially dissolving it. One type is recombinant Tissue Plasminogen Activator (rTPA).

focus or foci   A cardiac cell or group of cells that function as an ectopic beat.

frequent PVC   Six or more PVCs per minute.

G

gain   A control on the ECG machine that increases or decreases the size of the ECG tracing.

galvanometer   An instrument is used to detect electrocardiograph waves.

H

healthcare provider   The scope of practice of each healthcare provider will determine the extent of the interpretation and treatment of each of the cardiac dysrhythmias or conditions. Each specific scope is determined by the licensure of each state. For example: Prescribing a medication is the responsibility of the physician. But some state practices allow nurse practitioners and physician assistants to prescribe medication under the guidance of the physician.

hepatitis   Inflammation of the liver usually caused by a virus.

HIV (human immunodeficiency virus) The virus that causes AIDS (acquired immune deficiency syndrome).

Holter Proper name given to one type of ambulatory monitor, named after Norman Holter, inventor of the procedure and machine.

Holter monitor An instrument that records the electrical activity of the heart during a patient's normal daily activities; also known as an *ambulatory monitor*.

homeostasis The state of balance the body attempts to maintain by the regulation of body processes.

hypercoagulopathy An increased ability of the blood to form clots.

hypertension High blood pressure.

hypertrophy Abnormal thickening of the ventricular wall due to chronic pressure overload; is often caused by hypertension.

hyperventilation To breathe at an increased rate and depth of inspiration and expiration.

hypotension Condition in which the patient's blood pressure is not adequate to maintain good blood supply to the vital organs.

I

ICU Intensive Care Unit; a specialized patient care location for patients who require monitoring and constant patient care.

indirect contact A mode of transmission of infection involving fomites (objects) or vectors (person, animal, or microorganism).

infarction A lack of oxygen to body tissue due to a blocked blood vessel.

inherent rhythm The patient's own heart rhythm.

inhibited Electrical current is stopped from being sent to the myocardium.

input Data entered into an ECG machine, usually through electrodes on the skin surface.

intercostal space (ICS) The space between two ribs.

interpolated PVC A PVC that occurs during the normal R-R interval without interrupting the underlying rhythm.

interval The period of time between two activities within the heart.

interventricular septum A partition or wall (septum) that divides the right and left ventricles.

invasive Procedure that requires entrance into a body cavity, tissue, or blood vessel.

ischemia Lack of blood supply to an area of tissue due to a blockage in the circulation to that area.

isoelectric The period when the electrical tracing of the ECG is at zero or a straight line, no positive or negative deflections are seen.

isolation precautions Steps taken to prevent the spread of infection; some examples include separating the infected patient from others and using personal protective equipment.

IV fluid challenge Administration of IV fluid (i.e., 0.9% NaCl) with the intent of offsetting the effect of administered medication or to treat for hypovolemia. Often referred to as a fluid resuscitation.

J

J point A point on the QRS complex where the depolarization is completed and repolarization starts.

junctional escape rhythm

L

leads Covered wires that conduct the electrical impulse from the electrodes to the ECG machine.

left anterior descending artery One of the primary branches of the left main coronary artery supplying blood to the anterior wall of the left ventricle.

left atrium The left upper chamber of the heart, which receives blood from the lungs.

left ventricle The left lower chamber of the heart, which pumps oxygenated blood through the body. It is the biggest and strongest chamber, known as the workhorse of the heart.

limb An arm or a leg.

loss of capture The pacing activity continues to occur without evidence that the electrical activity has depolarized or captured the myocardium.

M

malsensing The pacemaker does not recognize or sense the patient's own inherent heartbeats.

maximal exercise Target heart rate of 220 minus the age of the patient.

midaxillary line An imaginary vertical line that starts at the middle of the axilla (armpit) and extends down the side of the chest.

midclavicular line An imaginary line on the chest that runs vertically through the center of the clavicle.

midscapular line Imaginary line on the back that runs vertically through the center of the scapula.

mitral (bicuspid) valve Valve with two cusps or leaflets located between the left atrium and left ventricle; it prevents backflow of blood into the left atrium.

mm (millimeter) A unit of measurement to indicate time on the ECG tracing. The time is measured on the horizontal axis.

multichannel recorder An ECG machine that monitors all 12 leads but records three leads at once and switches automatically, recording each of the four sets of three leads.

multifocal Varied shapes and forms of PVCs.

mV (millivolt) A unit of measurement to indicate voltage on the ECG tracing. Voltage is measured on the vertical axis.

myocardial Pertaining to the heart (*cardia*) muscle (*myo*).

myocardial infarction (MI) (heart attack) A blockage of one or more of the coronary arteries causing lack of oxygen to the heart and damage to the muscle tissue.

myocardial injury Reduction or interruption of blood flow persists for a few minutes, the affected myocardium will transition from myocardial ischemia to a worsened state.

myocardial ischemia A reduction or interruption in blood flow and oxygen to the myocardium, possibly for a short period of time.

N

neurological Pertaining to the nervous system, its diseases, and its functions.

neuropathy Common cause is chronic diabetes mellitus. May cause vascular and autonomic nervous system problems, with loss of ability to maintain blood pressure and loss or impaired sensation.

noninvasive Procedure that does not require entrance into a body cavity, tissue, or blood vessel.

non-ST segment elevation MI (NSTEMI) A type of heart attack in which the classic signs and symptoms are not present. Caused by incomplete occlusion of a coronary artery. The patient often has vague complaints (e.g., fatigue), and inspection of the 12-lead ECG does not reflect the classic ST segment deviation or presence of pathologic Q wave. This type of patient requires further testing and assessment.

normotensive Normal blood pressure.

O

occasional PVC More than one to five premature ventricular contractions per minute.

oscilloscope A monitor or television-type device that shows the tracing of the electrical activity of the heart.

output display The part of the ECG machine that displays the tracing for the electrical activity of the heart, usually in a printed form on a 12-lead ECG machine.

oversensing The pacemaker senses electrical current from other muscle movements or electrical activity outside of the body as the patient's heart electrical current.

oxygenated blood Blood having oxygen (oxygen-rich blood).

P

pacemaker Refers to a natural or man-made source of electrical current causing depolarization of the myocardium.

pacemaker competition Competition between the pacemaker generator and the heart's inherent rate over control of the myocardium.

pacemaker malfunctioning The pacemaker fails to send an electrical impulse to the myocardium at the predetermined interval.

pacing spike A mark on an ECG tracing shown when a patient has a pacemaker.

pallor Pale skin.

palpitations Fast, irregular heartbeat sensation felt by the patient, which may or may not be associated with complaints of chest pain.

paraspinous line Imaginary line on the spine that runs vertically through the side of the spine.

parasympathetic A division of the autonomic nervous system (ANS) that prepares the body for rest.

pathologic Q wave ECG evidence of myocardial infarction. A pathologic Q wave must measure 0.04 second or wider in duration and/or be greater than or equal to 1/3 the height of the R wave in that lead. Must be seen in two or more contiguous leads to be clinically meaningful. Absence of Q waves does not eliminate the possibility of MI.

percutaneous coronary intervention (PCI) Another name for angioplasty. This minimally invasive procedure is performed with a sheath and catheter to inject dye for flouroscopic examination to determine the specific location of a narrowed or occluded artery. Once this portion of the procedure is performed, a catheter with a balloon is inserted, and the balloon is placed at the location of the obstruction and inflated. The intent is to outwardly compress the plaque and re-establish blood flow to the region of tissue distal to the occlusion.

percutaneous transluminal coronary angioplasty (PTCI) Similar to PCI, but now it is specific to a coronary vessel. A catheter with a balloon is inserted, placed at the location of the obstructed coronary artery, and inflated. The intent is to outwardly compress the plaque and reestablish blood flow to the region of tissue distal to the occlusion.

perfusion Supplying nutrients and oxygen to the organs and tissues by way of blood flow through the vessels.

pericardium A two-layered sac of tissue enclosing the heart.

personal protective equipment (PPE) Equipment designed to protect the user from the transfer microorganisms. Some examples include mask, gloves, and gown.

pharmacologic stress test A type of chemical stress test performed for patients unable to exercise in a more traditional manner. Medications are administered to the patient which cause either an acceleration of heart rate (mimicking exercise) or dilation of the coronary blood vessels.

physiologic Q wave Also known as a normal Q wave, it will measure less than 0.04 second in duration and less than 1/3 the height of the R wave in that lead.

polarization The state of cellular rest in which the inside is negatively charged and the outside is positively charged.

posterior axillary line Imaginary line on the back that runs vertically from the shoulder down on the outer edge of the rib cage.

posterior descending artery One of the primary branches of the right main coronary artery providing blood to the posterior wall of the heart.

precordial A type of lead placed on the chest in front of the heart; known as a V lead.

pulmonary artery Large artery that transports deoxygenated blood from the right ventricle to the lungs. This is the only artery in the body that carries deoxygenated blood.

pulmonary circulation The transportation of blood to and from the lungs; blood is oxygenated in the lungs during pulmonary circulation.

pulmonary edema Abnormal collection of fluid within the pleural space (lungs) due to congestive heart failure (left venricle).

pulmonary embolism A blocked artery in the lungs, usually caused by a blood clot.

pulmonary semilunar valve A valve found in the pulmonary artery that prevents backflow of blood into the right ventricle during pulmonary circulation.

pulmonary vein Transports oxygenated blood back into the left atrium of the heart.

Purkinje fibers The fibers within the heart that distribute electrical impulses from cell to cell throughout the ventricles.

Purkinje network Spreads the electrical impulse throughout the ventricles by means of the Purkinje fibers.

Q

quadgeminy Pattern in which every fourth complex is a premature beat.

R

R on T PVCs: PVC occurs on the downslope of the T wave or the vulnerable period of the ventricular refractory period.

rales (crackles) caused by retained airway secretions. When caused by pulmonary edema, the sound may be described as inspiratory very short, soft, high-pitched lung sounds.

renal Pertaining to the kidneys.

renal infarction A lack of oxygen to lung tissue due to a blocked blood vessel.

repolarization When heart muscle cells return to their resting electrical state and the heart muscle relaxes.

restenosis When a blood vessel that has been treated with angioplasty returns to a blocked state or becomes reoccluded.

retrograde moving backward

rhythm The regularity of an occurrence such as the heartbeat.

right atrium The right upper chamber of the heart, which receives blood from the body.

right marginal branch One of the primary branches of the right main coronary artery providing blood to the inferior wall of the left ventricle.

right ventricle The right lower chamber of the heart, which pumps blood to the lungs.

S

segment A portion or part of the electrical tracing produced by the heart.

seizure An interruption of the electrical activity in the brain that causes involuntary muscle movement and sometimes unconsciousness.

semilunar valve A valve with half-moon-shaped cusps that open and close, allowing blood to travel only one way; located in the pulmonary artery and the aorta.

septal artery Branch from the left anterior descending artery providing blood to the interventricular septum.

SICU Surgical Intensive Care Unit; a specialized patient care location for care of patients after surgery.

signal processing The process within the ECG machine that amplifies the electrical impulse and converts it to a mechanical action on the output display.

single-channel recorder An ECG machine that records one lead tracing at a time.

sinoatrial (SA) node An area of specialized cells in the upper right atrium that initiates the heartbeat.

skin rasp A rough piece of material used to abrade (scrape) the skin prior to electrode placement.

somatic tremor Voluntary or involuntary muscle movement; also known as body tremor.

speed A control on the ECG machine that regulates how fast or slow the paper runs during the tracing.

ST segment elevation MI (STEMI) Classic MI with expected ST segment deviation and development of pathologic Q wave. Occurs 75%–80% of the time. Caused by complete occlusion of a coronary artery.

standard precautions Procedures, such as wearing gloves, used with all patient that are designed to prevent the spread of infection.

stat Immediately.

stent A small, metal mesh tube that opens up inside a coronary artery to keep it patent.

stress ECG Another name for exercise electrocardiography.

submaximal exercise Target heart of 220 minus the age multiplied by a percentage between 60 and 85.

suprasternal notch The dip you feel at the anterior base of the neck just above the manubrium where the clavicle attaches to the sternum.

supraventricular An ectopic focus originating above the ventricles in the atria or junctional region of the heart.

sympathetic A division of the autonomic nervous system (ANS) that prepares organs for fight-or-flight (stressful) situations.

syncope Condition when the patient loses consciousness (fainting).

systemic circulation The pathways for pumping blood throughout the body and back to the heart.

systole The contraction phase of the cardiac cycle, during which the heart is pumping blood out to the body.

T

tachycardia A fast heart rate, usually greater than 100 beats per minute.

target heart rate (THR) Heart rate measurement needed to truly exercise the heart.

technician An individual who has the knowledge and skills to carry out technical procedures.

technologist An individual who specializes in a field of science.

telemetry The transmission of data electronically to an unattached or distant location.

thrombolytic agent Medications administered intravenously that posses the ability to lyse or dissolve a clot.

thrombus A blood clot that forms on the inside of an injured blood vessel wall.

TJC The Joint Commission (formerly the Joint Commission on Accreditation of Healthcare Organizations, or JCAHO): organization that establishes patient safety goals for healthcare facilities.

tricuspid valve Valve located between the right atrium and right ventricle; it prevents backflow of blood into the right atrium.

trigeminy Pattern in which every third complex is a premature beat.

triggered Electrical current is sent from the pacemaker generator to the myocardium to cause the depolarization of the myocardial tissue.

tunica adventitita Tough, fibrous, outermost layer of the artery, responsible for keeping the vessel open.

tunica intima Innermost layer of the artery; single-cell layer of endothelial cells that comes in direct contact with the blood.

tunica media Middle layer of the artery; comprised of smooth muscle. This layer is responsible for dilation and constriction of the vessel walls so plays a major role in maintaining blood pressure.

U

underlying rhythm Occurs before the next expected sinus impulse, causing an irregularity.

unifocal Early complex that has shape suggesting only one irritable focus present.

unipolar A type of ECG lead that measures the flow of electrical current in one direction only.

unstable angina (pre-infarction angina) A warning sign that the disease that has been causing angina has worsened. Signs and symptoms associated are less predictable, last longer, and are more painful than previously experienced.

V

vagal tone Condition in which impulses over the vagus nerve exert a continuous inhibitory effect upon the heart and cause a decrease in heart rate.

venae cavae Largest vein in the body, which provides a pathway for deoxygenated blood to return to the heart; its upper portion, the superior vena cava, transports blood from the head, arms, and upper body; and its lower portion, the inferior vena cava, transports blood from the lower body and legs.

volume expander IV solution administerred to fill fluid volume or replace the space that blood normally takes up. The context referred to in this book is referring to inert fluids, specifically 0.9% NaCl. It is given to increase blood volume in the hypotensive or potentially hypotensive patient in an effort to maintain homeostasis.

W

wandering baseline Also known as baseline shift. Occurs when the tracing drifts away from the center of the graph paper.

widow maker Proximal occlusion of the left main coronary artery leads to potential for anterior, lateral, and septal wall MI. It has been long-associated with cardiogenic shock and death.

Photo Credits

Chapter 1

Figure 1.1: Image: © Texas Heart Institute www.texasheartinstitute.org; **Figure 1.2**: © Total Care Programming, Inc; **Figure 1.4**: © Comstock Images/PictureQuest RF; **Figure 1.5**: Courtesy of Aerotel, Inc.; **Figure 1.6**: © Philips Medical Systems; **Figure 1.7**: © Total Care Programming, Inc; **Figure 1.8**: Courtesy of Aerotel, Inc.; **Figure 1.9 (left)**: © The McGraw-Hill Companies, Inc./Jill Braaten, photographer; **Figure 1.9 (right),1.10**: © Total Care Programming, Inc.

Chapter 3

Figure 3.7: © Total Care Programming, Inc; **Figures 3.8, 3.9**: Courtesy of GE Healthcare Systems; **Figure 3.11 (both)**: © Philips Medical Systems; **Figure 3.12a**: © Total Care Programming, Inc; **Figure 3.12b**: Courtesy of Tempo Medical Products; **Figure 3.13**: © Total Care Programming, Inc.

Chapter 4

Figures 4.1, 4.5 (both), **Figure 4.10**: © Total Care Programming, Inc.

Chapter 5

Figures 5.1, 5.2: © Total Care Programming, Inc.

Chapter 11

Figure 11.1: © Total Care Programming, Inc; **Figure 11.2**: Image: © Texas Heart Institute www.texasheartinstitute.org.

Chapter 12

Figures 12.1, 12.2: Courtesy of Aerotel, Inc.; **Figures 12.3–12.5**: © Total Care Programming, Inc; **Figure 12.6**: © Total Care Programming, Inc. **Figure 12.7 (both)**: © Card Guard AG/Life Watch Holdings Corp; **Figures 12.8, 12.9**: Courtesy of Aerotel, Inc.; **Figures 12.10, 12.12**: © Total Care Programming, Inc.

Chapter 13

Figure 13.9: © Dynamic Graphics/Jupiter Images; **Figure 13.10**: Imagestate RF; **Figure 13.11**: © Phototake; **Figure 13.14**: © Vasomedical, Inc. All Rights Reserved. EECP is a registered ® trademark of the Vasomedical, Inc.

Index

Page references followed by *f* indicate figures; *t*, tables.

A

Abbreviations (A-Z listed), medical, 375–389
ABCs of prevention (AHA), 2*t*
Accelerated idioventricular rhythm, 213–214, 213*f*
Accelerated junctional rhythm, 172–174, 172*f*
ACE (angiotensin-converting enzyme) inhibitors, 364
Acetylcholine, 39
Acronyms (A-Z listed), medical, 375–389
Action potential of heart, 42
Acute coronary syndrome (ACS), 315–317
Acute myocardial infarction (AMI), 344
Adenosine (Adenocard), 257, 367
Advanced cardiac life support (ACLS), 210, 219, 221
Agonal rhythm, 210, 210*f*
Alcohol and stress test, 263, 269
Alligator clips, 102, 102*f*
Alternating current (AC) interference, 96*t*, 98–99, 99*f*
Ambulating, 280
Ambulatory monitoring
   described, 280–283, 281*f*, 282*f*
   in doctor's office/ambulatory care, 8–10, 9*f*
   educating patient for, 288–292, 289*f*, 290*f*, 291*t*
   outside healthcare facility, 10–13, 10*f*, 12*f*
   preparing patient for, 292–293
   reasons for using, 282–283
   reporting results of, 296–298
   variations/functions of, 283–287, 285*f*, 286*f*, 287*f*
Ambulatory monitors
   applying, 293–296, 294*f*, 295*f*
   handling, 284
   removing, 296–298
   voice-activated, 284
American College of Cardiology, 316, 322–324
American Heart Association (AHA)
   ABCs recommended by, 2*t*
   on acute coronary syndrome, 315–316
   frequency of ECG recommendation by, 6
   immediate care guidelines by, 322–324
Amlodipine (Norvasc), 363
Amputee and ECG, 105
Anatomical landmarks, 87, 87*f*
Anatomically contiguous lead, 343
Angina pectoris
   assessing symptoms of, 311–312
   exercise electrocardiography and, 255
   medications for, 363, 364, 366
Angina, unstable, 312–313, 313*t*
Angiogram, 269

Angioplasty, 5, 327, 328*f*
Angle of Louis, 87, 87*f*
Anorexia in ventricular failure, 318
Anterior axillary line, 87, 87*f*
Anterior infarction, 341*f*
Antiarrhythmic therapy, 283, 364
Anticoagulants, 329, 364
Antiplatelet agents, 323, 365
Aorta, 31–32, 32*f*, 33, 34*f*, 36*f*
Aortic-semilunar valve, 31–32, 31*t*, 32*f*, 34*f*
Apnea, 219, 221
Arm leads; *see* Limb leads
Arrhythmias; *see* Dysrhythmias (arrhythmias)
Arteries
   in cardiovascular system, 32*f*, 33, 34*f*, 35
   coronary, 33, 36*f*, 309, 309–310*f*
   layers of, 309, 310*f*, 311
Artifact filter, 65–66, 263
Artifacts
   correcting, 96*t*
   electronic pacemaker and, 234, 235*f*
   reducing potential for, 86
   troubleshooting, 95–100, 96*t*, 99*t*
Ascites, 319
Aspirin (Bayer), 323, 365
Asystole, 219–221, 219*f*
   differentiating from fine fibrillation, 219
   sinus arrest and, 140
Atenolol (Tenormin), 363
Atherosclerotic plaque, 314
Atorvastatin (Lipitor), 366
Atria, heart, 32, 32*f*, 34*f*
   depolarization of tissue of, 172
   quivering, 157
Atrial dysrhythmias, 149–159
Atrial fibrillation (A fib), 157–159, 157*f*, 177, 178*t*, 363, 364
Atrial flutter (A flutter), 154–157, 155*f*, 177, 178*t*
Atrial kick, 43
   in atrial dysrhythmias, 156, 158
   in complete heart block, 196
   electronic pacemaker and, 234
   in ventricular dysrhythmias, 213, 214, 215
Atrial pacing, 233, 235*f*
Atrial rate, determining, 126
Atriobiventricular pacing, 234, 235*f*
Atrioventricular (AV) block
   differentiating types of, 193, 193*t*
   first degree, 188–189, 188*f*

Atrioventricular (AV) block—*Cont.*
  second degree
    Mobitz I/Wenckebach, 189–192, 190*f*
    Mobitz II/Hay, 192–194, 192*f*
  third degree (complete), 194–197, 195*f*
Atrioventricular (AV) node/junction
  described, 39–40, 40*t*, 41*f*
  dysrhythmias originating from, 169–180
  impulses delayed/blocked to, 188–190
Atrioventricular (AV) valves, 31–32, 31*t*
Atrioventricular delay, 235
Atrioventricular pacing, 233–234
Augmented leads, 57–58, 58*f*
Automatic external defibrillators (AEDs), 11–12, 11*f*
Automaticity, 38, 154, 206
Autonomic nervous system (ANS), 39
AV dissociation, 196
aVF lead, 57–58, 57*f*, 58*f*, 60*f*
  anatomically contiguous, 343
  infarction areas identified by, 339*f*
  portions of heart viewed by, 338*f*, 338*t*
aVL lead, 57, 57*f*, 58*f*, 60*f*
  anatomically contiguous, 343
  infarction areas identified by, 339–340*f*
  portions of heart viewed by, 338*f*, 338*t*
aVR lead, 57, 57*f*, 58*f*, 60*f*, 106
Axis deviation, electrical, 345, 346*f*, 347, 347*t*, 348*f*

B

Baseline shift; *see* Wandering baseline
Basic life support (BLS), 210
Bathing and ambulatory monitoring, 291
Batteries and electronic pacemaker, 239
Bed and ECG, 86, 93
Behavior, standards of, 19
Benazepril (Lotensin), 364
Beta blockers, 260, 324, 363
Bicuspid valve; *see* Mitral (bicuspid) valve
Bigeminy pattern of complexes, 208*t*
Billing, 101
Biphasic waveform, 149
Bipolar leads, 57
"Bizarre" complexes; *see* Complexes, ECG
Blocked electrical impulses, 189
Blood pressure
  assessing, 324
  exercise electrocardiography and, 255, 262, 267
  heart regulation and, 39
Blood thinners, 329, 364, 365
Blood vessels, 33
  cardiac, 34*f*, 309–310*f*
  collateral, 330
  layers of, 309, 310*f*, 311
  placement of, in CABG, 329, 329*f*
Body mechanics, 13, 14*t*, 92, 94
Body tremor; *see* Somatic tremor
Bolus, 324
Bradycardia, 126
  ECG machine alerting of, 67
  sinus, 132–134, 132*f*

Breast implants and ECG, 105
Breath sounds, 317–319
Bruce protocol, 265*t*
Bundle branch block dysrhythmias, 241–243, 242*f*
  differentiating types of, 349–350, 349–350*f*
  electronic pacemaker and, 235
Bundle branches, 39–40, 40*t*, 41*f*
Bundle of His (AV bundle), 39–40, 40*t*, 41*f*, 195
"Bunny branch block," 349
Burn dressings and ECG, 106

C

Caffeine and stress test, 263, 269
Calcium channel blockers, 363–364
Calcium ions, heart regulation and, 39
Calibration (standardization) mark, 65, 66*f*, 71, 95
Calipers, 124–125, 124*f*, 125*f*, 128
Captopril (Capoten), 364
Capture
  loss of, 239, 240*f*, 240*t*
  pacemaker and, 234
Cardiac arrest, 108, 221, 367
Cardiac care unit (CCU), 7
Cardiac control center of brain, 39
Cardiac cycle, 36–37
Cardiac enzymes (markers), 323, 345
Cardiac glycosides, 363
Cardiac output
  absent, 218, 221
  average/adequate, 35, 131
  decreased, 35–36
    signs and symptoms of, 132*t*
    in atrial dysrhythmias, 150, 156, 158–159
    in heart block dysrhythmias, 191–192, 193, 196
    in junctional dysrhythmias, 170, 176, 178, 180
    in sinus node rhythms, 131, 134, 135–136
    in ventricular dysrhythmias, 208–209, 210, 213, 214, 215
Cardiac output parameters, 189
Cardiac patient
  assessing, 320, 321*f*, 322*f*
  immediate care of, 322–324
  additional tests for, 324–325
  further treatment of, 326–330
Cardiac symptoms; *see also specific symptom*
  atypical, 313–315, 314*t*, 317
  reporting, 322
  typical, 311–313, 313*t*
Cardioactive drugs, 257, 367
Cardiolite, 256, 367
Cardiologist, 256, 281, 296
Cardiopulmonary resuscitation (CPR)
  ECG technician and, 5
  exercise electrocardiography and, 263
  for ventricular dysrhythmias, 217, 219, 221
Cardiotonics, 367
Cardiovascular Credentialing International (CCI), 396, 400, 405

Cardiovascular disease, 2, 2*t*
Cardiovascular system, 28–42
    blood circulation of, 33–36
    cardiac cycle of, 36–37
    conduction system in, 38–41
    electrical stimulation and, 41–42
    heart anatomy in, 29–33
Cardioversion, electrical, 326
Carvedilol (Coreg), 363
Centers for Disease Control and Prevention (CDC), 14–15, 94, 313
Cerebral vascular accident (CVA), 2
    ABCs to reduce, 2*t*
    atrial dysrhythmias in, 159
    exercise electrocardiography and, 261
Certified Cardiographic Technician (CCT), 400–405
Certified Rhythm Analysis Technician (CRAT), 396–400, 405–409
Chaotic/disorganized tracing, 217, 217*f*
Chemical stress test and agents, 256–257, 367
Chest leads/electrodes, 59, 59*f*
    anatomical landmarks for, 87, 87*f*
    applying, 88–90, 89*f*, 89*t*
    placement for 15- or 18-lead ECG, 106–107, 108*f*
    right-side placement of, 106, 106*f*
    shaving/clipping hairs for, 263, 292, 294
Chest pain/discomfort
    assessing, 311–312
    exercise electrocardiography and, 264, 266, 267
    in myocardial ischemia, 312, 314
Chest pressure, 312
Child; *see* Pediatric patient
Cholesterol-lowering agents, 366
Cialis (tadalafil), 367
Circulation, blood
    coronary
        defined, 33
        major vessels/valves in, 33, 34*f*, 36*f*
        principles of, 35
    electrocardiogram and, 29
    pulmonary, 33–34, 35*f*
    systemic, 33, 34, 35*f*
Circumflex artery, 309
Clinical management
    assessment, 320, 321*f*, 322*f*
    immediate care, 322–324
    additional tests, 324–325
    further treatment, 326–330
Clinical triad of ventricular failure, 319, 319*f*
Clopidogrel (Plavix), 365
Clostridium difficile, 18
Clot busters, 326–327, 365–366
Clothing and ambulatory monitoring, 290–291
Code Blue
    for bundle branch block dysrhythmias, 243
    check patient before declaring, 218
    ECG during, 7, 108
    for heart block dysrhythmias, 193–194, 193*t*, 196
    for sinus arrest, 139
    for ventricular dysrhythmias, 217
Collateral blood vessels, 330

Communication; *see* Patient education/communication
Complete heart block (CHB), 194–197, 195*t*
    bundle branch block and, 243
    second degree AV block and, 193
Complexes, ECG
    calculate heart rate using, 73*f*, 74
    running, with lead codes, 95
    in sinus arrest, 138
    trigeminy pattern in, 150
    wide/bizarre, 42, 43*t*, 206, 207, 207*f*, 210, 210*f*, 211, 212*f*, 213, 213*f*, 214, 215, 215*f*
    widening, for interpretation, 65
Computerized interpretation; *see* Interpretation, rhythm strip
Conduct, rules of, 18
Conduction system, heart, 38–40, 41*t*; *see also* Pacemaker of heart; Rhythms, cardiac
    control of heart rate and, 206, 233
    delay in, 188
    pathways for, 39–40, 40*t*, 41*f*
    recording activity in; *see* Waveform, ECG
    regulation and, 39
    unique qualities in, 38–39
Conductivity, 38
Confidentiality, 19, 268
Congestive heart failure (CHF), 154, 262, 363, 364, 366
Consent, implied/informed, 20, 259
    handling problems obtaining, 21, 259*t*
    narcotics and, 324
    patient refusal of, 85, 259*t*
    sample form for, 260*f*
Continuous monitoring, 104–105
    in hospital (acute care), 7
    outside healthcare facility, 13
    patient's responsibility in, 283
    technician's responsibility in, 5, 6*f*
Contractility, 38
Contraction, heart
    in cardiac cycle, 36–37, 37*f*
    in conduction system, 38
    depolarization and, 42
    heart output and, 35
    myocardium and, 31
    recorded in ECG waveform, 42, 43*t*, 44*f*
Contraction-relaxation pattern, continuous, 215
Coronary angiography, 324, 325*f*
Coronary arteries
    blockage of, 311–312
    in cardiovascular system, 33, 35, 36*f*
    in clinical management, 309, 309–310*f*, 311
    vasodilation of, 367
    12-lead ECG views of, 338*t*
Coronary artery bypass graft surgery (CABG), 327, 329, 329*f*
Coronary artery disease (CAD), 2
Coronary care unit (CCU), 7
Coronary circulation, 33, 35, 36*f*
Coronary vascular disease (CVD), 255, 366
Coumadin clinic, 329
Coumadin (warfarin), 364, 365

Coupling of premature complexes, 208*t*
Crash cart, 219, 261
Critical thinking skills, 20–21

D

Death
  due to coronary artery occlusion, 327
  due to ventricular dysrhythmias, 217*f*, 218, 219*f*, 221
  mixing medications and, 367
  risk of, and non-classic signs, 317
  of tissue, 344–345
Defibrillation in clinical management, 326
Defibrillator, 11, 217
Deflections (EGC waves), 42–43
  changing height of, 64–65, 67
  positive, 106
Deoxygenated blood, 33
Depolarizations, 42
  absence of, 219, 219*f*
  dissociative, 194
  with electronic pacemaker, 234, 235, 239
  no delay between, 215
  retrograde, 172
  series of rapid, 177
Dextrocardia, 106, 106*f*
Diabetes, cardiac symptoms and, 314–315
Diagnostic code (ICD-9), 101
Diary, patient, 289–292, 290*f*
  documenting/labeling, 296
  if patient forgot, 297
Diastole, 37, 37*f*
Digital monitor/monitoring, 12–13, 282*f*, 296
Digital storage system, 62–64
Digoxin (Lanoxin, Digitek), 363
Diltiazem (Cardizem), 363
Dipyridamole (Persantine), 257, 367
Dissociative depolarizations, 194
Diuretics, 366
Dizziness
  ambulatory monitoring and, 283
  in dysrhythmias, 137, 139, 159, 209
  exercise electrocardiography and, 262, 264, 267
  in myocardial ischemia, 312
Dobutamine (Dobutrex), 257, 367
Doctor's office, use of ECG in, 8–10
Documentation, 20, 20*t*; *see also* Patient information/
    records
  in ambulatory monitoring, 291, 291*t*, 296
  of ECG rhythm/tracing, 100–101, 132
  of heart block dysrhythmias, 197
  of intervention (i.e., oxygen therapy), 157
  of patient diary/tape/disk, 296
  of patient medications, 83
  of repeat ECGs, 108
  of seizure, 108
  of special patient considerations, 105–106
  of speed/gain change, 64, 65
  of ventricular dysrhythmias, 210, 217, 219
Dot matrix paper, 69, 70*f*

Drug toxicity, atrial dysrhythmias and, 151
Dying heart in ventricular dysrhythmias, 210, 210*f*
Dysrhythmias (arrhythmias), 4
  ambulatory monitoring and, 284
  analyzing tracing for, 123–130
  atrial, 149–159
  defibrillator for, 11
  heart block, 187–197
  junctional, 169–180
  medications for, 283, 364
  re-entry, 177
  rhythm strip to check, 105
  sinus, 136–137, 137*f*
  ventricular, 206–221

E

e-ICU, 8, 285*f*, 286*f*
Echocardiogram, 269
Echocardiography, 324, 325*f*
Ectopic impulse, 149
Education, patient; *see* Patient education/communication
Einthoven triangle, 56–57, 57*f*, 58*f*
Einthoven, Wilhelm, 4, 42
Elderly patient; *see* Geriatric patient
Electrical activity of heart; *see* Conduction system, heart
Electrical impulses
  blocked/non-conducted, 189
  triggered, 239
Electricity
  electrocardiograph machine and, 4
    AC current interference and, 98–99
    grounding for safety with, 92–93
    patient's fear of, 85
  electronic pacemaker and, 233
Electrocardiogram (ECG) tracing, 2–3
  artifacts on
    correcting, 96*t*
    reducing potential for, 86
    troubleshooting, 95–100, 96*t*, 99*t*
  electronic pacemaker and
    complications relative to, 239, 240*f*
    evaluating function of, 234–236
  15- or 18-lead, 106–107, 108*f*
  interpreting; *see* Interpretation
  patient information on, 66, 67*f*, 83–84
  recommended frequency of routine, 6
  recording
    applying electrodes/leads for, 88–90, 89*f*, 89*t*, 91*f*
    during cardiac arrest, 108
    communicating with patient for, 85–86
    emergencies during, 108
    identifying anatomical landmarks for, 87
    operating machine for, 95
    preparation for, 83–84
    during respiratory arrest, 108
    safety/infection control in, 92–94, 93*t*, 94*t*
    during seizure, 108
    special considerations for, 105–107, 108*f*
  reporting completed, 100–101, 131–132

serial (multiple) and repeat, 97, 108
size settings for, 64–65, 66*f*, 67
speed settings for, 64, 65, 70
voltage measurement on, 64, 71, 72*f*
12-lead, 60*f*, 61
  heart views of standard, 337–338, 338*f*, 338*t*
  infarction areas identified by, 339–341*f*
  right-side, 106, 106*f*
  transtelephonic, 287, 288*f*
Electrocardiograph (ECG) machine/instrument, 2, 3*f*,
    61–64
  controls on, 64–67
  electricity and, 4, 85, 92–93, 98–99
  functions of, 61–62
  graph paper for; *see* Graph paper
  lead wires for; *see* Lead wires
  maintenance/care of, 101–102, 103*f*
  operation of, 95
  types of, 6–13, 61, 61*f*
    in doctor's office/ambulatory care, 8–10
    in hospital (acute care), 7–8
    outside healthcare facility, 10–13
    technological advances in, 4, 62–64
Electrocardiographer, role of, 5
Electrocardiography
  history of, 4
  skills/knowledge to perform, 13–20
    patient education/communication, 16–17
    safety/infection control, 13–16, 14*t*, 15*f*, 16*f*, 17*t*
    troubleshooting, 20–21
  uses for, 6–13, 8*t*
    in clinical management, 323, 325
    in doctor's office/ambulatory care, 8–10
    in hospital (acute care), 7–8
    outside healthcare facility, 10–13
Electrocardiology, 4
Electrodes, 55
  chest
    anatomical landmarks for, 87, 87*f*
    placement, 89*f*, 89*t*
    shaving/clipping hairs for, 263, 292, 294
  disposable, 68–69, 68*f*, 102
  dried, rhythm if, 217
  in Einthoven triangle, 56–57
  on geriatric patient, 294
  limb, 88
  for longer use, 69
  loose/disconnected, 288
  mixing types of, 68
  for pediatric patient, 104
  placement of
    for ambulatory monitoring, 293–296, 295*f*
    for electrocardiography, 88–90, 91*f*
    for exercise electrocardiography, 263, 264*f*
    special considerations for, 105–107, 106*f*, 108*f*
  reusable, 102
  wandering baseline and, 98
Electrolytes, 39, 216, 366
Electronic devices and ECG, 86, 93
Embolism in atrial dysrhythmias, 159

Emergencies, medical, ECG and
  during cardiac arrest, 108
  communication during, 219
  in complete heart block, 193–194, 193*t*
  determining heart rate during, 126
  during exercise electrocardiography, 254, 262*t*
  in extended sinus arrest pause, 139
  in hospital (acute care), 7
  during seizure, 108
  in ventricular dysrhythmias, 210, 213, 217, 218–219, 221
Emergency room (ER), 7
Emphysema, atrial dysrhythmias in, 154
Enalapril (Vasotec), 364
Endocardium, 30, 30*t*, 31*f*
Enhanced external counter pulsation (EECP), 330
Enoxaparin (Lovenox), 364, 365
Epicardium, 30, 30*t*, 31*f*
Erectile dysfunction, medications for, 367
"Escape beats" (PVCs), 216
Escape rhythm, 170–172, 170*f*
Ethics; *see* Legal/ethical issues
Event marker, 283
Excitability, 38, 44*f*
Exercise electrocardiography, 8–9, 9*f*
  described, 253–254, 253*f*, 254*f*
  performing, 263–264, 264*f*
  period following, 268–269
  preparing patient for, 257, 258–259*t*, 260–261
  prior to ambulatory monitoring, 283
  protocols for, 265–266*t*, 265–267
  reasons for using, 255–256
  reporting
    patient symptoms during, 264, 267
    results of, 268
  sample consent form for, 260*f*
  variations of, 256–257

F

f (fibrillatory) waves, 157, 157*f*
Fainting; *see* Syncope
False positive stress testing, 269
Fears of patient, 85, 266, 292
Fetal position and ECG, 106
Fibrillation
  atrial (A fib), 157–159, 157*f*, 177, 178*t*
  ventricular, 217–219, 217*f*,
Fibrinolytic therapy, 326–327, 365–366
1500 method of calculating heart rate, 72, 74*f*
"Fine" fibrillation versus asystole, 219
First degree atrioventricular (AV) block, 188–189, 188*f*,
    193, 193*t*
Flatline, straight, 219, 219*f*
Flatline tracing, 99–100
Flutter (F) waves, 155, 155*f*
Flutter-to-flutter waves, 155
Fluttering sensation
  in junctional dysrhythmias, 176, 178
  in sinus node rhythms, 136
Focus, ectopic, 150

G

Gain control setting, 64–65, 66f, 67
Galvanometer, 4
Gel/paste, electrode, 68f
   dry, 69, 217
   removing buildup of, 102
   wandering baseline and, 98
Geriatric patient, 106, 294, 315
Graph paper
   checking/loading, 84, 84f
   handling/changing, 69–70, 71f
   measurements on, 71
   speed of, 64, 70, 174
   types/size of, 69, 70f
Grid paper, 69
Ground electrode, 56
Grounding ECG machine, 92–93

H

Hand hygiene
   before/after ECG, 92, 94
   practices/procedures, 15, 15f, 17t, 18, 369–370
Handheld monitor, 284–285, 287f
Hay rhythm, 192–194, 192f
Healthcare providers
   scope of practice by, 6, 178, 290, 322
   use of ambulatory monitor by, 281–282
   use of ECG by, 6, 253–254
Health Insurance Portability and Accountability Act
   (HIPAA-1996), 18
Hearing impaired patient, 18
Heart
   anatomy of, 29–33
      chambers/valves, 31–32, 31t, 32f
      circulation, 33, 35, 36f
      layers/function, 29–30, 30t, 31f
      location, 30f
      size/weight, 29
      vessels, 32f, 33, 34f, 36f, 309, 309–310f, 311
   blood pathways through, 33–34, 34f
   conditions requiring alternate tracings, 106–107, 106f,
      108f
   conduction system of; see Conduction system, heart
   contraction of; see Contraction, heart
   dying, 210, 210f
   as a pump, 29, 35–36, 38, 42
   ready phase of, 42
   reenergizing phase of, 42
   relaxation phase of
      in cardiac cycle, 36–37, 37f
      recorded in ECG waveform, 42, 44f
   views of, on 12-lead tracing, 337–338, 338f, 338t,
      339–341f
Heart attack; see Myocardial infarction (MI)
Heart block dysrhythmias, 188–197
   differentiating types of, 193, 193t
Heart Card, 287f
Heart disease; see Cardiovascular disease

Heart failure, 317–319, 318f, 319f
   atrial dysrhythmias in, 154
   electrical pacemakers for, 234
   exercise electrocardiography and, 262
   medications for, 367
Heart fluttering; see Palpitations
Heart rate
   in atrial dysrhythmias, 149, 150, 152, 152f, 153,
      155, 157
   in bundle branch block dysrhythmias, 243
   calculating, 72, 73f, 74, 74f
   changing speed for rapid, 65
   control of, 206, 233
   determining atrial/ventricular, 126, 127t
   exercise electrocardiography and, 267
   in heart block dysrhythmias, 190, 192, 195
   in ischemia/injury/infarction, 342
   in junctional dysrhythmias, 169, 171, 172, 174, 176, 178
   setting limits (alarm) for, 67
   in sinus node rhythms, 130, 132, 133, 135, 137, 139
   in ventricular dysrhythmias, 207, 210, 211, 213, 215,
      217, 219
Heart rate calculator, 127t
Heart sounds, 37, 44f
Heartbeat
   abnormal; see Dysrhythmias (arrhythmias)
   in cardiac cycle, 36–37, 37f
   focus functions as ectopic, 150
   rate/sounds of, 37, 44f
   regulation of, 39
Heartsite.com, 327
Heparin, 364, 365
Herrick, James B., 4
History, medical; see Patient information/records
Holter monitor
   in ambulatory monitoring, 281, 281f
   in doctor's office/ambulatory care, 8, 9f, 10
   5-lead, 295f, 297
Holter, Norman, 281
Hospital (acute care), use of ECG in, 7–8
Hypercoagulopathy, 329
Hypertension, 262, 363, 364, 366
Hypertrophy, 347
Hyperventilation, 262
Hypotension
   assessing, 324
   in junctional dysrhythmias, 170
   mixing medications and, 367
   in right ventricular failure, 319
   in sinus node rhythms, 139

I

ICD-9 code, 101
Identification, patient; see Patient information/records
Idioventricular rhythm, 211–213, 212f
   accelerated, 213–214, 213f
Imaging agents, 256, 367
Impulses; see Electrical impulses, blocked/non-conducted

Infant; *see* Pediatric patient
Infarction; *see* Myocardial infarction (MI)
Infection control
    before/after ECG, 92–94
    maintaining ECG equipment, 102
    precautions, 14–16, 15*f*, 16*f*, 17*t*, 18, 93*t*, 94
Inferior infarction, 339*f*
Information, patient; *see* Patient information/records
Inherent rhythm, 235
Injury; *see* Myocardial injury
Inotropic agents, 367
Input data, 62
Intensive care unit (ICU), 7
Intercostal space (ICS), 87, 87*f*
Intermittent monitoring, 284, 287*f*
Interpolated premature complexes, 208*t*
Interpret-TIP
    atrial dysrhythmias, 150, 151, 153, 155, 158
    bundle branch blocks, 243
    computerized QRS measurement, 129
    heart block dysrhythmias, 188, 191, 193, 195
    junctional dysrhythmias, 170, 172, 174, 176, 178
    pacemaker rhythms, 234
    sinus node rhythms, 131, 133, 135, 137, 139
    variables affecting QT interval, 126
    ventricular dysrhythmias, 206, 207, 210, 213, 214, 215, 217
Interpretation, rhythm strip
    of ambulatory monitoring, 296–298
    change of speed/gain and, 64, 65
    computerized machine, 4, 62
        from ambulatory monitor, 281, 296
        if artifact, 66
        of PR interval, 128
        of QRS duration, 129
    of exercise electrocardiography, 268–269
    5-step process of, 123–130, 342
Intervals, ECG, 42, 43*t*, 125*f*; *see also specific types of*
Interventricular septum, 31, 32*f*, 34*f*, 40, 41*f*
Invasive procedure, 257
Ischemia, 139; *see also* Myocardial ischemia
Isoelectric line, 42, 342
Isolation (transmission-based) precautions, 15, 92, 93*t*, 94, 371–374
Isosorbide dinitrate (Dilatrate-SR, Isordil), 366
Isosorbide mononitrate (ISMO), 366
IV fluid challenge, 324

J

J point, 45, 125*f*, 128, 129*f*
Jaw pain, 311, 312
Jewelry and ECG, 86
Joint Commission (TJC), The, 85, 389
Jugular vein distention, 319
Junctional dysrhythmias, 169–180
Junctional escape rhythm, 170–172, 170*f*
Junctional rhythm, accelerated, 172–174, 172*f*
Junctional tachycardia rhythm, 174–176, 174*f*, 178*t*

L

Labetalol (Normodyne, Trandate), 363
Laboratory tests for assessment, 323
Lateral infarction, 340*f*
Law/ethics; *see* Legal/ethical issues
LCD (liquid crystal diode) display, 66, 67*f*, 84
Lead circuits, 56–57
Lead codes on tracing, 55–56, 60*f*, 95
Lead selector, 67
Lead wires; *see also* Electrodes
    for ambulatory monitoring, 295–296
    attachment of, 90
    care/safety of, 93, 102, 103*f*
    continuous monitoring and, 105
    identification of, 55–57, 55*t*, 56*f*, 91*f*
    multiple (serial) ECGs and, 97
    placement of, 91*f*
    rhythm if poorly connected, 217
    stress loops for, 295*f*
    types of, 57–59, 58*f*, 59*f*
Leads I, II, and III, 57, 57*f*, 58*f*, 60*f*
    AC interference and, 99*t*
    anatomically contiguous, 343
    continuous monitoring and, 105
    infarction areas identified by, 339–340*f*
    portions of heart viewed by, 338*f*, 338*t*
    rhythm strip and lead II of, 105
Left anterior descending artery, 309
Left atrium, 31, 32*f*, 34*f*
Left bundle branch block (LBBB), 241, 242*f*
    differentiating, 349, 349–350*f*
    electronic pacemaker and, 235
Left ventricle, 31, 32*f*, 34*f*
    12–lead ECG views of, 338, 338*f*, 338*t*
    failure of, 317–318
    problems requiring alternate tracings, 106–107, 108*f*
Left ventricular hypertrophy (LVH), 347, 351–352, 351*f*
Leg leads; *see* Limb leads, standard
Legal/ethical issues, 18–20
    consent and narcotics, 324
    documentation of procedure, 132, 296
    informed consent, 259
    knowledge of equipment before using, 297
    liability and medical records, 85
    maintaining patient records, 71
    privacy of patient information, 19
    scope of practice, 178, 290
    securing patient information, 268, 296
"Lengthen, lengthen, drop equals Wenckebach," 193
Levitra (vardenafil), 367
Lewis, Sir Thomas, 4
Liability, professional, 19, 85
Libel, 20
Limb electrodes, applying, 88
Limb leads, standard, 57, 58*f*
    AC interference and, 99*t*
    continuous monitoring and, 105

Limbs, 55
Lisinopril (Prinivil, Zestril), 364
Loop-memory monitor, 286–287
Loss of capture, 239, 240f, 240t

M

MAC 550 resting ECG analysis system, 63f
Malfunctioning pacemaker, 239, 240t
Malsensing pacemaker, 239, 240t
Mastectomy and ECG, 105
Medications
   affecting electrocardiography, 83, 260
   antiarrhythmic, 283
   cardioactive, for stress test, 257
   for clinical management, 323–324, 326–327, 329
Metoprolol (Toprol XL, Lopressor), 363
Midaxillary line, 87, 87f
Midclavicular line, 87, 87f, 90
Midscapular line, 107, 108f
Mitral (bicuspid) valve, 31–32, 31t, 32f, 34f
Mitral valve regurgitation, acute, 154
mm/sec (millimeters/seconds), 64
Mnemonics for remembering
   cardiac patient assessment, 320, 321f, 322f
   Wenckebach rhythm, 193
Mobitz I (Type I/Wenckebach) rhythm, 189–190, 190f,
   193, 193t
Mobitz II (classical) rhythm, 192–194, 192f
Mobitz, Woldemar, 190
Modified chest lead (MCL), 105
Morphine IV, 324
Multichannel recorder, 61, 61f
Multifocal atrial tachycardia (MAT), 152–154, 152f
Multifocal premature complexes, 208t
Muscle movements and ECG, 97, 108, 217
MUSE Cardiology Information System (GE Healthcare),
   62–64, 63f
mV (millivolts), 64
Myocardial cells, 38
Myocardial infarction (MI), 2, 344–345
   ABCs to reduce, 2t
   acute, 344
   alternate tracings for type of, 106–107, 108f
   assessing symptoms of, 311–312
   atrial dysrhythmias in, 159
   ECG changes predictive of, 4, 316–317, 316f
   exercise electrocardiography and, 261
   junctional dysrhythmias in, 176
   leads identifying areas of, 339–341f
   outside healthcare facility, 10–11
Myocardial injury, 344
Myocardial ischemia, 343–344
   assessing symptoms of, 312
   exercise electrocardiography and, 255, 256f
   medications for, 313t, 323–324, 366
   premature ventricular complexes and, 207
   ST segment and, 43
   supraventricular tachycardia and, 180

Myocardium, 30, 30t, 31, 31f
   progression of damage to, 343
   quivering, 217
Myoview, 367

N

Narcotics and consent, 324
National Center for Competency Testing, 409
National Health and Nutrition Examination (2006), 311
National Healthcareer Association (NHA), 390
National Heart Attack Alert Program, 106
National Institutes of Health (NIH), 311
National Library of Medicine (NLM), 311
Naughton protocol, 266t
Neurological influences on atria, 149
Neuropathy, 314–315
Nifedipine (Adalat, Procardia), 363
Nitrates, 366–367
Nitroglycerin (Nitro-Dur, Nitrolingual, Nitrostat), 313t,
   323–324, 366
Non-conducted electrical impulses, 189
Non-ST segment elevation MI (NSTEMI), 316–317
Noninvasive procedure, 253
Nuclear isotope, 256

O

O-P-Q-R-S-T, 320, 321f
Order form, 83–84
Oscilloscope, 5, 6f, 7, 62, 296
Output display, 62
Oversensing pacemaker, 239, 240f, 240t
Oxygen therapy
   in clinical management, 323
   and ECG, 156
   for ventricular dysrhythmias, 209
Oxygenated blood, 33, 34, 35

P

P-P interval
   in atrial dysrhythmias, 149, 155, 157
   in heart block dysrhythmias, 188, 190, 192, 194, 195
   in heart rate calculation, 126, 127t
   in junctional dysrhythmias, 171, 172, 174
   in rhythm calculation, 65–66, 99t, 125, 125f
   in sinus node rhythms, 132, 135, 137
   in ventricular dysrhythmias, 207, 210, 211, 213, 215,
   217, 219
P wave, 42–43, 43t, 125f
   configuration of, 126–127
      in atrial dysrhythmias, 149, 150, 151, 152, 153, 155, 157
      in bundle branch block dysrhythmias, 242f, 243
      in heart block dysrhythmias, 188, 190, 192, 195
      in ischemia/injury/infarction, 342
      in junctional dysrhythmias, 170, 171, 173, 174, 178
      in rhythm calculation, 96t, 124–125, 125f

in sinus node rhythms, 130, 132, 135, 137, 139
  in ventricular dysrhythmias, 207, 210, 211, 213, 215, 217, 220
  with electronic pacemaker, 234
  inverted, in junctional dysrhythmias, 169f, 170, 170f, 172, 174, 176
  missing, in ventricular dysrhythmias, 206, 207, 207f, 210, 210f, 211, 212f, 213, 214
Pacemaker, electronic (artificial), 5
  artifact filter for spikes due to, 66, 70f
  for bundle branch blocks, 243
  complications of, 239, 240f
  evaluating function of, 234–236, 283
  external, for heart block, 194, 196–197
  implanted, 233f
  monitoring, 8, 13
  rhythms stimulated by, 232–234
  for sinus bradycardia, 131f, 134
  temporary, 243
Pacemaker of heart, inherent
  backup, 169
  in complete heart block, 196
  electrical impulses initiated by cells of, 38
  failed, 210, 211
  normal, 39, 130
  pathways of, 39–40, 41
  regulatory function of, 39
  shifting, 150, 152f
  unique qualities of, 38–39
  in ventricular dysrhythmias, 197, 210, 211
Pacing, cardiac
  types of, 233–234
  for ventricular dysrhythmias, 213, 214
Pacing spike, 234, 235, 235f
Pain scales, 321f
Pallor, skin, in ventricular failure, 318
Palpitations
  ambulatory monitoring and, 283
  in junctional dysrhythmias, 176, 178
  in myocardial ischemia, 312
  in sinus node rhythms, 136, 137
Paper; see Graph paper
Paraspinous line, 107, 108f
Parasympathetic nervous system, 39
Parietal pericardium, 29–30, 30t, 31f
Pathologic Q wave, 344
Patient; see also Cardiac patient
  markings on, for serial ECGs, 97
  muscle movements of, 97, 108, 217
  positioning of, 86, 106
  reporting complaints of, 264, 288
  symptoms of; see Cardiac symptoms
  tracings for special conditions of, 105–107, 106f, 108f
Patient diary, 289–292, 290f
  documenting/labeling, 296
  if patient forgot, 297
Patient education/communication
  abnormal blood pressure, 255
  for ambulatory monitoring, 288–292, 289f, 290f, 291t

before/during ECG procedure, 16–17, 85–86
  in emergency situations, 219
  for exercise electrocardiography, 257, 258–259t, 260–261, 268
  if patient child, 85, 103, 292, 293
  if patient fearful, 85, 266, 292
  if patient hard of hearing, 18
  if patient nonresponsive, 86
  if patient on medications, 83
  if patient refuses ECG, 85, 259t
  knowledge of machine prior to, 65, 84
Patient information/records; see also Documentation
  entering data about, 66, 67f, 84
  identifying/verifying, 85, 86, 92, 103
  liability and, 20, 85
  maintaining, 71, 100–101
  obtaining medical history for, 258t, 261
  order form and, 83–84
  protecting/securing/labeling, 18–20, 268, 296
  required information for ECG, 20t
Pause, length of, in sinus arrest, 139
Pediatric patient
  ambulatory monitoring for, 292, 293
  electrocardiogram of, 85, 103–104, 104f
Percutaneous coronary intervention (PCI), 327
Percutaneous transluminal coronary angioplasty (PTCI), 327
Pericardium, 29–30, 30t, 31f
Personal protective equipment (PPE), 15, 16f, 370–371t
Pharmacologic stress test, 257
Physician order, 83
Physiologic Q wave, 344
"Picket fence" atrial pattern, 155, 155f
Polarization, 41–42
Portable monitor, 10–11, 10f
Positioning of patient, 86, 106
Posterior axillary line, 107, 108f
Posterior descending artery, 309
Posterior infarction, 341f
Posterior leads, 107, 108f
Postsymptom event monitor, 284–285, 287f
Potassium ions, heart regulation and, 39
PR interval, 42, 43t, 44, 45f, 125f
  in atrial dysrhythmias, 150, 151, 152f, 153, 155, 157
  in heart block dysrhythmias, 188, 190, 191, 192, 193, 195
  in ischemia/injury/infarction, 342
  in junctional dysrhythmias, 170, 171, 173, 175, 178
  measuring, 128, 128f
  in sinus node rhythms, 131, 133, 135, 137, 139
  Stress test, 243
  in ventricular dysrhythmias, 207, 210, 212, 213, 215, 217, 220
Pravastatin (Pravachol), 366
Precautions
  isolation (transmission-based), 15, 92, 93t, 94, 371–374
  standard (universal), 14–16, 15f, 16f, 17t, 92, 368–370
Precordial leads, 59, 59f
  right, 106–107, 108f

Pregnant patients and ECG, 106
Premature atrial complexes (PACs), 149–150, 149*f*
Premature junctional complex (PJC), 169–170, 169*f*
Premature ventricular complexes (PVCs), 207–209, 207*f*
   medications for, 363
   troubleshooting, 216
   types/patterns of, 208*t*
Preparation
   for ambulatory monitoring, 288–293, 291*t*
   for ECG procedure, 83–84
   for exercise electrocardiography, 257–262, 258*t*, 260*f*
Privacy of patient, 19, 85, 86, 93
Professionalism, 19
Propranolol (Inderal), 363
Pulmonary artery, 31–32, 32*f*, 33, 34*f*
Pulmonary circulation, 33–34, 35*f*
Pulmonary edema, 317–318
Pulmonary embolism, atrial dysrhythmias and, 159
Pulmonary semilunar valve, 31–32, 31*t*, 32*f*, 34*f*
Pulmonary veins, 32*f*, 33, 34*f*, 36*f*
Pulse
   electronic pacemaker and, 234
   in ventricular dysrhythmias, 215, 219, 221
Pulse oximetry, 323*f*
Purkinje fibers (network), 30, 40*t*
   in conduction system, 39–40, 41*f*
   in heart block dysrhythmias, 195
   in ventricular dysrhythmias, 206

Q

Q wave, 42, 43
   physiologic/pathologic, 344, 345*f*
QRS complex, 42, 43, 43*t*, 45*f*
   duration/configuration of, 125*f*, 128–129, 129*f*
      in atrial dysrhythmias, 150, 151, 152*f*, 153, 155, 157
      in bundle branch block dysrhythmias, 241, 242*f*,
        243, 349, 349*f*
      in heart block dysrhythmias, 188, 190, 191, 192,
        193, 195
      in ischemia/injury/infarction, 342
      in junctional dysrhythmias, 170, 172, 173, 175, 178
      in sinus node rhythms, 131, 133, 135, 137, 139
      in ventricular dysrhythmias, 206, 207, 210, 212, 213,
        215, 217, 220
   with electronic pacemaker, 234, 235
   missing, 193, 217, 219
   P wave configuration and, 126–127
   in rhythm calculation, 124–125
   sawtooth pattern between, 155, 155*f*, 215
   wide/bizarre; *see* "Wide/bizarre" complexes
QT interval, 42, 43*t*, 44, 45*f*, 125*f*, 126
Quadgeminy pattern of complexes, 208*t*
"Quivering" atria/myocardium, 157, 217

R

R-on-T PVCs, 208*t*
R-R interval, 45, 125*f*
   in atrial dysrhythmias, 149, 155, 157, 158
   calculating heart rate from, 72, 73*f*

   in heart block dysrhythmias, 188, 190, 192, 194, 195
   in heart rate calculation, 126, 127*t*
   in junctional dysrhythmias, 171, 172, 174, 177
   in rhythm calculation, 124, 125
   in sinus node rhythms, 132, 135, 137
   in ventricular dysrhythmias, 207, 210, 211, 213, 215,
      217, 219
R wave, 42, 43, 130, 208*t*
Rales, 318
Rate pressure product (RPP), 267
Re-entry dysrhythmias, 177
Records, patient; *see* Patient information/records
Reference electrode, 56
Regadenoson (Lexiscan), 257, 367
Relaxation of heart
   in cardiac cycle, 36–37, 37*f*
   recorded in ECG waveform, 42, 44*f*
Remote monitoring; *see* e-ICU; Telemedicine monitoring;
      Telemetry monitoring
Renal infarction, atrial dysrhythmias and, 159
Repolarization, 42, 342
Respirations
   exercise electrocardiography and, 255
   in left vs. right ventricular failure, 317–319
Respiratory arrest, 108
Restenosis, 327
Retrograde depolarization, 172
Rhythm strip
   documenting, 100–101, 132
   5-step process to interpret, 123–130, 342
   special uses for, 105
Rhythms, cardiac
   in atrial dysrhythmias, 149, 150, 152, 152*f*, 155, 157
   in bundle branch block dysrhythmias, 243
   in heart block dysrhythmias, 188, 190, 192, 195
   heart rate and, 126, 127*t*
   inherent vs. pacemaker, 235–236
   in ischemia/injury/infarction, 342
   in junctional dysrhythmias, 169, 171, 172, 174, 177
   regularity of, 124–125, 124*f*, 125*f*
   from sinoatrial node, 130, 132, 135, 137, 138
   underlying, 169
   in ventricular dysrhythmias, 207, 210, 211, 213, 215,
      217, 219
   in ventricular tachycardia, 206
Right atrium, 31, 32*f*, 34*f*
Right bundle branch block (RBBB), 241, 242*f*
   differentiating, 349, 349–350*f*
Right ventricle, 31, 32*f*, 34*f*
Right ventricular failure, 319, 319*f*
Room conditions, 83, 86
Rosuvastatin (Crestor), 366
RV1 to RV6 leads, 106, 106*f*

S

S-A-M-P-L-E, 320, 322*f*
S wave, 42, 43
Safety, 94*t*
   ambulatory monitors, 284
   angina assessment, 312

body mechanics, 13–14, 14*t*, 92, 94
crash cart, 219
elderly patients, 294
electricity
    and electrocardiograph, 4, 92–93
    and electronic pacemaker, 233
electrodes, 68
exercise electrocardiography, 254, 261–262, 262*t*, 263
infection control; *see* Infection control
lead wires, 93, 102, 103*f*
patient identification, 85, 86, 92
reporting symptoms, 322
ST segment elevation, 345
"Sawtooth" pattern
    in atrial flutter, 155, 155*f*
    in ventricular tachycardia, 215, 215*f*
Scanner
    ambulatory monitor, 10, 282
    bar code ID, 67*f*
Scope of practice, 6, 178, 290, 322
"Scribbles" atrial pattern, 157, 157*f*
Second degree atrioventricular (AV) block
    Type I (Mobitz I/Wenckebach), 189–192, 190*f*
    Type II (Mobitz II/Hay), 192–194, 192*f*
Segments, ECG, 42, 43*t*, 125*f*; *see also specific types of*
Seizure, 108
Semilunar valves, 31–32, 31*t*
Sensors; *see* Electrodes
Septal infarction, 340*f*
Shortness of breath
    exercise electrocardiography and, 264, 266, 267
    in myocardial ischemia, 312, 314, 315
    in ventricular failure, 318
Signal processing, 62
Silver electrodes, 69
Simvastatin (Zocor), 366
Sinoatrial (SA) node, 39–40, 40*t*, 41*f*
    rhythms delayed from, 188–189
    rhythms originating from, 130–140
    rhythms overriding, 149–159
Sinus arrest, 137–140, 138*f*
Sinus bradycardia, 132–134, 132*f*
Sinus dysrhythmia, 136–137, 137*f*
Sinus rhythm, normal, 130–131, 131*f*
Sinus tachycardia, 135–136, 135*f*, 178*t*
6–second method of calculating heart rate, 73*f*, 74, 126
Skin rasp, 263
"Skipping" sensation, 209
Slander, 20
Somatic tremor, 96*t*, 97, 97*f*
Sotalol (Betapace, Sotalex), 363
Speed control setting, 64
    graph paper and, 70
    increasing, for junctional tachycardia, 174
    troubleshooting, 65
ST segment, 42, 43, 43*t*, 45*f*, 125*f*
    exercise electrocardiography and, 256*f*
    in ischemia/injury/infarction, 342–344, 342*f*, 345
ST segment elevation MI (STEMI), 316, 316*f*
Standard limb leads, 57, 58*f*

Standard (universal) precautions, 14–16, 15*f*, 16*f*, 17*t*, 92, 368–370
Standardization (calibration) mark, 65, 66*f*, 71, 95
Stat ECG, 7, 8, 101, 108
Statins, 366
Stent, 327, 328*f*
Stress test
    false positive, 269
    pharmacologic, 257
    prior to ambulatory monitoring, 283
    protocols for, 265–266*t*, 265–267
    treadmill, 8–9, 9*f*, 253*f*, 254*f*
        with nuclear isotope (chemical), 256, 367
Stroke; *see* Cerebral vascular accident (CVA)
Stroke volume, 35
Suprasternal notch, 87, 87*f*
Supraventricular, 177
Supraventricular tachycardia (SVT), 177–180, 177*f*, 178*t*, 364
Surgical intensive care unit (SICU), 7
Sweating, 312, 314, 315
Symbols (A-Z listed), medical, 375–389
Sympathetic nervous system, 39
Symptom-based telemedicine monitoring, 13
Symptoms, cardiac
Syncope, 139
    ambulatory monitoring and, 283, 287
    exercise electrocardiography and, 262
    in myocardial ischemia, 315
Systemic circulation, 33, 34, 35*f*
Systole, 37, 37*f*

T

T wave, 42, 43, 43*t*, 44, 125*f*
    in ischemia/injury/infarction, 343, 344*f*
    in ventricular dysrhythmias, 208*t*
Table, exam, 86, 93
Tachycardia, 67, 126
    exercise electrocardiography and, 255
    junctional, 174–176, 174*f*
    sinus, 135–136, 135*f*, 178*t*
    supraventricular, 177–180, 177*f*, 178*t*
    ventricular, 215–217, 215*f*
Tachydysrhythmias, 177, 367
Target heart rate (THR), 267
Technician, electrocardiograph/monitor, 5
    certification of, 396, 400, 405
    exam content outline for, 409
    knowledge of machine by, 65, 84
    NHA correlation chart for, 390–396
    remaining calm, 8
Technologist, cardiovascular, 5
Telemedicine monitoring, 12–13
Telemetry monitoring, 5, 7, 284, 285*f*, 286*f*
Telephonic monitoring; *see* Transtelephonic monitoring
Thallium, 256, 367
Third degree atrioventricular (AV) block (complete), 194–197, 195*f*
Three-channel recorder, 61
Thrombolytic therapy, 326–327, 365–366

Thrombus, atrial dysrhythmias and, 159
"Thump" sensation, 209
Ticlopidine (Ticlid), 365
Time, representation of, 71, 72f
Tissue death, 344–345
Tobacco and stress test, 263, 269
TP segment, 125f
Tracing; see Electrocardiogram (ECG) tracing
Transmission-based precautions; see Isolation (transmission-based) precautions
Transtelephonic monitoring, 12, 12f, 284–287, 286f, 288f
Treadmill stress test, 8–9, 9f, 253f, 254f
   with nuclear isotope (chemical), 256, 367
Treatment; see Clinical management
Tricuspid valve, 31–32, 31t, 32f, 34f
Trigeminy pattern of complexes, 150, 208t
Triggered electrical impulses, 239
Troubleshooting, 20–21
   artifacts, 95–100
   asystole, 140
   consent, 21
   ECG tracing speed, 65
   electrodes, 288
   flatline tracing, 100
   gain (deflection height), 67
   graph paper, 70
   heart block dysrhythmias, 193
   heart rate calculation, 74
   lead wire, 56
   midclavicular line, 90
   multiple (serial) ECGs, 97
   patient diary, 292, 297
   patient symptoms versus tracing, 131
   premature ventricular complexes, 216
   reporting problems, 264
   stress, 8
Tunica adventitia/media/intima, 309, 310f, 311
12–lead tracing; see Electrocardiogram (ECG) tracing

U

U wave, 42, 43t, 44
Unconsciousness
   in heart block dysrhythmias, 196
   in ventricular dysrhythmias, 213, 215, 219, 221
Underlying rhythm, 169
Unifocal premature complexes, 208t
Unipolar leads, 57
Universal/standard precautions, 14–16, 15f, 16f, 17t, 92

V

V1 to V6 leads, 59, 59f, 60f
   anatomically contiguous, 343, 343f
   applying, 88–90, 89f, 89t
   identifying landmarks for, 87, 87f
   infarction areas identified by, 339–341f
   pediatric patient and, 104
   portions of heart viewed by, 338f, 338t
   right-side placement of, 106, 106f

V3R lead for pediatric patient, 104f
V4R to V6R leads, 107, 108f
V7 to V9 leads, 107, 108f
Vagal tone, 136
Vagus nerve, 39
Veins, 33–34
   cardiac, 32f, 34f, 36f, 309–310f
   layers of, 309, 310f, 311
Vena cava, superior/inferior, 32f, 33, 34f, 36f
Ventricles, heart, 31–32, 32f, 34f
Ventricular dysrhythmias, 206–221
Ventricular failure, left/right, 317–319, 318f, 319f
Ventricular fibrillation, 217–219, 217f
   differentiating fine, from asystole, 219
Ventricular hypertrophy (LVH), left, 347, 351–352, 351f
Ventricular pacemaker, 233
Ventricular pacing, 235, 235f
Ventricular rate, determining, 126
Ventricular tachycardia, 215–217, 215f
Verapamil (Calan, Isoptin), 363
Viagra (sildenafil), 367
Visceral pericardium, 30, 30t, 31f
Vitamin K, 329
Voltage on ECG tracing, 64, 71, 72f
Volume expander, 324

W

Waller, Augusta D., 4
Wandering atrial pacemaker (WAP), 150–151, 152f
Wandering baseline, 96t, 98, 98f
Warfarin (Coumadin), 364, 365
Waveform, ECG
   analyzing, in rhythm strip; see Interpretation
   biphasic, 149
   calibration mark as first, 66f
   chaotic/disorganized pattern of, 217, 217f
   of chaotic scribbles, 157, 157f
   components of, 42–45, 43t
   electrical stimulation and, 41–42, 44f
   measurements of
      using calipers, 124–125, 124f, 125f
      using graph paper, 71, 72f
   normal, 7f, 45f
   production/recording of, 54–59, 60f
   regulating height of, 64–65, 66f, 67
   sawtooth pattern in, 155, 155f, 215, 215f
   widening, for interpretation, 65
Wenckebach, Karel Frederik, 190
Wenckebach rhythm, 189–190, 190f
   differentiating, 193t
   mnemonic for remembering, 193
"Wide/bizarre" complexes; see Complexes, ECG
"Widow maker," 327
Women's cardiac symptoms, 313–314, 314t, 315
Wound dressings and ECG, 106
Wrist monitor, 284–285

Rhythm Identification

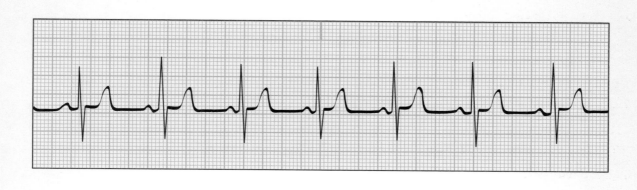

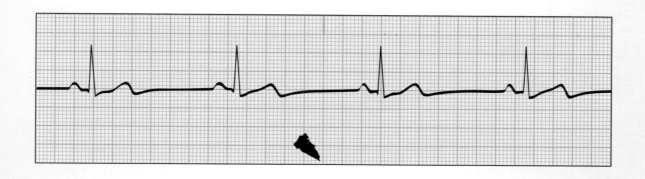

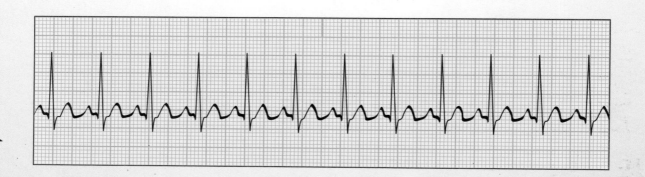

Sinus Rhythm is the only rhythm for which all five steps are within normal limits.

Sinus Bradycardia, the heart rate is less than 60 and all other measurements are within normal limits.

Sinus Tachycardia, the heart rate is greater than 100 and all other measurements are within normal limits.

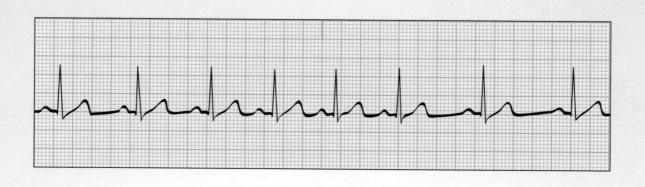

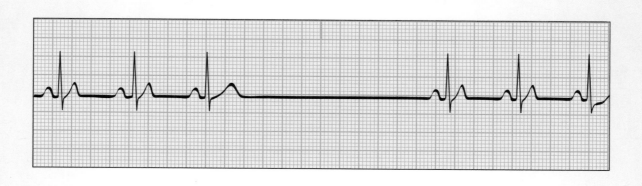

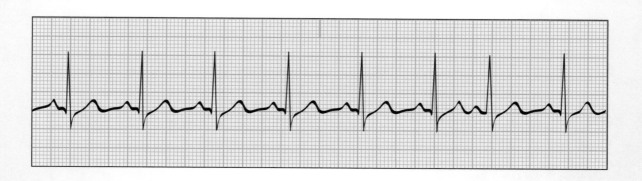

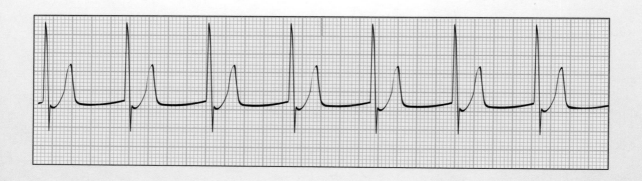

Sinus Dysrhythmia, the P-P and R-R intervals will progressively widen then narrow following the patient's breathing pattern.

Sinus Arrest has regularly occuring PQRST's both before and after the arrest period. No electrical activity during the arrest period.

Remember to report frequency and duration of Sinus Arrest!

A Premature Atrial Complex (PAC) is a complex that occurs sooner than it should with a positively deflected P wave.

Remember to analyze and report the underlying rhythm along with the PAC.

Wandering Atrial Pacemaker (WAP) has at least three different shaped P waves. The rhythm may be regular or irregular. Rate is typically between 60 – 100 bpm

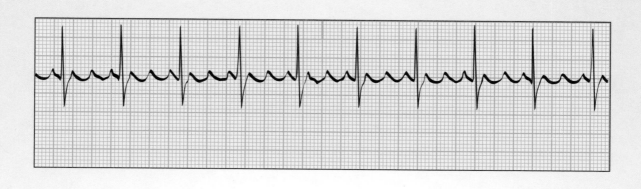

Atrial Flutter has a "sawtooth or picket fence" atrial pattern (no P waves, F-waves instead that may be in a ratio) between the QRS complexes.

Atrial Fibrillation has "chaotic" atrial electrical activity (no P waves, f-waves instead) with irregular R – R intervals.

PJCs cause the rhythm to be irregular. The P wave is inverted if it can be seen. It may occur before, during or after the QRS. If the P wave occurs during the QRS, the P wave will not be seen due to its low voltage.

Junctional Rhythm may have an inverted or absent P wave. The P wave may occur before, during or after the QRS complex. The rate for this rhythm is 40 – 60 bpm.

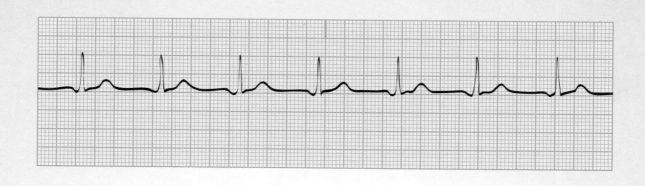

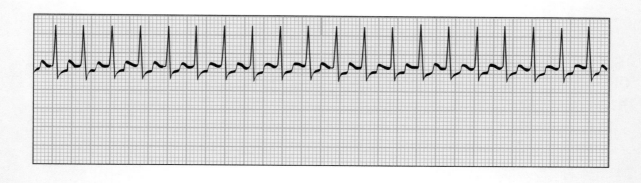

Accelerated Junctional Rhythm may have an inverted or absent P wave. The P wave may occur before, during or after the QRS complex. The rate for this rhythm is between 60 – 100 beats per minute.

Junctional Tachycardia Rhythm may have an inverted or absent P wave. The P wave may occur before, during or after the QRS complex. The rate for this rhythm is between 100 – 180 bpm

Supraventricular Tachycardia presents with a "normal - narrow" appearing QRS complex and a rate of greater than 150 beats per minute. Remember for heart rates approaching 150 and higher, it will be very likely that the P wave will be buried. Be prepared to increase the paper speed for this rhythm.

First Degree AV Block, the PR interval is constant and measures greater than 0.20 second.

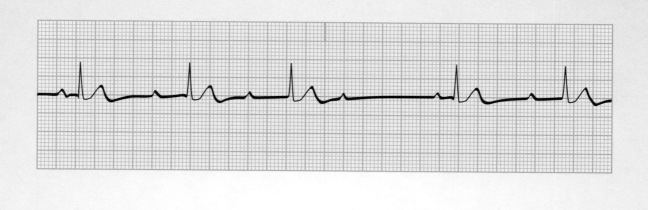

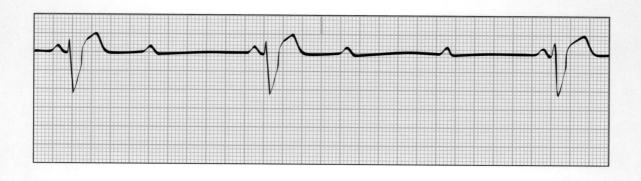

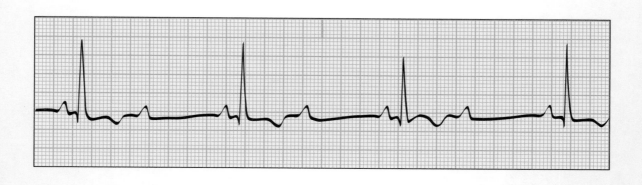

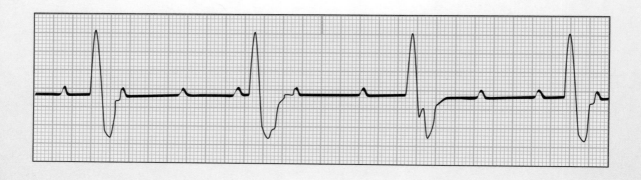

Second Degree AV Block Mobitz I (Wenckebach) has a cyclical prolonging PR interval until the QRS is dropped. Then the cycle begins again. ***Remember the clue "lengthen, lengthen drop Wenkebach"

Second Degree (AV) Block, Mobitz Type II has a constant PR interval with blocked QRS complexes

Second Degree (AV) Block, Mobitz Type II has a constant PR interval with blocked QRS complexes

Third Degree (Complete) Heart Block, the P-P and R-R intervals are regular (constant) but firing at different rates.

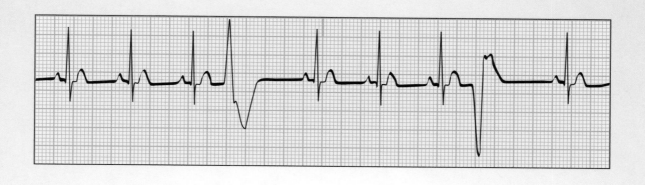

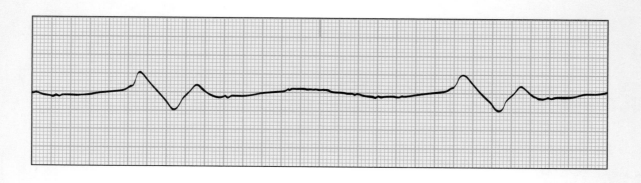

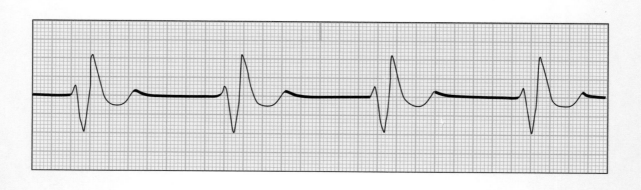

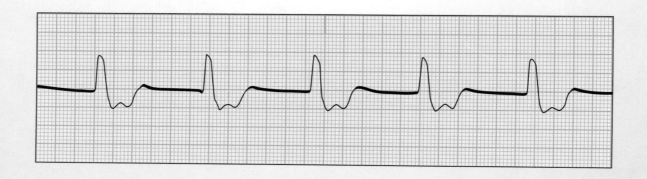

A PVC is an early QRS complex that is wide (0.12 second or greater) and has a bizarre appearance. There is no P wave. PVC's may come in different shapes – describe them appropriately. Remember to identify the underlying rhythm when providing the interpretation.

Agonal Rhythm has an absence of P waves, a ventricular rate of less than 20 beats per minute, and wide-bizarre QRS complexes

Idioventricular Rhythm has an absence of P waves, slow ventricular rate of 20 to 40 beats per minute, and wide-bizarre QRS complexes.

Accelerated Idioventricular Rhythm has an absence of P waves, a ventricular rate of 40 to 100 beats per minute, and wide-bizarre QRS complexes.

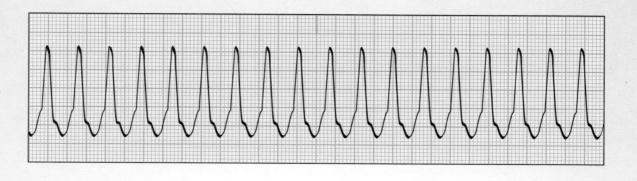

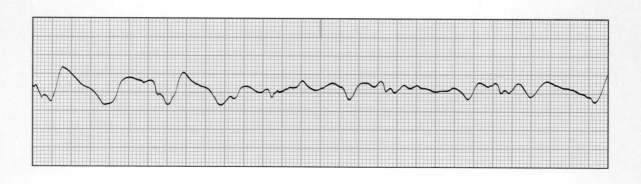

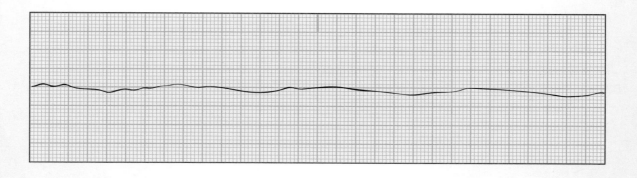

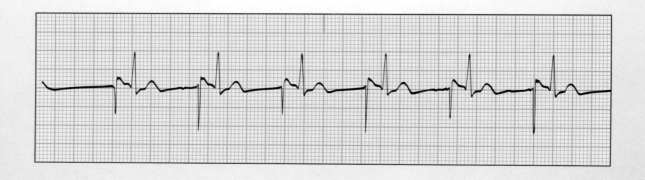

Ventricular tachycardia has wide and bizarre QRS complexes with a classic "sawtooth" appearance, a rate in excess of 100 beats per minute, with, no P wave.

Ventricular fibrillation is the absence of organized electrical activity. There are no P waves, QRS complexes or T waves. The tracing has a chaotic or disorganized appearance.

Asystole is absence of ventricular activity and depolarization. Often this is called "the straight or flat line" of rhythms. No electrical activity is present. This rhythm is neither regular nor irregular. It is simply absent!

Atrial Pacemaker Rhythm is identified by the presence of a pacing spike immediately prior to the atrial depolarization (P wave)

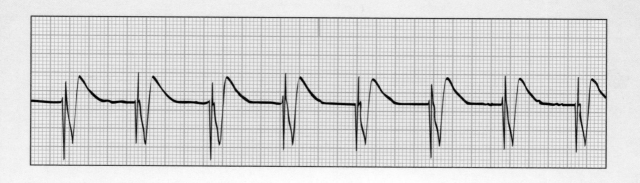

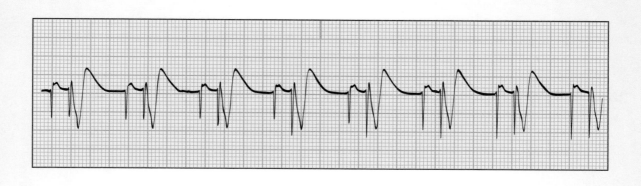

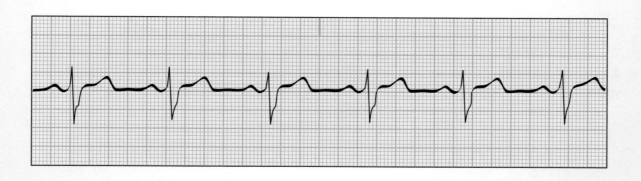

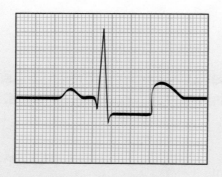

Ventricular Pacemaker Rhythm is identified by the presence of a pacing spike immediately prior to the ventricular depolarization (QS complex)

Atrioventricular Pacemaker Rhythm is identified by the presence of a pacing spike immediately prior to the atrial depolarization (P wave) and the ventricular depolarization (QS complex).

A rhythm containing **Bundle Branch Block** will retain its own usual features with the only change being the QRS complex now measures 0.12 second or greater

An ST segment below the isoelectric line is known as **ST segment depression** and may indicate myocardial ischemia.

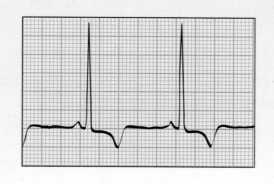

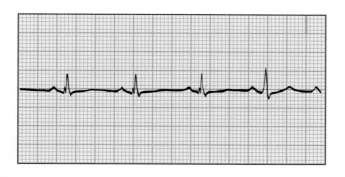

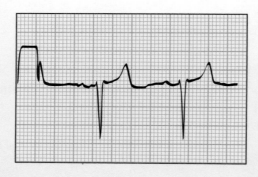

T wave inversion, or a negatively deflected T wave indicates ischemia and is usually seen with ST segment elevation.

T wave inversion with ST elevation on a 12-lead ECG is considered myocardial injury, acute injury pattern, or acute MI (AMI). It means the problem is happening right now.

Physiologic Q wave is normal and the width measures less than 0.04 second and the depth measures less than one-third of the height of the R wave in that lead.

Pathologic Q wave indicates tissue death (infarction) and is defined as measuring 0.04 second and/or greater than or equal to one third the height of the R wave in that lead tracing.

Cardiovascular Medications

Beta Blockers

Atenolol (Tenormin®)

Metoprolol (Toprol XL®, Lopressor®)

Many end with an *ol*. Treats angina, HBP, rhythm disturbances such as Afib and PVCs (Antiarrhythmic)

Beta Blocker

Beta Blocker

Propranolol (Inderal®)

Sotalol (Betapace®, Sotalex®)

Labetolol (Normodyne®, Trandate®)

Carvedilol (Coreg®)

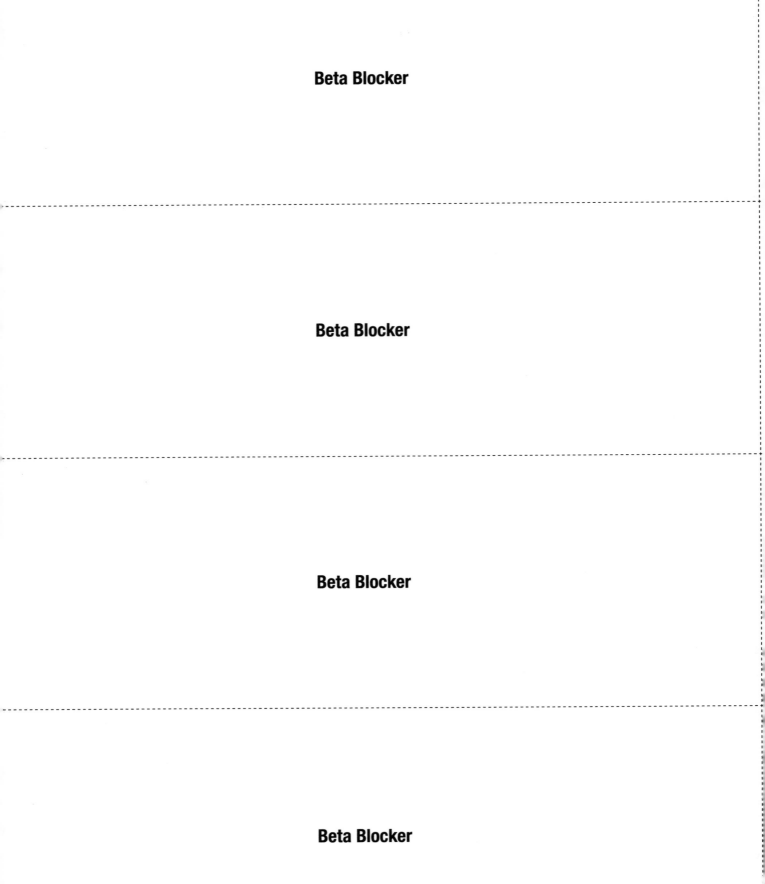

Beta Blocker

Beta Blocker

Beta Blocker

Beta Blocker

Cardiac Glycosides

Digoxin (Digitek®, Lanoxin®)

Calcium Channel Blockers

amlodipine (Norvasc®)

Increases the force of the heart's contraction and slows the heart rate. Side effects including depression of the ST segment.

Cardiac Glycosides - increases the force of the heart's contraction and slows the heart rate. Side effects including depression of the ST segment.

Treats angina, HBP, rapid rhythm disorders (Afib, SVT), coronary artery spasms. (Antiarrhythmic)

Calcium Channel Blocker

diltiazem (Cardizem®)

verapamil (Calan®, Isoptin®)

nifedipine (Adalat®, Procardia®)

Ace Inhibitors

Calcium Channel Blocker

Calcium Channel Blocker

Calcium Channel Blocker

**Many end with _il_. Block conversion of antiotensin I to II. Treats
CHF and HBP**

Enalapril (Vasotec®)

Lisinopril (Prinivil®, Zestril®)

Captopril (Capoten®)

Benazepril (Lotensin®)

Ace Inhibitor

Ace Inhibitor

Ace Inhibitor

Ace Inhibitor

Antcoagulants

Warfarin (Coumadin®)

Heparin

Enoxaparin (Lovenox®)

Stop blood from clotting, prevent clots from forming or enlarging.

Oral anticoagulant

Injectable anticoagulant

Injectable anticoagulant

Antiplatelet Agents

Aspirin (Bayer®)

Clopidogrel (Plavix®)

Ticlopidine (Ticlid®)

Keeps platelets from clumping and inhibits clot formation.

Antiplatelet

Antiplatelet

Antiplatelet

Sodium Channel Blockers

Potassium Channel Blockers

Fibrinolytics

Diuretics

Antiarrhythmic

Antiarrhythmic

Dissolves clots to treat heart attack, stroke, pulmonary embolism or prosthetic heart valve.

Remove salt and water from the body. Treats HBP and CHF.

Cholesterol-Lowering Agents

Atorvastatin (Lipitor®)

Rosuvastatin (Crestor®)

Simvastatin (Zocor®)

Statins

Statin - lowers cholesterol

Statin - lowers cholesterol

Statin - lowers cholesterol

Nitrates

Nitroglycerin (Nitor-Dur®, Nitrolingual®, Nitrostat®)

Isosorbide dinitrate (Dilatrate-SR®, Isordil®)

Isosorbide mononitrate (ISMO®)

Vasodilators that treat chest pain. Do not handle with bare hands. Do not mix with medications taken for erectile dysfunction.

Nitrate (vasodilator)

Nitrate (vasodilator)

Nitrate (vasodilator)

Inotropic agents (Inotropes)

Adenosine (Adenocard®)

Dobutamine (Dobutrex®)

Persantine (Dipyridamole®)

Affect the contractile force or pumping action of the heart.

Inotropic and chemical stress testing agent

Inotropic and chemical stress testing agent

Chemical stress testing agent

Regadenoson (Lexiscan®)

Cardiolite®

Thallium®

Myoview®

Chemical stress testing agent

Imaging agent for cardiac stress test

Imaging agent for cardiac stress test

Imaging agent for cardiac stress test